ADOPTION AND THE FAMILY SYSTEM

ADOPTION
and the
Family System

Strategies for Treatment

MIRIAM REITZ, PhD, LCSW
KENNETH W. WATSON, MSW, LCSW

THE GUILFORD PRESS
New York ⌐ London

To Klaus Baer, in honored memory of our chosen and cherished relationship.

Miriam Reitz Baer

To Barbara Watson, my island of tranquility in an all too hectic world.

Kenneth W. Watson

© **1992 The Guilford Press**
A Division of Guilford Publications, Inc.
72 Spring Street, New York, NY 10012

Printed in the United States of America

This book is printed on acid-free paper.

Last digit is print number: 9 8 7 6 5 4 3 2 1

Library of Congress Cataloging-in-Publication Data

Reitz, Miriam, 1935–
    Adoption and the family system: Strategies for treatment
/ Miriam Reitz and Kenneth W. Watson.
        p.   cm.
    Includes bibliographical references and index.
    ISBN 0-89862-797-4   0-89862-033-3 (pbk.)
    1. Adoption — United States.   2. Family social work — United States.
3. Family psychotherapy — United States.   I. Watson, Kenneth W.,
1929-   . II. Title.
HV875.55.R45   1992
362.82'98'0973 — dc20

91-44266
CIP

Preface

This book presents a practice model for providing therapy to members of the "adoption triangle" (adopted persons, birth parents, and adoptive parents). For a combined total of more than 60 years, we have observed under what circumstances they have asked for help and what the recurrent issues have been. We have applied family systems concepts to our understanding and experimented with family therapy interventions, noting which were most effective with the special features of adoption. The outcome is a model distilled through our clinical training, knowledge, and skill into practice wisdom.

Despite the proliferation in recent decades of the literature on both family therapy and adoption, there has been little focus on the *treatment* of families involved with adoption. We offer our approach both as one sample of the current state of the practice art and as a way to generate hypotheses. Little definitive, formal research on adoption and family therapy has been done. Where research findings are available, we have cited them; we believe, however, that findings from practice are valid field research. The clinician's skills in observing recurrent themes and patterns resemble those of the formal researcher who looks for patterns in statistical data. Both clinicians and researchers must then interpret their findings.

More research will be urgently needed in the decades ahead. Not only should the hypotheses of clinical practice continue to be tested, but information is also needed about the outcomes of all the current changes and alternatives in family building. In particular, we will need to learn about the experience of individuals who enter families through new procedures in adoption or through newly developed birth technologies.

Our main interest is in providing a basis for informed clinical practice with families linked in adoption. We are aware that some of our positions on systems concepts, premises about adoption, and treatment approaches may meet with disagreement. We welcome discussion that will benefit clinical services to all members of the adoption triangle.

We offer this book to help clinicians become more aware of common issues and useful techniques in helping families involved with adoption. At the same time, we recognize that adoption affects individuals and familes in many different ways. We respect the rich variety of experiences within the adoption framework. Our goal is to help clinicians respond to the unique experiences of all members of the adoption triangle. If adopted persons and other members of their dual families also find this book useful in any way, that is a bonus.

Our collaboration began in 1986, when The Family Institute of Chicago sponsored a 2-day conference, *Helping Families with Issues around Adoption.* The conference was opened by Charles Kramer, MD, founder of The Family Institute of Chicago and a pioneer of family therapy. One of the speakers, Ann Hartman, remarked, "Adoption is a subject that always evokes passion." The response of the audience proved her correct. From the passion of that conference, the idea of this book was born.

Kenneth W. Watson has spent his entire social work career in child welfare, for many years as the assistant director of the Chicago Child Care Society. His specialties are adoption and foster care. He early integrated family systems concepts with child developmental theory, so that whole families involved in child placement might be better served. He has done extensive training and has contributed to the development of state and national adoption policies.

Miriam Reitz also began her social work career in a child welfare agency, but in the area of family counseling. With the founding of The Family Institute of Chicago in 1968, she moved to the practice and training of others in family therapy. She has maintained a special interest in families who have added children through adoption or foster care, and has continued to consult with agencies on these subjects.

Neither of us has been directly involved in the adoption experience. When we looked to our extended families and our circles of friends, however, we had ample personal contact with all members of the adoption triangle. We believe that the same is true of most clinicians, for adoption touches almost everyone.

All case material cited in this book is derived from real clinical experience. To protect the confidentiality of the family members, all identifying facts have been changed. In many instances, there are symbolically equivalent substitutions or combinations of several cases. The disguises are sufficiently impenetrable that even a participant would not recognize more than the resonance that goes with universal human themes.

Finally, we thank the people who have encouraged the production of this book. Most especially, we are grateful to all those people who opened their lives and shared their experiences around adoption with us. Some are represented in the case material, but all, we hope, are well represented in every line.

Miriam Reitz
Kenneth W. Watson
Chicago

Contents

PART II. BIRTH FAMILIES

PART III. FORMING AN ADOPTIVE FAMILY

PART IV. THE ADOPTIVE FAMILY
IN TREATMENT

PART V. THE LIFETIME IMPACT
OF ADOPTION

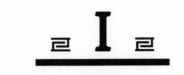

OUR APPROACH
TO FAMILIES LINKED
IN ADOPTION

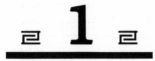

Premises

Myths of Adoption from Ancient Times to the 1960s

Adoption is a powerful experience that touches upon universal human themes of abandonment, parenthood, sexuality, identity, and the sense of belonging. In mythology and folklore, adoption is usually presented as a way to rescue a child from parents who are unable to protect the child from harm (e.g., Moses) or from parents who would themselves harm the child (e.g., Oedipus). A common theme of these early stories is that although the adoption enables a child to be reared in safety, it does not forestall the need for the adopted child to work out a destiny in the context of his or her origins.

From the beginnings of human history until now, adoption has served a variety of functions—from providing a royal family with an heir, to adding "indentured" hands to make a family financially self-sufficient, to emptying the orphanages to save community dollars. Although adoption down through the ages appears to have been primarily intended to meet the needs of those adopting, it has generally been described as an act of kindness intended to save children from harmful environments. In more recent times, the primary function of adoption has been to meet the needs of infertile couples who wanted to experience parenting, and many adoption agencies came into existence to "solve" the infertility problems of those affluent enough to support such agencies.

The rescue fantasy persisted, however, so with this shift adoption was viewed not only as a solution for infertility, but also as a means of saving children from their poor environments. To justify the separation of children from their birth parents, a third function

3

of adoption was identified: to provide a solution for birth parents who were involved in premature, unintended pregnancies, and found themselves unable to rear their children. Not addressed in this highly romanticized version was the inherent pain of adoption. Adoptive families and adoption agencies collaborated to present adoption as what it can never really be — a chance for birth parents to go on happily with their lives, for children to grow up in trouble-free families, and for adoptive parents to fulfill themselves and find immortality through children to whom they have sole claim by virtue of the adoption.

The harsh reality is that adoption is a second-best plan. It is second best for children, who in an ideal world would always be reared by adequate birth parents; second best for the birth parents, who wish either that their pregnancies had never occurred or that they could rear the children themselves; and second best for adoptive families, whose decision to adopt is usually reached only after they have exhausted all efforts to have children biologically. No matter how positively anyone tries to present adoption to adopted children, or what language is used, the issue that confronts them is their abandonment by their birth parents to the care of strangers. And there is no "happily ever after."

Instead of confronting this situation, however, adoptive parents and adoption agencies for years directed their efforts to preserving the romantic myth. To do this, three conditions had to prevail: An adopted child had to approximate adoptive parents' fantasy of the child they might have had by birth; adoption had to be viewed as a static event with no developmental implications; and the reality of the adopted child's other family had to be denied by both the adoptive parents and the agency. The first condition was met by early placement and careful matching. The second was addressed by ignoring the impact of adoption on the way in which the child and the adoptive family developed. And the third condition was fulfilled by early placement and by developing ways of explaining the child's adoption that "avoided" the trauma.

As recently as a generation ago, adoption agencies were intent on duplicating for adoptive families the parenting experience they had been denied by nature. Every attempt was made to locate a child who matched an adoptive couple's physical characteristics, intellectual potential, and even talents and tastes. In order to allow the adoptive parents to experience parenthood as fully as possible, and to provide the infant with a continuous parenting experience, efforts were made to place each baby as early as possible. That meant that the matching was generally based upon what was known about the birth parents. The goal was placement direct from the hospital into the adoptive home. This was more often realized in adoptions in which there was no agency involvement. In some such situations, when a birth mother entered the hospital she used the adoptive parents' name; upon release from the hospital, the birth mother handed her child over to the adoptive parents. The birth certificate was already in their names. That subterfuge was unnecessary, because when an adoption decree is signed in most jurisdictions, a new birth certificate is issued giving the adoptive parents as the child's parents; this is still generally the case.

Once an adopted child was placed in the adoptive family, the adoptive parents were encouraged to treat the child as if he or she had been born into the family. The adoption was over once the judge signed the decree. The implications of the adoption for the subsequent development of the child or the family were either viewed as inconsequential or denied altogether. Thus, issues like the ongoing anxieties of the adoptive parents (a child learning about an undisclosed adoption or the possible reappearance of the birth parents) could remain undiscussed.

For the most part, adoptive parents were encouraged by agencies to tell their children about their adoption. This advice was based on the belief that secrets were a barrier to families' integrity, and that *not* telling children subjected them to the risk of learning traumatically from some other source. Since adoption practice was based in large measure on the premise that adoption saved children from a bad environment, the dilemma was how to discuss adoption with the children in a way that sanctioned the adoptive parents' pre-eminent right to parenthood by virtue of the rescue, yet did not reflect too badly on the birth parents and do damage to the children's self-esteem.

Adoptive parents and agencies rose to the challenge. Whatever the real circumstances of children's birth, some adoptive parents fabricated explanations for the adoption, such as that both birth parents had died in a tragic car accident. Other explanations were that the birth father was killed in war and the birth mother felt unable to rear a child alone; or that the parents loved each other very much, but were too young to get married; or that the birth mother was unmarried and wanted very much to keep the child, but felt that this would be a selfish act when a two-parent family was available to adopt.

Adoption agencies routinely denied the genetic and psychological importance of birth fathers. They seldom offered them services or even attempted to see them for information. They assured surrendering birth mothers that their children would indeed go to families that could offer more than they could. They counseled such mothers to sign a relinquishment and go on with their lives. They supported policies and laws that sealed off information and contact between birth parents and their children as a condition of adoption. They counseled adoptive parents to assure their adopted children that they had been "chosen" by their adoptive parents.

For those parents who elected to tell their children about their adoption, the telling was often viewed as a one-time experience. Many adoptive parents saw it as an unpleasant necessity — something to be gotten through as quickly as possible, so that the myth that their children were really theirs alone could be preserved. Most adoptive parents wanted to delay the telling as long as they could, but most professionals advocated introducing the word "adoption" early. They suggested that infants should first hear the word in story or song, perhaps while the parents were bathing, feeding, or rocking them. The positive regard the parents were demonstrating for their children would then become attached to the word "adoption." It would be one of the early words in the adopted children's vocabularies, and they would grow up feeling that it was a positive thing in their lives.

What was overlooked, of course, was the developmental impact of adoption on children at every stage of their lives. Adopted children must adjust to the stress of their adoption on a continuing basis. The issues of adoption have different meaning and impact to children as they develop, because their understanding and adjustment to adoption is influenced by their emerging cognitive capacity and their developing coping efforts (Brodzinsky, 1990). What adoption means to a child on any day depends on the child's developmental level. Most children under the age of 4, for instance, lack the cognitive capacity to understand an explanation of what adoption is. Introducing the word to them while they are affectually engaged with their caretakers may well be of value (Brodzinsky, 1990, p. 12), but telling children about adoption can never be a one-time event. As they face new life experiences and as their ability to deal with abstract concepts develops, adopted children will need to examine what adoption means over and over gain. For instance, most children are anxious when they face an early separation from their parents for day care, kindergarten, or school. For the adopted child, adoption, now has new meaning in the context of his or her capacity to understand and cope with the fear of separation. In adolescence, accepting that one is adopted takes on other dimensions as adopted teenagers struggle with the issues of identity, sexuality, and the responsibilities inherent in adulthood and independence.

At each developmental level, adoption complicates the tasks for an adopted child and for his or her adoptive family. As such a family goes through its developmental sequence, the dynamics of the family system are affected by the special way in which the family was formed and by its relationship to the birth family of the adopted child.

Challenges to the Myths

Although in the preceding section we have been critical of the practices that were spawned by the "conspiracy of denial" between agencies and adoptive parents, we must also point out that all parties believed they were acting in the best interests of children. The myth that adoption offered a happy solution for the presenting problems of all who participated has only been seriously challenged within the last 30 years. It is now generally acknowledged that although adoption offers a viable plan for some, it is not a problem-free solution for any. And it is acknowledged that all three parties to an adoption — birth parents, children, and adoptive parents — each have rights, needs, and a claim to community services. These three groups of participants in adoption make up the "adoption triangle" (also called the "adoption triad"), and an awareness of the impact of adoption on each is essential to sound adoption placements and effective clinical interventions.

Challenges to the old myths came from three sources: (1) Participants in earlier adoptions challenged traditional agency practices as they returned to agencies with their questions, their problems, and their wish to reunite with those from whom they had been separated by adoption; (2) agencies recognized the numbers of children who were not being served by adoption because of their race, their age, or their special needs, and began to shift their programs to focus on children needing adoptive homes rather than on families needing to adopt; and (3) a study of adoption published in 1964 by H. David Kirk, *Shared Fate* (see Kirk, 1984, pp. 89–90), challenged the conventional wisdom of denying the differences that adoption makes.

Increasingly over the past two to three decades, participants in adoption have been seeking those from whom they have been separated. Adults who had been adopted as infants sought out and found their birth parents, and birth parents found the children they had surrendered for adoption. They learned that earlier promises had often not been fulfilled. Adoptive families had not always been able to meet the needs of the children they adopted. They encountered the same range of problems of other families — divorce, alcoholism, illness, financial reverses — and, in addition, the potential for additional problems as a result of being adoptive families. As people searched, they sought information from agencies to help them. Some used agency support and assistance in the reunion process or in sorting out their future relationships with new-found family members. From the members of the adoption triangle who were living the adoption experience, agencies learned a good deal.

Adoptive families described the problems they experienced and for which they might have sought help along the way. Adoption agencies had often denied their service requests, claiming that the counseling they requested was not an appropriate agency responsibility. Some families had been referred to community mental health centers or private therapists. Often families found such therapists unfamiliar with the impact of adoption or the issues that it raised. Some had been advised that the adoption was irrelevant to their family difficulties, and others that the adoption was the source of all of the family problems. Some were even advised to see about "giving the child back" to the agency. Over the past several years efforts to sensitize therapists to some common issues that face adoptive families have increased (Bourguignon & Watson, 1987; Hartman & Laird, 1990; Winkler, Brown, van Keppel, & Blanchard, 1988).

Birth parents whose children had been adopted many years before helped agencies understand the continuing impact of that loss in many areas of their lives. Most wanted to know what had happened to their children; many hoped they would be found by their children; and some were themselves searching. Some told of seeking treatment for a variety of emotional problems and learning that the problems were related to their adoption experience. Many expressed anger toward the agencies because of the lack of services that might have helped them rear the children to whom they had given life. Others told of calls made to the adoption agencies to find out whether children they had surrendered had been placed in adoption, and of the agencies' responses that they were unable to share any information about children who had been relinquished.

From adults who were adopted as children, agencies learned about the fantasies and fears adopted children have about their origins. As small children, many recalled wondering why they were not living with their birth families. As adults they have shared with us three reasons that occurred to them: There was something wrong with them and their birth families did not want to keep them; there was something wrong with their birth parents and they could not keep them; or they were kidnapped by their adoptive parents. Each of these alternatives was unpleasant, and adopted children chose from among them according to which served them best at any given time. Each of the three courses complicated the children's relationships with their adoptive families; since in most instances the fantasies did not surface for family discussion, they placed a hidden burden on the adoptive parents as well.

The adults adopted as children also shared their childhood fantasies about who their missing parents might be. Could they really be the birth children of their adopted parents, or perhaps of one of them? If the children were old enough at adoption to remember former foster parents or social workers who were involved in their placement, could those persons really have been birth parents? Or, if other adults took an interest in the children, was it perhaps because they were biologically related to them? There are instances in which a birth parent has indeed taken such an interest, either as a part of a conscious effort to locate a child and unobtrusively enter that child's life, or as a matter of coincidence.

Marjorie was placed as an infant through an agency in Pittsburgh 20 years ago. Her adoptive parents were from West Virginia and moved back there immediately after the adoption. Marjorie returned to the Pittsburgh area to go to college. During her second year of college, a cousin who worked at the largest department store in Pittsburgh suggested that she apply there for part-time work. Following a routine employment interview, she was asked back for an interview with the director of personnel. She was initially apprehensive, and was relieved when the director of personnel simply wanted to verify her date and place of birth and her parents' current address. When she said that she had been born in Pittsburgh, the interviewer inquired about relatives in the area. Marjorie said that other than the cousin who had suggested the job to her, all of her relatives lived in West Virginia. She said that her parents had really only come to Pittsburgh to adopt her.

Marjorie was hired and soon became aware of the special interest the director of personnel had taken in her. When Marjorie was working, the personnel director often dropped by to see how she was doing. Marjorie was surprised when she remembered Marjorie's birthday and invited Marjorie to have lunch with her on that day. Marjorie talked to her mother about her new friend and how strange it was they seemed to get along so well, since there was such a wide difference in their ages. Marjorie's mother thought it a strange coincidence. She said nothing to Marjorie, but asked Marjorie's cousin to find out a little more about the personnel director. She turned out to be Marjorie's birth mother, who had noted Marjorie's birth date on the application and decided to follow up the unlikely possibility that Marjorie could be the child she had surrendered. The adoptive mother contacted the agency that had arranged the adoption, and with agency support arranged for contact with the birth mother and then a "family reunion" for Marjorie.

Adults adopted as children also shared with agencies and clinicians their worry about possibly marrying a biological relative. Although this also may seem unlikely, the odds are higher than they initially appear. Adopted children and young adults often seek out other adopted persons to be part of their intimate friendship group. Many adoptive families live in the same geographical area as the birth families of their children. Some birth parents have several children placed in adoption over a span of years, and the children may not know of one another's existence. An adopted person contemplating marriage to another adopted person is often spurred to search for or verify background information.

As agencies were rethinking their services because of feedback from earlier adoption clients, the increased focus on the adoption of special needs children lent additional impetus to change. The adoptive parents of a 6-year-old child, of a child who was physically or developmentally disabled, or of a family of several siblings could hardly deny the differences that adoption made. Many such children were adopted by the foster families with whom they lived. These families knew the children's history and had perhaps had contact with their birth families. Other children who were adopted by families in which they had not already lived brought to their new adoptive families experiences, memories, and "selves" that were already rooted somewhere else.

Finally, David Kirk's work provided a conceptual framework for understanding and assessing the differences that adoption makes to families. His seminal 1964 study explored the way in which adoptive parents perceived adoption along a continuum, one end of which was identified by the "rejection" of the differences that adoption makes, and the other by the "acknowledgment" of those differences. His conclusion was that the acknowledgment of differences was more conducive to good communication, order, and stability in adoptive families (see Kirk, 1984, p. 99).

Since Kirk's study first appeared, adoption practitioners and family clinicians have been struggling to conceptualize adoption in a new way. Fueled by the questions that those who had earlier experienced adoption were asking and by their own experiences with special needs children, they sought a framework that would encompass the complexities of the adoption experience for all members of the adoption triangle, and that would provide guidelines for effective service to them whenever their need arose. This book is an effort to further that process.

Adoption Redefined, and the Role of Family Systems

We begin with a new definition that reflects the realities of the adoption experience. *We define "adoption" as a means of providing some children with security and meeting their developmental needs by legally transferring ongoing parental responsibilities from their birth parents to their adoptive parents; recognizing that in so doing we have created a new kinship network that forever links those two families together through the child, who is shared by both.* In adoption, as in marriage, the new legal family relationship does not signal the absolute end of one family and the beginning of another, nor does it sever the psychological tie to an earlier family. Rather, it expands the family boundaries of all those who are involved.

This book is written primarily for clinicians. We hope that others interested in adoption will find it useful; our intent, however, is to help professionals who are trying to help members of the adoption triangle at any time in those people's lives. We believe that adoption can be a good plan for some children, for some birth parents, and for some adoptive parents. We also know of the ways it can complicate people's lives and of the pain it sometimes causes. It is our hope that by looking critically at the clinical issues involved, we can help adoption work better for those for whom it is the best option.

Some clinicians have identified a cluster of symptoms or character traits that they feel are common enough in adopted adults to be labeled the "adoption syndrome." We prefer to identify certain developmental tasks that adopted children may find more difficult as a function of their adoption. The issues of self-esteem, loss, and identity are the most obvious (cf. Brinich, 1990). Like all children, adopted children will face these tasks in a variety of ways, depending on their individual characteristics, the family systems in which they are operating, and the broader environment in which those systems function. Like all children, they will develop the capacity to respond to external stimuli in three ways: affectually, behaviorally, and cognitively. Independent of the fact that they are adopted, some will find one of these three modes more comfortable than the others. Depending upon their genetic makeup and their early experiences, they will develop their individual characteristics and personalities. They will become part of their immediate family systems, yet will always be a part of other family systems, too. They will reflect the impact of their adoption in a variety of ways, some of which may be problematic. The adoption themes are constant; the human variations are endless.

The best context within which to examine adoption is that of family systems. Every decision to place or to adopt and rear a child is made within the framework of the family systems of those involved, no matter how poorly this fact is perceived by them, by the adoption worker, or by the clinician. No decision to treat an adoption-related problem should be made outside the context of the extended family system created by the adoption.

This extended family system is made up of many other family systems: the family of origin of the child's birth mother; the family of origin of the child's birth father; the family created by the birth parents and their child; the adoptive family into which the child is placed, and the family of origin of each of the adoptive parents; and the families that each of the birth parents may form later if they choose not to marry each other. Neither the adoption worker involved in facilitating an adoption nor the clinician offering service to a birth parent at some later time will have an opportunity to work with members of all of these family systems. Although the family system for treatment remains the *primary* family system of the client at the point of the therapeutic encounter, it is essential to the provision of effective service that a professional work within the conceptual context of the many systems involved.

With so many family systems linked by every adoption, it is not surprising that so many people's lives are touched by adoption. Adoption is no small phenomenon that affects only the occasional person or family seeking help; rather, it is a factor that therapists would do well to explore routinely as they gather family history and formulate their assessments.

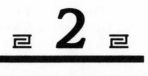

Assessment

Families linked in adoption come in as great variety as the range of human possibilities permit. Regardless of their particular link to adoption, they must deal with the universal human needs for attachment, generativity, and coping with loss. The only certain commonality among these families is that they have undergone fundamental loss experiences beyond those that any family can normally expect. No other common experiences can be assumed for all families linked in adoption. Nor can any similar assumptions be made about common experiences for any subgroup of members of the adoption triangle.

Families linked in adoption come from all socioeconomic groups and ethnicities, and live in both urban and rural settings. The members of these families come from families of origin that run the gamut of levels of functioning, values, developmental struggles, and symptoms. Their conditioning by their original families has, in turn, shaped their efforts to make good attachments with spouses and children.

What families of origin have taught and demonstrated about reactions to loss is particularly important as all of these individuals deal with the experience that links them to adoption. Often, difficulties with the loss related to adoption are the reasons why a family seeks counseling. The loss may be presented directly as the problem; more often, however, the effects of the loss have been hidden in the family dynamics, leading to a focus on some other problem. Thus, when faced with a problem presented by a family linked to adoption, a clinician needs a versatile framework for assessment. It must be comprehensive enough to include all family contingencies, but it also must help the clinician to understand a particular problem in the context of particular family dynamics. A three-dimensional schema (Reitz, 1982) that meets these needs is presented below (See also Glidewell, 1976; Reid & Epstein, 1972; and Simon, 1960).

For the therapist, assessment of a family requesting treatment is a cognitive process that begins from the first contact with a family member. Often the first contact is by telephone, but even then who calls, what is said, and how it is said provide initial clues. The therapist's responses and further questions about the problem and other family members provide additional assessment information and the beginnings of a therapeutic alliance. In each subsequent meeting, the therapist continues to develop a picture of the problem in relation to the family experiencing it. Every interaction with family members adds information for the continuing process of adding, correcting, and confirming the perceptions of the therapist. Out of this process emerges an assessment of the family's situation, which in turn guides the treatment.

As a therapist begins an assessment, it is useful to consider the following questions, which are discussed in detail in the remainder of this chapter.

- What is the presenting problem, and who is the symptom bearer?
- How has the family tried to solve the presenting problem? What has been the result?
- What is the life stage of the family? That is, have any major developmental changes just occurred, or are any impending?
- What is the function of the presenting problem in the dynamics of the family as a whole, and in those of the marital relationship in particular?
- How can the assessment guide the treatment plan, so that the two processes interact and refine each other?

What Is the Presenting Problem, and Who Is the Symptom Bearer?

Neither part of this question can always be answered on the basis of initial presentations. At the least, opening statements must be considered for the point at which family members locate the problem: outside the family (e.g., "The problem is the school"), in a particular family member (e.g., "We are here only because of Sue"), or in family relationships (e.g., "We are fighting all the time").

Some families offer a lesser problem at first. When they have gained some comfort with the therapist, perhaps already by the second meeting, they bring out the more important concern. Other families present such a list of problems that an order of priority must be created, and then the most pressing problem and/or the one most amenable to change must be selected.

Similarly, the answer to "Who is the symptom bearer?" may not always be as obvious or clear-cut as a family would have a therapist think. A lesser problem of another family member may be used for entry into therapy. In such a case, the family members may believe the presented problem to be most serious, or they may be shielding the person with a more serious symptom. Sometimes family dynamics can mislead a therapist at first, as when a family requests help for a flamboyant, favored child while ignoring a less favored, seriously depressed one.

In exploring the initial presentation of the problem, a therapist may learn that the family is experiencing a life- or system-threatening crisis. Life-threatening crises may take the form of potential suicide, potential homicide, or physical violence that may get out of control. Threats to the system mean that some family member is about to run away or be thrown out. When a therapist identifies any such serious risks, the niceties of thorough exploration and alliance building must be forgone. Instead, the strict focus must be on working out an immediate plan for ensuring the safety of all family members.

How Has the Family Tried to Solve the Presenting Problem?

Exploration of the family's attempts to solve the designated problem provides a reading of the family's resourcefulness, ability to communicate and cooperate, and type of organization. Since the request for help usually indicates that there has been a worsening of the situation, the answers to this question often reveal feelings of anxiety, anger, or helplessness in some or all family members. These emotions may result from lack of ideas or knowledge about what to do. Many times, however, attempts to solve the problem that have *not* made a difference are repeated with intensified effort, thus reinforcing the problem and making the organization more rigid. Alternatively, there may be lack of persistence in efforts that really could lead to change in the problems, thus promoting a looser organization or chaos.

What Is the Life Stage of the Family?

In the life of a family system, major developmental changes are those in which members are added to or leave the family. Partial additions (e.g., the family cares for a grandchild several hours per day) or leavings (e.g., the youngest child starts school) may also have an unsettling effect on the arrangement of relationships in the family. The "launching" stage of family life — that is, young adults' leaving home — is a most difficult stage for many families, because of multiple developmental changes across generations and alliance shifts that affect every member (McCullough, 1980). (For discussions of this and other specific stages of family life, see Carter & McGoldrick, 1980.)

Consideration of life stage issues is extremely relevant to most families linked in adoption. Concerns about adding a member apply to the family in which a teenage daughter is unexpectedly pregnant, to the infertile couple, to the family who adopts, and the adult adoptee. The issues of exiting a family are especially poignant for the birth mother who places her child in adoption, for that child sooner or later, and for the adoptive family that must launch young adults.

What Is the Function of the Presenting Problem?

Each of the "schools" of family therapy suggests some variation on defining the function of the presenting problem. The position taken here is that the presenting problem is an attempted but *paradoxical* solution to difficulty in the dynamic operation of the family. The paradoxical nature of the symptom is that it both distracts from and calls attention to the source of the problem in the relationships in the family.

The source of the problem in a family's relationships can best be understood by learning how relationships have been negotiated by the founding couples. These negotiations establish three key dimensions that define the original marital system. Further considerations are the ways in which these dimensions have shifted over the lifetime of the family — in particular, during each addition to and subtraction from the family. The final consideration, most important for assessment, is the form of the dimensions at the time of the symptom production, which leads to the family's presentation for treatment.

The three key dimensions of this assessment schema are

psychological, behavioral, and systemic in type. They can be pictured as concentric circles, as in Figure 2.1. The processes of development and assessment move in opposite directions through the three rings. Development of a relationship begins with the innermost ring, the psychological dimension. Assessment of a family relationship system must start with the outermost ring, representing regulation, or the degree of organization of the system. The middle circle represents the behavior/communication dimension. ("Behavior" and "communication" are used synonymously here, since behavior is nonverbal communication and verbal communication is behavior.)

The Psychological Dimension

Our elaboration of the three key dimensions follows the process of development. The innermost dimension, the psychological one, is the sphere of meanings, world view, emotions, perception, and cognition. The psychological theme of a relationship is identified by content that is consistently associated with intense emotions. Thus it is the least observable dimension and often must be elicited or inferred over time.

Individuals who form and stay in a relationship of sufficient duration to become a marriage have connected in the psychological realm. This means they have recognized in each other someone at

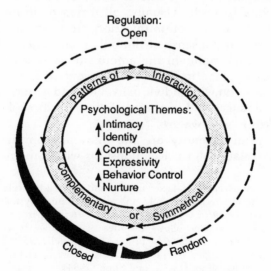

FIGURE 2.1. Three-dimensional model of marital systems.

an equivalent level of psychological maturation. Usually this derives from similar or equivalent experiences in families of origin which either supported or handicapped psychological maturation. Each partner hopes for a psychological exchange in the marriage that will enhance each one. The expected exchange may be based on replication of whatever was good in the original families. At the same time, there are usually wishes for reparation of whatever was painful.

Often the spouses' early experiences have put them on opposite sides of the same issue, so that they sense their equivalence but hope for an exchange that will move both toward wholeness. For example, a shy man may pair with an outgoing woman. Their exchange around expressivity of emotions may enable him to become more comfortable in social situations while she gains a steadying supporter.[1] Usually, current marital patterns can be clearly traced to the patterns of relationships learned in families of origin, including both positive and negative aspects.

The coming together or exchange in regard to similar developmental issues creates the "psychological theme" of a marriage. Psychological themes of relationships have been identified and adapted to parallel Erik Erikson's (1963) developmental tasks of the individual. Beginning with the earliest, they are as follows: basic nurture, behavior control, expressivity of emotions, role competence, gender identity/values, and intimacy.

Content indicating a theme of intimacy focuses on the nature of the relationship itself. Usually, all forms of intimacy—mutual respect, shared values, communication, and sexual contact—provide satisfaction and a sense of mutual enhancement. But a couple must identify and maintain the amount of closeness and distance desired by each person in all areas. The content indicating a theme of identity has to do with individual values and gender security, and the degree of successful accommodation of these factors into a marital sense of "who we are."

Intimacy and identity are the most appropriate themes for mature adult relationships. Relationships with a theme of intimacy

1. The concept that psychological exchange is fundamental to a relationship follows those theorists who view relationship history as important to systems development. Other theorists emphasize the "here and now" of systems operations and disregard history. This practice model follows the idea of exchange based on individual psychological need, first articulated by Fisher and Mendell (1960). Similar concepts have been further developed by Jackson (see Lederer & Jackson, 1968), Sager (1976), Ziegler and Musliner (1977), and Slipp (1984).

are rarely in need of treatment. When such couples do come for therapy, it is usually for adjustment in their closeness–distance arrangements, which can readily be achieved on a short-term basis. Relationships with a theme of identity are also not prevalent in the clinical population, but are seen most often at two life stages. Couples with this theme may either seek help with initial difficulties in forming a marital identity or request therapy at midlife, when the changing values of at least one spouse have dislocated the previous sense of marital identity. Couples who are marrying at midlife may request help with both aspects.

Content indicating a marital theme of competence has to do with adequacy in carrying out social roles, especially those of spouse and worker, and perhaps that of parent. This is the appropriate theme for the marriage of young adults. Spouses who make a good exchange on this theme struggle through the issues, support each other's sense of competence, and move on to a firm sense of identity as a couple. Other young adults come to marriage and establish this developmentally appropriate theme, but have so much anxiety about their competence that they remain mired in the issues indefinitely.

Since the theme of competence is developmentally appropriate for marriages of young adults, the way in which this stage works out is crucial to the future of the marriage. A couple's marriage may either develop into the more mature themes or bog down on the theme of competence, which becomes increasingly inappropriate as they age. Yet another possibility is regression to one of the early, truly out-of-phase themes. Thus, when a marriage with this theme is presented to a therapist, the life stage of the spouses has special relevance for assessment and outcome of treatment. This theme also commonly combines with any possible readings of the other two dimensions. Perhaps because the theme of competence is pivotal to development and to level of functioning, it is frequently the theme of marriages presented for treatment. The complementary form of behavior that reflects a theme of competence has even acquired a name of its own: the "overadequate–underadequate" relationship. (This relationship type was first discussed and named by Bowen, 1978.)

The pivotal theme of competence also has particular relevance to families linked in adoption. For example, an adolescent may test social competence in relation to the opposite sex, and the result may be an unplanned pregnancy. Whether the situation at all supports or only does damage to the individual's sense of competence or to the relationship with the sexual partner depends on the reactions of important people around them. In a very different but related sense, the spouses who are ready to go on to the developmental stage of becoming parents but are thwarted by infertility have surely experienced a blow to their sense of competence; adoptive parents suffer lifelong grief from their inability to assume the parental role biologically. Finally, adoptees frequently report that factors of adoption cause them continuing doubts about their adequacy in social roles.

The theme of expressivity is shown by content related to the handling of emotions. When this is the marital theme of young adults, the developmental lag is not yet severe; for older adults, it suggests that they are "stuck" on emotional issues that reflect their experience of relationships in families of origin. How couples with a theme of expressivity respond to treatment depends on their life stage and degree of emotional trauma. The variations on this theme are well represented in clinical populations. Therapists are very familiar with one complementary arrangement indicating a theme of expressivity: the partnership of a obsessive–compulsive male who is underexpressive with a hysteric female who is overexpressive.

The content of the theme of behavior control, as its name suggests, has to do with ensuring the "correct" form of behavior. In a complementary arrangement, one spouse often becomes parent and director of the other. In a symmetrical arrangement, spouses may fight about proper behavior, or may join an organization such as a religious or political group that prescribes a code of behavior.

The theme of nurture has to do with basic emotional supplies; its issues are expressed in terms of attention, security, food, money, and basic bodily functions. Although this theme may seem to overlap with the theme of intimacy, it is qualitatively quite different. For example, at this level sex is either avoided, sought for body contact, or used for compulsive reassurance rather than for true sexual exchange.

The themes of behavior control and basic nurture embody the issues of infancy. When these are still the themes of adult relationships, the discrepancy in age-appropriateness is a clue to dysfunction. Adults who still struggle with very early issues generally experienced severe deprivation in their early attachments; therefore, they remain needy in regard to these issues and find mates in equivalent positions, with whom they create dysfunctional relationships. The individuals in marriages with psychological themes of behavior control or nurture usually fall within the individual diagnostic categories of narcissistic personality disorder, borderline personality disorder, or various psychoses.

The Behavioral Dimension

As spouses come together and create a psychological theme, there are myriad interactions and negotiations (often not in conscious awareness) as to what behavior is permissible. From this cumulative process, the operating rules of the relationship develop. These in turn shape a consistent, identifiable "pattern of interaction" — the behavioral dimension for assessment. For a couple, two broad gestalts are possible for the pattern of behavior: "symmetrical" and "complementary." (These terms are adapted from Watzlawick, Beavin, & Jackson, 1967.)

A symmetrical pattern of behavior is one in which both partners behave in similar ways. The most common clinical example of this behavior pattern is the conflictual pair who fight in an exquisitely tit-for-tat fashion, staying exactly equal even as they escalate; *what* they fight about provides the content of their psychological theme.

A complementary pattern is one in which each partner behaves in different ways, which together form a whole gestalt. For example, a leader and a follower need each other to fulfill their roles, which consist of quite different behavior. The very different behavior of spouses in complementary behavior patterns may distract from awareness of their common psychological theme. The behavioral differences in complementary spouses' connection to the theme can be thought of in this way: One person acts out the theme while the other defends against it. A common clinical example of this arrangement is that of the caretaker and the symptomatic spouse. The nature of the symptoms may provide a clue to the underlying psychological theme. The symptoms may be of any type — anxiety attacks, phobias, depression, violent behavior, substance abuse.

The Regulation Dimension

The third dimension develops from the other two. As the psychological and behavioral exchanges are negotiated, the dynamic structure of the relationship system emerges. Since dynamic structure is maintained by rules of operation and permissible deviation, this dimension is called "regulation." Here, regulation is defined as the degree of organization of the system and the operating rules that maintain this degree of structure.[2] The regulation dimension is seen as a continuum of predictability versus unpredictability. It is manifested in a family's uses of time, space, and energy. (These concepts are adapted from Kantor & Lehr, 1976.) The continuum ranges from "closed" through "open" to "random" types of regulation (See Figure 2.1).

Closed regulation of a system is indicated by predictable use of time, space, and energy, with little spontaneity. The family with extremely closed regulation has a highly predictable organization: How, when, and where activities are done are strictly prescribed for each member. Little or no spontaneous deviation is permitted before some correction takes place. For example, in a family with closed regulation everyone returns home at appointed times. Then dinner is served daily at the stroke of 6:30 to a washed and waiting family. After dinner, all members watch the same television shows together. In such a family, if a teenager lingers behind closed doors after dinner to listen to music, very few minutes will pass before someone worries and tells the teen to return to the family.

From this extreme of closed regulation, a family system may fall at a point along the continuum with a decreasing gradient of predictability and increasing amounts of permissible spontaneity. A regulation is considered close to the open range when the generally predictable use of time, space, and energy is nearly balanced by the possibility of deviation. When regulation is only a little into the closed range, for example, dinner may be served at about the same time each day with all family members expected. Activities before and after dinner may have some routine, but each person has some freedom of choice. Only a serious deviation, such as someone not showing up for dinner, will bring a correction.

For a designation of open regulation, the organization of the system must be balanced between stability and flexibility. There must be enough stability to maintain the integrity of the system through the inevitable developmental changes. But there also must be enough flexibility to permit changes, especially when these are

2. Although the term "regulation" is conceptually related to the definitions of "structure" and "boundary" in other systemic models, it is not defined identically and is considered more dynamic. However, similar concerns with how family systems maintain integrity in the face of developmental and other inevitable changes are integral to the research of Beavers and of Olson. Furthermore, both have investigated the different kinds of family organizations and the implications for treatment. See for example, Beavers (1976, 1982), Beavers and Voeller (1983), and Olson et al, (1983).

needed to accommodate the maturation of family members. (All human systems technically are "open," since anything alive must undergo change. Thus the terms used here are relative.) This is not to say that open regulation makes it easy for a family to accommodate developmental change. But open regulation *does* mean that a family, despite the inevitable stress, will work out the accommodations needed to support the developmental needs of all members. In a small example, a parent walks away and leaves a child at kindergarten, even though the parent is crying and the child is not.

Random regulation is the designation for organizations at the other end of the continuum, as shown in Figure 2.1. Random regulation indicates degrees of lesser organization, with decreasing amounts of predictability. On the continuum between open and random organization, but closer to open, a household has some predictable schedule; however, this is readily overthrown for spontaneous use of time, space, and energy. At the extreme of random organization, a family has no regular time or place for eating, sleeping, or being together. Often the activities and whereabouts of family members may be unknown. At this extreme, the system may be described as "unorganized" or "chaotic," but even this is a type of organization.

Finally, the gap between the two extremes of the continuum can be closed by overlapping the ends, as shown at the bottom of Figure 2.1. Thus, a category of regulation is created that includes some of the features of both extremes. When the regulation of a family system is in part very rigidly predictable and in part very unpredictable, communication is likely to be rife with double-bind messages. The content of communication focuses on basic nurture, the earliest theme, thereby adding the discrepancy of infantile issues held by adults. Thus, in these most dysfunctional (probably psychotic) systems, incongruities are prevalent in all dimensions.

The Three Dimensions as Guidelines for Assessment

These three dimensions cannot be taken as discrete categories, because living systems defy such labeling. The dimensions are useful only as guidelines for making observations and putting them into a coherent assessment. When a clinician is forming an assessment from dimensional readings, the regulation dimension is the key to the level of dysfunction in the family. Thus the reading of the regulation dimension is crucial for evaluating the potential for change, as well as for guiding intervention.

Theoretically, any readings of the behavioral dimension or of psychological themes can combine with open regulation to produce more functional systems. Conversely, in theory, any reading of the behavioral or psychological dimensions could combine with either extreme of regulation to produce a most dysfunctional system. In reality, for reasons of development described earlier, more mature themes are most likely to be found with some degree of open regulation; the earliest themes combine with the extremes of regulation, producing the most dysfunctional family systems. The pivotal midrange themes can be more or less anxiety-ridden, thus possibly combining with any degree of regulation. Symmetrical or complementary patterns of behavior can be either functional or dysfunctional, depending on how they are regulated.

Assessment of the Roles of Children

By the time of their marriage, most spouses have negotiated the dimensions of their relationships, so that the relationship can be considered a formed system. Any child who arrives is introduced to the dimensions of the system as it exists. Whether or not the marital system is functioning to the satisfaction of the couple, the child must find a place in relation to the marital system already in operation, as well as to whatever role has been prepared for him or her . Each successive child in turn must respond to the larger pre-existing system and must negotiate a place.

A child, even a newborn infant, is a full negotiator in establishing his or her role in the family. Yet a child cannot be considered a founding contributor to the dimensions of the system in the same way as parents are. The maturational level of parents, as reflected in the psychological theme and regulation dimensions of the marriage, has shaped the system that a child confronts. Since parents are only able to induce a child to take on roles that they know and expect, maturational assets and deficits are passed on and shape the child's development.

When spouses in the most functional marriages decide to have a child, the decision is mutual, even though one spouse may be more enthusiastic than the other. It is based on readiness to extend their sense of well-being, try on the next developmental role as parents, and provide another generation of the family. The spouses engage in both individual and joint preparation, which includes dreams and expectations for the child, as well as expectations of how they will be parents together. Optimally, the preparations provide for a continued strong alliance between spouses, while allowing each parent to have a nurturing relationship with the child.

But even the best-functioning and best-prepared parents may confront the unexpected, which strains the operation of their system. The child may arrive with a temperamental or physical problem (such as prematurity, a handicap, or an illness) that affects the initial attachment process. Other parents may make comfortable arrangements for new members up to a particular number and then find the family system's resources overloaded. Still others can adjust their systemic arrangements as needed for new members, but then experience difficulty when affected by events beyond their control. Such events may include illnesses, deaths, economic reverses, or even later developmental stages of family life.

Couples whose developmental themes are appropriate but loaded with anxiety from past experiences are more vulnerable. Depending on their amount of personal and interpersonal conflict, the regulation of their systems may be somewhat, moderately, or severely closed or random. Under the pressure of any unsettling events, their regulation tends to move toward one extreme or the other. In particular, the addition of one or more children may strain such families' ability to nurture members. All subsequent developmental stages may pose a threat, especially when children's development affects the issues of the psychological theme (i.e., unresolved issues of the parents' development). Other unexpected factors, such as a "surprise" child, health problems, or losses, can have a heavy impact and can overload such systems.

Some marital systems never develop an exchange satisfactory to the spouses and/or never approach an appropriate psychological theme for an adult relationship. In these dysfunctional systems based on early themes, the needs and expectations of each partner are too much for the other, who is needy at the equivalent level. These spouses generally have had a family background in which there were severe deficits in parental giving of nurture and/or training in behavior control.

When these individuals want children, the desire reflects the wish for another chance for nurture to self. A child joining such a couple receives an induction to a pre-established role of caretaker, in one of several possible forms, to one or both parents. Any attempts by a child in such a role to develop appropriate autonomy brings the threat of change into the arrangements, thus intensifying anxiety. (See also Wynne, Ryckoff, Day, & Hirsch, 1967.)

Several variant family structures that include the same two parents are possible only through adoption. These occur when parents adopt several older children serially, adopt a sibship, or add children both by adoption and by birth. In these instances, the

normal anxiety inherent in adding family members can be compounded in the effort to foster attachments with children of
different ages, temperaments, and traumatic experiences. Furthermore, each child's maturation, timing of arrival, and subsequent
testing of placement may be out of sequence with normal individual
and family development.

The diagnostician who tries to understand the dynamics of such
a family surely needs a picture of the family's growth. The sequence
of arrivals should be traced in detail with these questions: "What was
it like before? How did the next arrival come about? What happened
then?" In the most complex situations, the interaction of multiple
factors may best be charted on paper.

Assessment of a Single-Parent Family

In the assessment of a single-parent system, it is as important to learn
the origins of the arrangement as it is to know the beginning of a
two-parent system. Several factors are important to assessment in
such a case:

1. The age and maturity of the parent, and whether the person
is a single parent by choice or by default.

2. The relevant system in which to view the single parenthood.
This could be the family of origin, a failed marriage, and/or the
network of a single adult who has chosen to become a parent. Such
a network may include medical and/or child welfare organizations.

3. The relationship and attitude of the single parent to family
of origin and to the missing parent. In the case of the single adoptive
parent, the attitude toward the other parents is relevant, (i.e. the
birth parents).

4. The ways in which all of these factors impinge on the role of
a child, or variously on the roles of several children, by age, birth
order, or gender.

The factors of age, maturity, and choice are directly related to
the individual's life stage and psychological needs at the time of
becoming a parent. Whether an adolescent becomes a single parent
accidentally or deliberately can have long-term positive or negative
effects on emancipation. If adolescents develop an intense relationship (perhaps leading to marriage) in order to escape the original
family, having children may also be a means to shore up individuation. If such a relationship subsequently breaks up, the single

parent's ongoing needs and attitudes to the ex-partner and to the family of origin will directly affect the roles of the child or children.

Even a person who comes to marriage and parenthood dealing with appropriate young adult issues of competence may still experience a floundering marriage and become a single parent. Here the assessment questions are whether the person has chosen the separation or feels abandoned, whether the other parent is still available and to what extent, and whether there is appropriate support from the family of origin (neither too little nor too much). Each of these factors affects the role development between parent and child.

Finally, some adults, often in their 30s or 40s, have concluded that they will not marry but want to become parents. Often these people are successful in careers and are sufficiently affluent to be able to provide comfortable physical care for children. They may fall anywhere on the developmental continuum, but their level of maturity is basic to their motivation to become single parents by choice, either by birth or by adoption. At the most optimal level is the person who is capable of and has experienced strong, well-functioning relationships but for some reason has decided not to marry. Such a person may be motivated for and capable of nurturing a child, but has usually also developed a good support system, sometimes with a designated "second parent" or "family." At the other extreme is the adult who has been disappointed in love experiences (perhaps from the original family on) and now wants a child who can permanently fulfill the unmet needs.

When a single parent adopts a child, most often the child is older than an infant and has special needs. In this circumstance, both persons have needs, expectations, and prior relationship experiences to bring to the negotiation of the new relationship. Here the potential pitfalls require considerable support, which is often supplied (at least initially) by the social worker who facilitates the placement. This role of the social worker is usually crucial to the formation of the family and may be integral to the new system, and therefore must be considered in an assessment.

Regardless of the circumstances of becoming a single parent, the parent must make some personal resolution of the "story" of this circumstance. The working out of such a "story" parallels the way in which two parents work out their decision for a child, and becomes preparation or shaping of a role for the child. Whether the single parent has been divorced or is in or out of contact with the other parent or parents, the personal resolution is important. It shapes attitudes and expectations, as well as what is actually told to a child. Thus the parent's resolution helps to create family beliefs about the situation. The story about the empty role in the household has a shaping effect on the parent–child relationship and on the child's identity formation. This effect can occur *regardless* of whether the position of the other parent is in fact still filled by the other parent or parent substitute outside the home.

Assessment of Variant Family Types and Roles

Therapists are increasingly faced with the need to assess the complex family systems of remarried families, in which children participate in two households with two sets of parents. Whenever there is an adoption within a remarried family, the fact of birth parents adds still another set. These systems must be viewed as parts of earlier systems, which come together in new marriages with generational anomalies. Assessment must consider the strength and duration of the current marriage(s) in comparison to the strength and duration of the pre-existing parent-child relationships. (For more specific discussion of the treatment of variant family forms, see Chapter 13 of this volume.)

Any family, regardless of type or level of functioning, can be struck by events (developmental or some other kind) that overwhelm its ability to operate by its usual rules. At such times of anxiety, the operations of a system often fluctuate, intensify, and/or reach a crisis state. As members of such a system attempt to solve the situation, they may work their way through to more satisfactory operations, and perhaps to more open regulation. In other cases family members redouble their efforts, so that the operations return to the prior arrangements or become more rigidly regulated. In still other cases family members flail helplessly in all directions, with the result that regulation becomes looser. But at such times, the operations of many families are rebalanced through the development of symptoms.

Most families have a member who is considered a little different from the others, whether in appearance, talents, interests, temperament, or health. In families where all of the children or all but one are the same gender, the "other" parent or child is obviously different. Sometimes having the same birth order position as a parent or resembling a special parental sibling may give a child a unique role.

Some special roles are based on behavior that creates expectations about replication. For example, an unplanned teenage pregnancy in a parent's family of origin can transfer to concern about a teenage daughter. Adoption into a family can surely create this aura of differentness. Also, the first child born to an adoptee automatically has a special role, if the child is the first birth relative the adoptee has ever known.

When family members' usual ways of coping are overwhelmed, the somewhat "different" one can be induced to take on or can volunteer for the role of symptom bearer. Symptoms offer a paradoxical solution to a family's anxiety: A person's behavior symbolizes and focuses the anxiety, while at the same time distracting the family from the original source. (See also Vogel & Bell, 1967.) A symptom, the end result of a family's process of dealing with anxiety, is what is presented to the clinician. Because the presenting problem is what has brought the family to the clinican's office and what they want help for, it must be the starting point. Knowing that a problem is the result of a whole family's process of coping with anxiety arms the therapist for what is a considerable assessment task.

The therapist not only must engage family members in exploring the problem, but also must gain understanding of the problem in relation to the family dynamics. The process begins with the elicitation of details about the most recent instance of the presenting problem. By asking about each family member's knowledge, attitude, and reaction to the incident, the therapist creates a bridge from the problem into the family dynamics. On hearing from each family member, the therapist can begin to hypothesize about the arrangements of the three dimensions.

After getting all the details of the presented instance of the problem, the therapist solicits details of other instances. On the basis of similarities or differences in the episodes, the therapist can confirm hypotheses, adjust them, or formulate new ones. In this process the therapist takes a reading of each of the three key dimensions of the family relationship system. Particular attention is given to the regulation dimension, in order to determine the level of family functioning and the assess possibility of change.

How Can the Assessment Guide the Treatment Plan?

The early reading of the regulation dimension suggests the initial approach to intervention. If relatively open regulation is evident, the therapist may focus upon the patterns of interaction and the associated emotional content of the psychological theme. If moderately rigid or moderately loose regulation is seen, the focus needs to be on the issues of regulation and the patterns of behavior. If extremely closed or extremely random regulation is experienced, the therapist must focus directly and mainly on those features.

Open regulation is shown in a number of ways. Family members are able to take turns in telling their views and to listen to one another. Individuals acknowledge their own behavior and emotions, both positive and negative. They respond thoughtfully to clarifications and sometimes adjust their views on the spot. All these characteristics also apply to their interaction with the therapist, a stranger. They readily engage in the process and accept direction, but maintain boundaries appropriate to a first meeting. When a therapist hears someone say in a first meeting, "I never thought of it that way before," or "That's a new way of looking at it," these are good indicators of open regulation. Thus, full attention can be given to the pattern of behavior and the content of the psychological theme.

Families whose regulation is on the rigid side usually provide clues through their behavior, which is mirrored in the details of the presented problem. They are always on time for appointments, sit properly in their chairs (and always occupy the same ones), and may even hold their bodies very still. The regularity in the pattern of communication is soon obvious. Often there is a spokesperson who directs the pattern, or a sequence of speakers that varies little.

Here the therapist must engage the person or persons who have the power to bring the family back. Since this may not be the spokesperson, the therapist has the task of locating the power while listening to the problem. Furthermore, the degree of rigidity must be evaluated by trying to redirect interaction or inducing some novelty. How the family responds to a therapist's attempts to engage them is significant and determines whether the focus can move on to the pattern of behavior or must stay with attempts to loosen severe rigidity.

Features of random regulation are also usually felt immediately. Often the whole family or some member is late, sometimes to the point of missing most of a session. Once present, some or all family members may move around the room, talk at the same time, or interrupt one another; arguments that exclude the therapist may break out until firm action is taken. Under these circumstances, a therapist must induce structure to the session and attempt to engage each individual. Rules may be laid down, such as "Only one may talk at a time," reinforced with the explanation that such rules are needed if the therapist is to help them. How family members respond to structure in the session determines whether the focus can move on to the patterns of behavior. If not, the focus must stay on maintaining structure in the session, so that the members can tell their story and the therapist can determine whether a contract can be developed. At least some members of such families may engage quite amicably with a therapist, but a positive response does not ensure that they will return.

Case Illustrations of Assessment

Several case vignettes are provided to illustrate assessment of the dimensions through the presenting problem, and the subsequent development of a treatment plan.

> A husband and wife in their mid-30s come for help at an important decision point in the medical treatment of infertility. They can choose another surgery for the wife followed by more powerful medication. They can try *in vitro* fertilization, but that will cause a severe financial burden. Furthermore, they have considered, and have conflicting feelings about, adoption or remaining childless. Both spouses are pleased about their relationship and struggling with what any of the options would mean for them as a couple.
> As they tell the therapist their situation, each participates, looks at the other and the therapist, and shows appropriate affect. Both are equally clear about own conflicts and where there is a difference with spouse. They respond readily to the therapist's questions and express gratitude for being understood.

Assessment: There is open regulation, symmetrical pattern of behavior, and a problem in the developmental stage of becoming parents. This is affecting their sense of identity as a strong couple who would be good parents.

Treatment Plan: The therapist should get the history of the infertility and the relationship, with special emphasis on eliciting the importance of children, grief, and stress. Finally, all the options should be thoroughly reviewed.

Prognosis: The possibility of working out a decision that is satisfactory and enhances the marriage appears excellent.

> A husband and wife in their early 20s apply for therapy, saying that their marriage has been troubled since the recent birth of their

first child, a daughter. Both say that their relationship before the birth was good, even though their jobs kept them apart frequently, but now the wife is at home. The husband's complaint is that his wife has become a full-time mother: She seems to exclude him from a relationship with the baby and has no time for him.

The wife admits that her attitude has changed a little, but says that it has to do with her background. She never felt valued in her family — in fact, she was adopted. Now that she has a child, she will show her adoptive mother and her birth mother just what a good mother should be! When the husband asks, "What about me?", the wife gets defensive and says that now she has company when he is on the road. Promptly, they trade accusations about all the times each has let down the other.

Assessment: The system is in flux at the developmental stage of adding a child. The relationship has been a little loosely regulated, with a symmetrical pattern and a theme of competence. There is potential for the regulation to become looser (with the couple more distant) or more predictable (in a conflictual style).

Treatment Plan: The therapist should focus on the pattern of interaction and its shifts after the birth of the baby. Also the expectations of marriage and being parents should be clarified between the spouses, with particular reference to how each was raised and the wife's adoption.

Prognosis: The outcome depends on the depth of emotional investment each has in the marriage versus the baby, as well as on whether the marriage is strong enough to work through conflicts, which may be basic and serious.

A mother and father apply for family therapy because of concerns for their 8-year-old son, who is adopted. They also have an adopted 6-year-old daughter, who is a thriving first-grader. The son is doing poorly in school, often seeming lost in daydreams, but otherwise not disruptive.

The mother reports that the boy recently asked her some questions about where he came from. The mother, acknowledging that she is very emotional, says that she tried to be frank with him but tears sprang into her eyes; the boy hastily withdrew to his room. That evening at dinner, the father tried to talk to the boy about school and his questions. When the boy refused to talk, the father yelled at him for being so obstinate and said that sometimes he too wondered where the boy came from. At that point the boy ran back to his room; the girl burst into tears, as did the mother. The father admits that this sort of scene has happened ever since the boy began having school problems — the father wants to help, but he just does not understand what is going on or why the boy cannot just shape up.

Assessment: The system demonstrates somewhat closed regulation and a complementary marital pattern of interaction in regard to expressivity; both children are allied more with the mother than with the father.

Treatment Plan: The therapist should promote openness of expression about adoption, supporting the children's right to ask. At the same time, the therapist should encourage the mother to discuss her emotions with some restraint, while helping the father to identify the emotions behind his anger.

Prognosis: The outlook is quite good, in that the closed qualities of regulation are not severe and the parents have expressed willingness to improve the situation.

A woman of 42, who has never married but has risen to become a department head in a large business, applies for help with the 11-year-old daughter she has just adopted. She reports that both she and the girl enjoyed the planning, the preplacement period, and the early days of living together. But the carefully planned placement took place during the summer, when the mother had taken a 2-month leave of absence and the daughter was not in school.

Within days of the opening of school and the mother's return to work, there have been problems. The daughter is clingy and does not want mother to go to work or to go to school herself. Frequently the mother receives phone calls that the daughter is sick at school and needs to go home. When both are at home, the daughter does not let the mother out of her sight. She eats huge amounts and also hoards sandwiches and cookies in her room. The girl prefers evenings together in front of the television. She often tries to curl up on the mother's lap, which in fact she is too big to do very successfully.

The mother tearfully reports that she knew the daughter had come from a deprived, neglectful background. Eventually she was abandoned and then was placed in several foster homes over a 2-year period. Even though the social worker explained that the daughter has much catching up to do, the mother believed that love and care would soon make the difference. Now she is not so sure. She has tried being firm about appropriate behavior, using methods that were successful for her parents. But the daughter just cries and continues the same behavior. The mother feels not only ineffective, but guilty because she unexpectedly feels smothered. Furthermore, she wonders whether this child is much more disturbed than she realized or can handle.

Assessment: This older, inexperienced mother probably came from a more orderly family system (with somewhat closed regulation) and established a successful work and life style based on independence and competence. She has adopted an undernurtured child from a family system that became so random in regulation that the system disintegrated and the child was abandoned. The two of them have no common experience to guide mutual expectations or even understanding.

Treatment Plan: the therapist should help this mother and daughter negotiate a new system in which the operating rules are appropriate to the different generational roles and needs. In addition, they should be educated about developmental lags based on deficits in nurture, which must be addressed but need not be pathological. They should also be helped to work out what is age-appropriate behavior and the circumstances in which it is required and when it is not.

Prognosis: The prognosis must be guarded until the strength of the attachment, mutual commitment, and motivation to work it out can be assessed. All these aspects of relationship development are likely to be severely tested in the next stage of placement. If the mother has sufficient commitment, energy, and support to withstand the testing, the prognosis will be good. A positive outcome will be aided if the child has some ability not to push beyond the mother's ability to cope.

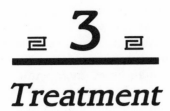

Treatment

Often with no more warning than a brief phone call, the family therapist is confronted with a family that has a problem to be fixed. The therapist is offered the final, evolutionary product of intricate and complex interactions of family development. At the outset, all that the therapist can be sure of is that someone is feeling pain. Regardless of what has led to the decision to make contact, some sort of discomfort has brought the family to a therapist. This pain, and the family's way of explaining it, are presented to the therapist as "the problem." The therapist must begin by listening to and exploring this offering, because this is the only approach that will make sense to them.

Whereas assessment is a cognitive process of the therapist, treatment is an interactive process between the therapist and the family seeking help. But these processes are not separable, and both go on throughout the course of a therapy. Ordinarily, assessment takes more conscious effort at the beginning, when a therapist must learn about the family members and what has brought them. But also from the start, every question or empathic response of the therapist shapes a family's experience of therapy.

Later, after a contract has been established, the emphasis is on intervention. Even then, the family's responses to interventions feed back to assessment and result in continual refinement of it. Thus the therapist is always engaged in a circular process. This process involves tracking what goes on in a family's interactions, adding the observations to assessment, and then using that to inform the next move with the family.

Furthermore, this circular process applies not only to cognition but also to affective aspects of therapy. The affective aspect first has to do with creating rapport, so that family members are engaged in a therapeutic alliance. Then the alliance must be monitored and maintained in well-balanced, working order with *all* family members. This is no easy task when family members may be at odds with each other or with the therapist over any topic. Thus the therapist must also track the nuances of therapeutic alliance and use this information to inform each succeeding move. In effect, this complex role of the therapist means negotiating and monitoring a new system — that is, the therapy system — while remaining in charge of a change process in the family's system.

Strategies for Initial Contacts

The interactive processes begin with the initial phone call. But they come to bear fully on the first interview, from the moment a therapist lays eyes on a family and decides how to open the session. After introductions, if a family waits politely for the therapist to talk (already an item of assessment), two approaches can be considered. If anxiety among family members seems at an ordinary level for first meetings, the therapist may open with a reference to the phone call. Adding that it is important to know each person's point of view, the therapist can ask the phone caller to begin by reviewing what was said. While the first person talks, the therapist picks up clues from nonverbal responses about whom to ask next. Such a beginning plunges a family into the process, thus alleviating anxiety about what therapy will be like. Such a beginning also establishes immediately that the therapist is interested in every person and role in the family. To ensure that this message gets across, the therapist must take care that the initial poll of views about the problem is completed. Even if family members refuse to speak, the invitation stands.

An alternative approach can be used when the anxiety level seems extraordinarily high. In such situations, it is preferable to begin by asking *how*, not *why*, the family has come. What may emerge is that someone has been coerced into coming by other family members, or that the whole family is resentful because of an involuntary referral by school, police, or court. A third possibility is that the family is in crisis and the anxiety is appropriate to a serious concern. In any of these cases, the source of the high anxiety must be addressed immediately.

Some families plunge in, opening the session without waiting for the therapist. This may be a clue to the level of their anxiety and/or their typical dynamics. Extremes of regulation are typically made known promptly. For example, a first meeting may be opened by a father who first questions the therapist's credentials. Then he pulls out a sheaf of notes about the problem, which he proceeds to read at length. Meanwhile, his wife and child sit quietly with downcast eyes. This picture suggests extremely closed regulation. By contrast, extremely random regulation is indicated by the family that comes in with everyone talking at the same time. Children may be running around the room, demanding toys or trips to the bathroom. In any case where a family takes over, the therapist must find a means to take charge of the session.

Whatever the opening, the therapist needs to use the first session to find out each family member's view of the presenting problem. Where each person locates the problem, as well as whether there is agreement among family members, must be noted. Problems may be located in family relationships, in the behavior of one member, or outside the family, perhaps with the referral source. The family may absolutely agree that the problem is the fault of the school or the fault of Mary alone. Members of another family may disagree about whether there is a problem or what it is, or they may join in coalitions with opposing views.

After tracking the initial process of problem presentation, the therapist can give comments on observations. This conveys the ability to hear and accept each person; it also gives the family members information about how the therapist reacts to their situation. When family members feel accepted rather than judged (as they might have anticipated), hope for a positive outcome and the therapeutic alliance are both fostered.

After responding to the initial poll about the problem, the therapist asks for details of the most recent occurrence of the problem. Since people tend to generalize or offer their conclusions, each must be asked to describe his or her own connection to the incident in specific, experiential terms — what was personally observed, said or done. As each person does this, behavior, emotions, motives, and assumptions are articulated, often for the first time. Each time the therapist responds with an empathic new inquiry, the perspective of the receiver as well as of the other family members may be affected. As the therapist takes in these verbal and nonverbal reactions, the focus of inquiry may shift.

After the initial presentation, further instances of the presenting problem are elicited. In hearing these episodes, the therapist continues to inquire into the reactions of each family member. Particular attention is given to any attempts to improve the situation and what resulted. Such efforts may range from parents taking a new approach to discipline to a little sister's warning that the mother is angry. Giving credit to attempts to help, whether or not useful, establishes the therapist's interest in solutions, not just problems. Furthermore, hearing about what was tried and what happened provides information about the regulation dimension.

Sometimes during early discussions of problems, anger and blame burst forth. The therapist must interrupt any attack or blaming match as quickly as possible, directing the speaker to talk only about his or her own feelings. If the person is unable to do so, even with the therapist's help, that individual is directed to tell it to the therapist. The therapist can then listen calmly and give understanding to the emotions, without agreeing with the judgment or blame of the other.

During these early discussions, the counselor may see or hear clues about important developmental events affecting the family. Clues may be obvious, as when the symptom bearer is a junior or senior in high school (especially if the teen is the oldest, the youngest, an only, or an adopted child). Other developmental issues may not be so obvious. For example, a father may turn 50 and may be upset about what he considers a failed career. Or perhaps a mother feels anxious about her daughter's 16th birthday, because she cannot stop thinking about the child she placed into adoption when she was 16 herself. When developmental change is basic to the problem, the family may introduce it as such. If the family does not mention an obvious transition, the therapist can ask about it, with a comment that developmental complications are normal and common. When unsure whether or what developmental issues may lurk, a therapist may fish into possibilities.

Through noting repetitive patterns and intensities of affect, the therapist takes a reading of the dimensions of assessment and the function of the problem for the system. For example, the presenting problem may be that 12-year-old Johnny has been caught several times at school smoking cigarettes in the washroom or skipping classes. In hearing about instances of phone calls from school, the therapist's formulation will develop quite differently under these differing circumstances:

1. The mother always handles the situation without telling anyone.
2. The mother pours out her upset to Johnny's older sister, but neglects to tell the father.
3. The mother gets anxious and calls the father home from work.

4. The mother's and father's roles are reversed in 1–3.
5. The mother attacks Johnny for being bad like his father, from whom she is divorced.
6. After every phone call from school, Johnny's adoption is discussed at length over dinner.

Discussions of the presenting problem should lead to sufficient understanding between therapist and family to underpin the therapeutic alliance and a contract. A therapeutic contract is a clearly verbalized agreement between therapist and family members about what the work is to be about. It is the therapist's responsibility to offer a contract statement as soon as feasible. This may occur toward the end of a first session or after as many as eight. If the contract cannot be agreed upon in the first session, the therapist should ask for a temporary contract for further exploration.

When the therapist first offers the contract statement, it must somehow include everyone who is to be involved in the treatment. The contract statement may be an inclusive, general statement or one with a specific element for each person. An example of a general statement is as follows: "So far, this is what I hear—all of you, parents and big boys, are upset and fighting among yourselves more ever since you adopted baby Joan. We can work together to stop the fighting and make things more comfortable for everyone, including the baby."

An example of a contract statement specific to each member is the following: "What I understand is that after years of wanting a baby, Mary, it is much harder to be alone with a newborn than you ever expected, and John is unsympathetic. John, you have such a good time with the baby that you can't understand why Mary is so angry with you. We can talk over what each of you is going through and how that affects your relationship, so that you can get back to happier times and become cooperative parents."

If family members agree to the offered contract statement, the contract is in place, the family feels understood, and the therapeutic alliance is reinforced. If any family members do not agree, they are asked for their reasons. The reasons are clarified and used to build a more accurate contract statement. Once the contract is agreed upon, the schedule of appointments, the expected duration, and membership can be specified.

Sometimes family members do not agree among themselves or with the therapist on any contract. Other times a family may insist on a contract unacceptable to a family therapist, most commonly "Fix this wild child and leave us parents entirely out of it." In any of these situations, the therapist recognizes the dilemma aloud and requests more time to mediate a contract statement acceptable to both family and therapist. If the difficulty cannot be resolved, this is acknowledged with the conclusion that this therapist and this family cannot work together. When sessions continue without an agreed contract, therapy is likely to lack direction, to be stalemated, or to be terminaed abruptly.

The contract is also a statement of goals. The contract statement provides a direction to the therapy and a means of measuring progress toward the stated goals. From the point of contract, the focus shifts from assessment to interventions that lead to the goals. By the time a contract is established, the therapist has made a preliminary assessment of the three dimensions. Using this assessment as a guide, the therapist considers which strategies, in what sequence, are most likely to be effective with the particular family.

Treatment of Families with Open Regulation

The features of open, flexible regulation, reflective of more functional families, are evident from the first contact. Individuals are expressive, thoughtful, and responsive to the views of other family members and therapist. Often the problem is so well described that the central pattern of behavior supporting the problem can be identified at once. Such ready identification of the problematic pattern permits the therapeutic alliance and contract to be established in the first session. When there is open regulation that permits such ready identification of the problems, the treatment focus moves directly onto the central behavioral pattern. In discussing just how the interactions transpire, the therapist also elicits emotions that trigger each individual's initiating or responsive behavior. Such intense, consistent emotional and behavioral reactions and their meanings indicate the psychological theme. Clarification of these emotions, behaviors, meanings, and misunderstandings in communication, and then their renegotiation, are the main interventions.

Often the therapist can soon describe back to the family members the central pattern of interaction and the triggers that mark exchanges. This serves to aid their understanding and enlists their efforts in further clarification of the problems and negotiation of solutions. A therapist aids the process mostly by monitoring the focus, and offering occasional clarification and interpretation. Reinforcing the family's understanding of what each person contributes to problems as well as to positive experiences supports change in therapy and its maintenance afterward.

If emotions are escalated, the therapist may need to ensure that each family member speaks for himself or herself instead of blaming. Many times the therapist simply needs to provide basic direction to families with open regulation and then stay out of their way. Usually they work through the problems and move rapidly toward their contracted goals.

A more functional family may be satisfied with symptom reduction. But if the family members recontract for further work, the second stage of therapy focuses upon the connections between present and past family experiences of the couple. Specific patterns of behavior and emotional responses of the present are traced to relevant relationship experiences in families of origin. These are worked through for similarities and differences between the past formative relationships and the present marriage. When the connections are clear, spouses can decide what changes they want in the present. For a well-functioning family that comes to therapy for a problem or developmental snag that is quickly resolved, delving into backgrounds is optional. If the parents choose to do so, the reason is to enhance personal growth. For them, even an in-depth review of their emotional lives may only take some months.

Generally, it is a treat for a therapist to engage in therapy with a family where there is open, balanced regulation. But this pleasure also may create pitfalls. A therapist may want the members of such a family to stay longer or work on more ambitious goals than they want. Furthermore, if a therapist is fortunate to have a personal relationship that functions as well as theirs, it may be too easy to form a nontherapeutic alliance with one or both spouses. Or if a therapist is not doing as well personally, there may be envy, inappropriate interference, or even sabotage of the process.

The course of treatment with a family characterized by balanced, open regulation is illustrated by the following case.

A husband and wife in their early 50s, came for therapy because the husband was depressed. They were puzzled by his mood, because things were going well between them and in his business. The wife had her own candy-making business in their house. The husband said sheepishly that all he felt like doing was staying home with his wife.

At this, his wife laughed and wondered who needed to keep an eye on whom these days. Then they related that their only child, a daughter by adoption, had left for college in a distant state just a month before. The therapist commented on the sense of loss that is natural when a child leaves home, especially an only and adopted one.

In response, the couple stared at the therapist, as though stunned. Then emotions came tumbling out of both parents simultaneously: "I thought you'd be so upset when she left." "And I thought it would be worse for you." "I've been remembering all the years of infertility and adoption expectancy." "Did you realize that she went to college in the state where she was born?" "Has she talked about her birth parents lately?" "Could we lose her?" After that outpouring, the spouses realized that they were indeed mourning their daughter's absence and had fears about what was to come. Each had tried to protect the other, and the daughter, by not talking about the worries. A therapeutic contract was simple — these feelings had to be aired.

In the next two sessions, the spouses faced the concerns and their sources. Before marriage, they had discussed a mutual wish for children, so the awareness of infertility was very painful to both. Both partners had physical problems, which in combination made their chances of pregnancy very slim. Nevertheless, they had undergone medical treatment for 6 years, but in the last of those years they began adoption procedures. Just prior to the decision to pursue adoption, the wife had become quite discouraged and depressed. In relating this, both became teary. Suddenly, awareness clicked. Both had been afraid that when the daughter left, the wife would again become depressed. Somehow they had colluded so that the husband took on their mutual sadness. Then he stayed at home so that they could "keep an eye on each other."

In the next meeting, the husband reported that he was feeling better and was back at his office daily. They had continued discussions every evening, but still wanted to review their results with the therapist. In particular, they wished to prepare for talking with their daughter, and also wanted to bring her to a session the next time she was home.

When their daughter came to the session, the parents first reviewed together what they had learned in therapy. Then the father asked whether her choice of college was related to her birth parents. The daughter was teary as she hesitantly admitted that it was. She had not talked to them because she did not want to hurt them or spoil anything among them. When the therapist said that most adopted persons are interested in their origins, the daughter acknowledged that she had always wanted to know more and hoped to look into it. But she wanted her parents to know that she loved them as much as ever. With that, they all cried, affirming their attachments and acknowledging worries. Finally, they discussed what role each should have in the daughter's search, while agreeing that all would be open and sharing of emotions and facts.

About 2 weeks later, the couple came back one last time. The daughter had returned to school with a search plan in place. The parents felt fine again and were thankful for the help. They made the final observation that talking out the issues and supporting the daughter's search had had a paradoxical outcome: They felt a new level of attachment among the three of them, which eased the separation from their daughter and made them a family of adults.

Assessment: The marital (and family) system had open regulation. The marital pattern of interaction was symmetrical and centered around the theme of identity. The parents hit a snag at the developmental stage of launching their daughter and returning to being a couple alone together. The snag was caused by the actual separation from the daughter, which stirred up fears for the future related to the loss issues of adoption and infertility.

Treatment Outcome: In six sessions, the goals were well met. The presenting symptom had dissipated, the grief and separation issues were expressed, and family relationships returned to at least the previous level of functioning and perhaps better.

Treatment of Families with Midrange Regulations

Couples and families with midrange regulations may represent 50% or more of the clinical population. Because the regulations fall at some point on the middle ranges of the continuum described in Chapter 2, they may be found in association with any of the psychological themes, although usually not the very earliest or latest. Marital systems based at an appropriate developmental level or with modest lag, but loaded with anxiety from the past, usually have midrange regulations. The age of these couples at the time of treatment is significant because of the possibility of increased developmental lag.

Assessment of whether a midrange regulation is nearer to open regulation or to an extreme provides a challenge of fine-tuning. There are no obvious markers that immediately help the therapist assess the gradient of regulation, as there are for open or extreme regulations. Instead, the therapist must compare instances of the problem presentations and determine whether there is more or less predictability to the process. In addition, the degree of similarity between their reports and what the therapist observes in session is noted.

Thus, if the patterns (both in session and out) are so predictable that the therapist can soon anticipate the sequences, the regulation is quite far along the continuum toward closed. However, if the pattern of interaction in regard to the problem is quite predictable but with small variations in each round, the regulation is moderately closed. If each instance of the problem and the way it is told seem to have a somewhat different sequence, the regulation is moderately random. If the therapist sees absolutely no connections between incidents and wonders what will happen next (both in session and out), the regulation is far along the continuum toward the random extreme.

The gradient of regulation can be tested quite early in the assessment process. A therapist can devise an intervention that requires a small change in the presenting problem. For example, a mother may always tell her older son first about calls from the school regarding Mary. In the second session the mother is asked not to tell her son at all, but to call her husband and make a date to discuss it that evening.

Once a contract is in place, the family members are asked to select which part of the problem they wish to address first. As the therapist engineers an intervention, family members are asked to participate in choosing the exact terms of the plan. The therapist must monitor the process, making sure that the plan involves a small change for each member. It must be specific, clearly understood by all, and applicable daily or at least several times a week. Tasks that are too large or unclear set up the family members for failure, damaging their hope and willingness to return to therapy. If the family is unable to participate in making a plan, the therapist can use diagnostic information to suggest an idea. Then the potential participants are asked whether their roles are acceptable and if so, to take responsibility for the results. Thus the plan is not just the therapist's idea, which can be thwarted.

A family's response to this initial intervention distinguishes whether the regulation is more moderate or more extreme. Families with moderate regulations usually carry out the plan with complete or partial success. Families with more extreme regulation do not carry out the plan; they may depreciate it, or say that they know it would not have helped. When families have demonstrated moderate regulation by at least partially carrying out the first task, the results should be thoroughly reviewed. Each person is to discuss his or her own reaction, what was done or not, and why. Success is supported while failures are examined without blame. Then the plan can be tried again until it is solidly mastered. When it is, another element may be added to the plan, or a plan may be developed for another problem.

During these initial planned interventions, the therapist develops a specific reading of the pattern of interaction, the gradient of regulation, and way in which the problem is maintained. The reading of the pattern must include the marital exchange as well as the alliances with children. From this precise reading, the central focus of treatment moves to interventions geared to the specific parts of the interaction pattern that support the problem.

As the result of each intervention is reviewed, successes and positive changes are celebrated while pitfalls are reconsidered. In this process, the therapist generally encourages each person's responsibility for his or her own behavior, as well as for owning emotions and motives. While interventions are being reviewed, associated emotions and motives may spontaneously come out. If not, the therapist must note nonverbal clues and invite individuals to say what they are thinking and feeling. As the process moves along, a therapist may decide to coach improved communication between particular family members or about certain topics at issue. Until the therapist sees an improved pattern of communication in session, it should *not* be assigned as homework. A plan for communication (either verbal or physical), that is assigned before individuals are able to carry it out, damages progress.

The pace at which families move through a series of planned changes, and the amount of change accruing, vary with the gradient of regulation and the psychological theme. The pace of a family must be respected, but a therapist can lead just a little ahead of any family. This ensures movement toward the goals but without undue pressure. As emotions emerge, the therapist can assess the emotionally intense content (i.e., the psychological theme). A therapist may or may not be able to work directly with the issues, but may at least identify them for the family. Whether a family works directly on the sources of their emotions and motives depends on the members' ability to understand their processes. When they are willing and able to do so, the therapist should make the most of their abilities as a further means of reinforcing change.

The problems of most couples and families with midrange regulations have direct connections to attachment experiences in the families of origin. Often these issues are currently re-enacted with parents, spouses and/or children. Even if understanding is not a goal, the adults need to make at least broad connections between past and present family relationships. Just enough understanding is needed so that an adult is able to separate old emotions from current realities, without automatic transfer to spouse or children.

The process with families characterized by midrange regulation tends to move in notable steps forward followed by setbacks. When a setback occurs, the therapist can assure family members that it is temporary and that they can regain the lost ground. Once the therapist identifies the pattern of regressions and what triggers them, their occurrence can be predicted. Then, regardless of outcome, the family has gained a little more insight and control.

Families with a gradient of regulation closer to the open may move through the process of symptom change and understanding dynamics in a matter of a few months. If they decide to recontract for a second phase, it is for in-depth work on the connections to the families of origin. Usually a husband and wife decide to do this work by themselves, but sometimes the whole family is included. Other families with somewhat more extreme gradients of regulation may take many months to solidify change in symptoms and the supporting patterns of interaction. Many of these families do not opt for second-phase treatment; instead, they may return to therapy every few years. A family or just a couple may rework the prior issues or deal with new problems, perhaps arising from a new stage of development.

Since families with midrange regulations have reached appropriate developmental themes but are fraught with anxiety, they are likely to resonate in some way with therapists. There may be identification in regard to dynamics, sources of anxiety, gender, family roles, or particular symptoms. In order to monitor such identification, therapists need to be aware of their own vulnerabilities and responses. For example, therapists should know whether they relate most comfortably to their own gender or the other. Many therapists are also vulnerable to particular roles, such as wanting to rescue scapegoats. Certain interactions (e.g., loud arguing) can cause difficulty. Even more difficult are dynamics so familiar and comfortable to a therapist that they are missed as problematic to a particular family.

Such overlap of experiences between therapist and family holds the potential for "triangles." A therapeutic triangle is defined here as occurring when a therapist consistently supports particular family members while consistently confronting certain others. What makes this a triangle is that the therapist has lost the freedom of movement to support and confront every member as needed. A fixed triangle sabotages therapy. Conversely, if a therapist has awareness and control of vulnerabilities, such "inside" knowledge can lead to particularly helpful work.

The following example illustrates the treatment of a family with midrange regulation.

A wife phoned for an appointment for her husband. The serenity of their home life had been shattered by a phone call on behalf of the husband's birth mother. He ended the call quickly and then rushed out of the house; he came in at 3 A.M., very drunk for the first time in his life. Since then he had refused to talk about it. The wife sounded frightened when she asked for the husband to come alone because he needed help. However, she had not yet told him that she would make the request. In discussing how to talk to him, the wife also agreed to come with him, but definitely refused to bring the children. Both spouses were in their early 40s, and had a son aged 12, and a daughter aged, 9.

The spouses arrived early and sat quietly side by side in the waiting area; on being invited in, they sat the same way, looking at the therapist. When the therapist asked the wife to review the phone call, she took a quick look at her husband and then softly repeated the story. When the therapist asked the husband's reaction, he somewhat defensively agreed that her story was essentially correct. But, he emphasized, he had never been drunk before and would not be again, so there was no need to talk about it. The wife began to apologize until the therapist asked what had happened to her feelings about the situation. Then she could say that *she* was still very upset about what had happened, because the serenity of their home was shattered.

With that opening, the therapist asked what the "serenity" of their home was like prior to the phone call. Both spouses worked, and their schedules were very regular — a time for dinner, home-work, TV, and bed. Everyone in the family got along pleasantly, but no one was very talkative or "lovey-dovey." Weekends also had a plan — chores for everyone on Saturday, with an occasional outing planned well in advance. Sundays were occupied by church and alternating visits to the two sets of grandparents.

The mention of grandparents gave an opening to ask about the husband's relationship with his parents. He had always known about his adoption, but it was never talked about. His parents (now in their 80s) were never demonstrative, but he felt loved. Still, he always felt that there was some secret about his heritage that could not be talked about. His wife added that before they were married, when they discussed children, he had said that he might have a dark heritage. She agreed to marry him nevertheless;

after all, both were over 30, and they had already dated for 2 years.

While she talked, the husband hung his head and said that he always seemed to be behind schedule. That was true about finishing college, finding and keeping a good job, and getting married. Now, when things had finally been going smoothly for a few years, this had happened. Then he went on about how jumbled he felt since the phone call about his birth mother. Feelings he had never faced pounced on him. He did want to know about his birth parents, but he was afraid what this would do to his adoptive parents, wife, and children. Maybe there was a shameful secret or bad genes that he was passing on. Even if he might want to know, actually meeting his birth mother seemed unfathomable.

His wife quickly tried to soothe him, saying that they would just forget the whole thing and get back to normal. The husband said that he knew his drinking scared her because of her father, but *he* was scared, wondering if his bad genes had showed up. Then the wife said tightly, "Does that mean I can't trust your promise not to drink again?" At this point, the spouses agreed that they did have some issues and would come for four more appointments.

These sessions were used to open communication between the two, at first focused on emotions. First they were coached to tell each other in session any one thing each liked and one thing each disliked. After they practiced and could do this in session, the task was assigned as daily homework. The next plan was to make those daily comments about the other person. They carried out these plans precisely, and at first stiffly but with increasing ease.

In the third session, feelings about the husband's adoption were discussed, with homework to follow up on certain points with a 10-minute (the amount was chosen by them) conversation each evening. A discussion of his birth mother took up the fourth meeting, with emphasis on what contact with her could mean to him, her, the children, and all the grandparents. With so much still stirring, the scheduled contract was renewed and became open-ended. Over the next months, these timid people addressed their fears of being found inadequate as spouses, parents, and workers. The husband, in particular, worried about his adequacy as a human being who was adopted and could have "bad genes." The wife had to confront fears, derived from her childhood experiences with her father, that men could not be trusted. Her father had doted on her when sober but became unpredictably mean when drunk. As some resolutions were reached, the spouse's sense of competence was enhanced.

Then the children came to sessions for a while, so that they also would have an opportunity to learn more open communication on these vital matters. The husband was coached to talk with his adoptive parents about the call about his birth mother. They said very little, but as he promised to continue regular visits with them, they offered no objection. Eventually he decided to talk with his birth mother on the phone. She was only 60, had a large and boisterous family, and cried as she told of her longing for him all these years. The man was so touched by her joy that he agreed to meet her, but only with his wife present.

The family stayed in treatment for some months longer, dealing with all the repercussions of dual heritage as they affected three generations of families linked in adoption. When the family stopped therapy, communications were open and clear in regard to both content and emotions. Each member was working out comfortable roles with all the members of their dual extended family. The self-esteem of all four seemed improved, and there was also more energy, vitality, and flexibility of arrangements. On the whole, the household remained orderly and rather predictable.

Assessment: The marital (and family) system had moderately closed regulation, a symmetrical pattern of interaction (both spouses were subdued persons who defended against emotions), and a psychological theme of competence. Because the spouses were adults already past 40, the theme of competence represented a developmental lag, caused by much suppressed emotion left over from families of origin and the husband's adoption. The parental themes extended to the whole family, so that all four meekly went about their separate routines in most predictable ways. The phone call about the husband's birth mother, and his drunken response, unsettled the usual arrangements by taking the lid off emotions.

Treatment outcome: Eventually the changes were good. Communication was opened in regard to both spouses' fears about adequacy in general, and their fears about his adoption in particular. As a result, they reached more comfortable arrangements for the immediate family and for three generations of the families linked by his adoption.

Specific changes in the arrangements of the immediate family included a shift in the moderately closed regulation toward more openness. The symmetrical pattern of the spouses remained, but became more cooperative than distant. The adults' sense of competence improved, which in turn helped the children. The family moved toward the theme of identity: "We know who we are and what we can do, and we feel good about it!"

Treatment of Families with Extreme
Forms of Regulation

The extreme forms of regulation are made known at once—often during the initial phone conversation or in the waiting room. Either extreme becomes clearer yet during first sessions, through repetitions that make obvious the rigidity or lack of organization. The identification of extreme regulation is a cue that the therapist must make an early choice about what to offer: a short-term contract pertaining to one specific behavioral change, or a long-term attempt to change the basic arrangements of the organization. Although the therapist decides what to offer, the family ultimately chooses what it can or will accept. Often it is useful to offer an initial short term contract (four to six sessions) for work on one presented problem. Such a contract gives the therapist a chance to test the possibilities of treatment; the family, meanwhile, evaluates safety and possible gains from the situation. If a family wishes to continue after the initial contract, a series of short-term contracts can be added. Such a plan often leads into long-term work. Regardless of duration, the treatment of more dysfunctional families needs to remain problem- and behavior-focused.

Establishing a contract is quite a different matter with families characterized by either extreme of regulation. In a case where there is closed regulation, once the person with authority is engaged, the family attends sessions as requested, on time, and with all invited members. Therefore, when a therapist identifies closed regulation, the first consideration is to determine who has the power and then to engage that person or dyad. The site of power may not be obvious, such as when it is held by the person who cues the spokesperson or by the symptom bearer whose behavior controls the family.

Sometimes the need to engage the person with power requires the therapist to neglect alliances with other family members. If the therapist does engage this person, the family returns and the therapist has time to repair the neglected alliances. If the power is held by a symptom-bearing adolescent or child who refuses to return, the therapist can try to reinforce parental authority by inviting them to return without the youngster. When initial alliance building misses the person with authority in a family with closed regulation, the family does not return.

Contracting with a family where there is extremely random regulation is a haphazard endeavor. The looseness of this type of organization is such that no one has the power to bring the whole family in; these families may rarely or never do anything with all members present. Furthermore, agreements about attending sessions or about the content of contracts cannot be relied upon. When families have random regulation, a therapist must expect them to come late, miss appointments, and be unpredictable about who attends. A therapist must work with whoever shows up, because to refuse to see family members except as invited is to tell them to heal themselves before they can get help. Instead, the therapist holds to the planned structure of the therapy by commenting on who was expected and how to make it work next time. Having a whole-family session may become a goal in such a situation — one that is reached only after considerable structural change.

An assessment of extreme regulation indicates a general therapeutic approach most likely to be effective with each type. Often the presenting problem is directly related to the extreme regulation. The problem for a very rigid system may result from something unsettling the rigid arrangements, especially attempts at emancipation by the young. The situation may have escalated to a crisis or potential rupture of the system. With random regulation, the problem may be behavior that has drifted beyond the acceptable and that begs for controls, perhaps by community authorities.

The general therapeutic approaches with the two extremes have some similarities, but the purposes are opposite. In a closed system, regardless of the particular pattern of interaction being addressed, the effort always is to open and loosen arrangements. This is done by continually inviting and encouraging those family members to speak whose views are not permitted or valued, according to the operating rules of the family. In a system, where there is random regulation, by contrast, the general effort is always to build and increase structure. Thus, regardless of the specific behavioral task, the therapist is always encouraging each person to speak, but with some limits on the free-flowing communication (e.g., only one may speak at a time, a speaker is not interrupted but listened to, and speakers may not attack others but must speak for themselves).

Beyond these general approaches, a reading of an extreme regulation gives a therapist immediate information about the need to adjust expectations. The therapist must expect to limit goals, maintain a behavioral focus, stay in the here and now, work in concrete terms, keep a slow but steady pace, and contain (rather than elicit) emotions. The more extreme the regulation, the more the therapist limits expectations.

These general approaches to intervention with dysfunctional families constitute the basis of their treatment. The experience in the relationship with the therapist is what leads to change in their organizational difficulties. The process begins with the selection of one very small task that introduces change into the patterns surrounding the presenting problem. The therapist must take active charge of the selection process, while modeling respect for each person as well as direct, clear communication. Families with extreme regulation often have a very difficult time deciding where to begin. Rigid families tend to want global change, selected by their person with authority; families with loose regulation have trouble agreeing on anything or keep changing ideas.

In the process of selecting a problem, the therapist must ensure that each person not only chooses a contribution that pleases himself or herself, but makes a change in his or her usual role. Individuals functioning at this level may not be able to articulate their own needs. More often, however, they are so focused on themselves that they are unable to consider—much less respond to—the needs of others. Therefore, the therapist must appeal to the self-interest of each person, and secondarily teach the family members that benefits accruing to one person can also improve things for the others. Thus, these initial discussions already provide a therapeutic experience in relationship building through receiving and giving. For example, if a husband gives his wife the daily greeting in words that she wants, he is more likely to get the smile he wants, and vice versa.

When members of a dysfunctional system are successful in agreeing on which problem they will start with, there has already been some change in their arrangements. Then a small task can be developed for outside sessions wherein each person's role is specified in detail. Once a task is agreed upon, it is rehearsed in session so that each person's commitment to change is reinforced and pitfalls are worked out. The family must be able to do the task successfully in session before it is assigned as homework. The outcome of homework must be reviewed in detail in the next session. Every individual and cooperative success is praised; any part of the plan which did not work must be examined for what went wrong. The task may need to be simplified or made easier for some or all family members. In any case, the first plan should be solidly in place before any additional steps are undertaken.

With the most dysfunctional systems, working in small behavioral increments may need to continue for a long time. Each step should be designed to enhance the self-awareness and self-responsibility needed to meet the contracted goals. Emotions are elicited for discussion only after the individuals are able to talk in "I" messages, rather than blaming or projecting. When emotions escalate, the therapist must intervene immediately to contain them and to discourage outpouring. If someone becomes very anxious, the action must be stopped while the therapist soothes that person, acknowledging emotions but supporting self-control. Similarly, if there is unilateral or mutual blame, the therapist must intervene as soon as possible and before it escalates out of control. (Not only must a therapist keep the sessions safe; he or she also must provide an experience different from those that family members have at home.)

A useful way to interrupt blaming or conflict is to have each person talk to the therapist. The therapist in turn provides acceptance of the emotions and relates his or her own understanding of the message. Once the message is clarified with the speaker, the therapist turns to the other and delivers the message clearly. The second person is asked to respond to the therapist, who again offers understanding. When the second person's message is clarified, the therapist turns back to the first. Thus the therapist maintains tight control of the process by going back and forth between combatants, while ensuring that it remains constructive and safe. At the same time, the therapist is demonstrating and coaching better ways of speaking for oneself and listening to another. The therapist may use this intervention with various dyads in the family, while the others observe without comment until later. Often the observers learn as much as, if not more than, the participants.

Developmental deficits may be pervasive or go deeper than the issues of behavior control or the search for nurture. In such instances, a therapist may need to teach very basic perceptual skills, thereby providing what was missed at a very early age. Some individuals must learn how to read their own internal states, such as the physiological signs of particular emotions and their names. Others need to learn that their own and other people's behavior is interactive, as well as how to read the process.

Since the parents in dysfunctional systems usually have skewed or partial emancipation from their families of origin, these painful relationships are often still operating in the present. A report on a current difficult experience with a family-of-origin member can lead to a run-on about all such similar experiences, recent and past. Such an escalation may come from the person whose original family triggered the incident or from the spouse, but it can lead to the whole family's becoming embroiled. Similar effects can occur even when families of origin have been cut off or are otherwise gone. In such cases, an escalation can start when one spouse tells the other that his or her behavior is just like that of a (disliked or dysfunctional) parent.

Delving into past histories of parents in dysfunctional families is not useful and only distracts from current problems. A therapist may need a brief history in order to understand the three dimensions and the level of functioning. Otherwise, any material from the past should be acknowledged as to emotional content and then immediately tied to the issues of the present. This can be done either by describing it in terms of managing current relationships with the original families or by focusing on the controversy that has ensued between family members in the session.

First-phase treatment of the most dysfunctional families can go on for a long time. The work continues in very small increments, which cumulatively move their organizations away from the extreme. Although the issues of the psychological theme do not constitute a direct focus of discussions, they are addressed through the experience of treatment. Developmental deficits are modified by educating family members and supporting them in their efforts at maturation and self-management. When family members can take responsibility for themselves and choose within an appropriate range of behavioral and emotional responses, they have genuinely accomplished something; such achievements signal readiness for the second stage of treatment. In-depth work on the connections between present patterns and their origins in the past may or may not be within families' interests or abilities. A few recontract for this work; most are satisfied with meeting initial goals.

The early developmental deficits of dysfunctional adults require the therapist to take on the roles of model, teacher, and even substitute parent. Through these roles, a corrective experience is provided that balances nurture and regard with expectation and limits. The requirements of these roles are quite different from those of the role the therapist assumes with families that are more like himself or herself. At issue with dysfunctional families are the ways in which a therapist has personally resolved issues of dependency and authority. Generally, dysfunctional families pull hard for dependency but push hard against authority. They may try to run sessions, but ask for advice on what to do with their lives. A therapist must have it the other way: The therapist must stay in charge of sessions and hold family members responsible for what goes on outside. If a therapist is not clear or is conflicted about these issues, the therapy does not move. Thus, the therapist needs to have a grasp of his or her own abilities to nurture and to set limits, and then must monitor these as faithfully as the family's process.

Therapy with a family characterized by extreme regulation is illustrated by the following case.

A mother phoned for help regarding her 17-year-old daughter, who (the mother felt) was out of control. The daughter attended high school irregularly and hung out with a group that gathered nightly at an apartment. There, the mother feared, they drank, used drugs, and "who knows what else." The mother further reported that she was the only one in the family who was concerned—not the father, the daughter herself, or the two sons (one of whom was older and one younger than the daughter). When asked to bring in the family, the mother was not sure she could get anyone else to come. She was sure her sons would not, but she agreed to try for her daughter and husband.

The mother, an obese woman, and the daughter showed up 20 minutes late. The daughter was slender and dressed in very tight jeans, sweater, and boots. The mother said that they were late because the daughter would not come until she was bribed with the promise of new clothes. The daughter said airily that the promise was the only reason she came. Otherwise, there was nothing to worry about: "I can handle my own life. That's what everyone in the family always has to do anyway."

They permitted the therapist to follow up on that remark and explained that the family members mostly did go their separate ways. They were at home at different times, each eating and sleeping when they wished. The father often stopped at a local bar after work, so he too came home at different times. The mother had a part-time job processing orders at a small business and was free to leave when the daily intake was done. When she got home early, she spent the rest of the day cooking. Elaborate meals were left warming for her family while she took portions to her elderly mother and sister. Some evenings she did not cook, but ate supplies of her favorite foods by herself.

The parents spent little time together, but slept in the same bed. On occasion, the mother noticed the daughter coming home at an early morning hour, intoxicated. Then she turned to her husband, often by waking him and screaming about their daughter. The husband usually just went back to sleep, but he yelled at the daughter the next time he saw her and put down an impossible punishment. For example, he once said that she could not go out for a month, which was neither obeyed nor followed up. The next time the mother tried to talk to the daughter, she walked away.

The mother told most of the story, but her daughter interrupted from time to time to say "Don't worry," or to add some item for accuracy. The therapist strongly supported the mother in being concerned about her daughter, saying that it was appropriate for the mother to take responsibility and the father, too. The daughter looked intrigued that her father was invited to the next meeting but she was not. Then she protested that no one should come.

Only the mother and daughter showed up for the next session, again 20 minutes late. The mother said that the father was not interested , so she bribed the daughter again. This time the mother admitted that she was more upset about her daughter's presumed sexual activity than about substance abuse. The mother was afraid to ask the daughter what she was actually doing, but wanted her to abstain, not to use birth control. The daughter, in disgust, just said "Oh, Ma!" and refused to say any more. The mother said helplessly, "But you're so pretty, I just know you'll get in trouble." With this, the therapist renewed efforts to involve father by offering to phone him. Although he was initially reluctant, an appeal to the need for his opinion and help resulted in his agreement to come.

Both parents came to the next session, only 10 minutes late. The father was a husky man who came in his work uniform. He admitted to some concern for his daughter, but felt totally unable to deal with a young girl. But he knew what young guys were like! With that, his wife said, "Well, you should — after what you did to me." It emerged that when they were teenagers he had introduced her to beer and sex, resulting in a pregnancy that caused them to marry when she was 18.

Subsequently, the parents agreed to two more sessions in which to figure out what they wanted to do and could do to protect their daughter. What with changed and canceled appointments, it took a month for these appointments to occur. In the second session, the mother said that she thought the daughter was pregnant. The father yelled that he would kill her and the boy. The rest of this session was spent recognizing their emotions while trying to keep a calm discussion going about how to deal with the daughter. Finally it was worked out that the mother would talk to the daughter, and what she would say was decided upon. The father was not to be present or to interfere, but the mother was to tell him the outcome afterward.

Both parents and a scared-looking daughter came on time to the next session a week later. The daughter was indeed pregnant. The father yelled about rushing her off for an abortion, but the mother objected that this was against her religion. The father shouted that the daughter could not stay in his home with a baby. When the therapist asked the daughter for *her* reactions, she began to cry, saying, "I just can't even believe it's true."

Asking the parents to listen in silence, the therapist modeled talking to the daughter about her shock, fears, and confusion. Then she turned to her mother and said that she never wanted this to happen. The mother cried too, saying that she remembered how she felt; she told her daughter for the first time that she herself had been pregnant when married. With both women crying, the father said gruffly that he wanted to know what guy did this. That caused attention to turn to him and his anger. Again the therapist modeled acceptance and briefly elicited some tender concerns for his daughter.

Another session was planned for all three to discuss options, and especially for the daughter to think about choices. Instead, the mother showed up alone, 25 minutes late. She had worked out a plan with her own mother, whereby the daughter could be sent to relatives in another city. There she could have her baby and place it for adoption through the church agency. The father agreed; the daughter was given no choice, and was already gone. The mother had no idea how her daughter liked the plan. But now that the problem was "solved." she told the therapist, no further appointments were needed.

Assessment: The regulation of the family system was random, with considerable separateness and unpredictability in the behavior of all members, and unresolved issues of basic nurture. The marital pattern was complementary, but distant. The daughter followed a path of seeking nurture, attention, and limits, in ways apparently similar to those of her parents.

Treatment Outcome: The course of treatment was short and directly affected by the family's lack of organization. The daughter's pregnancy created some motivation for cooperation and change. Before long, however, the mother reverted to making a decision that resolved the situation to her satisfaction. The father reverted to concurrence. The daughter also was forced back on her own resources for resolving basic issues of nurture and autonomy. If the agency offered service beyond planning for her baby, developmental gains could be possible.

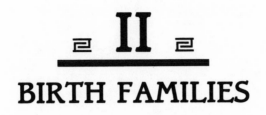

II

BIRTH FAMILIES

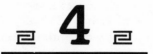

4

Fallacies about Birth Parents, and Factors in the Assessment Process

It is unfortunate that a discussion of members of the adoption triangle must begin with a discussion of the birth parents, because this tends to reinforce the perception that birth parents are offered services only to make adoptions possible. Although just a small number of parents lose their children to adoption, no adoption can take place without such a child, so adoption is inextricably linked to the services that those parents receive.

Children usually go into adoption because their birth parents fall into one of two groups. One group includes those who are young and unmarried, have become parents unintentionally, are unprepared to rear their children, and voluntarily release them for adoption as a way of providing them with secure and nurturing families. The other is made up of parents whose rights have been terminated involuntarily by court action because they have abused, neglected, or abandoned their children. Neither group of parents has generally been well served. Birth parents have been seen either as secondary clients who are entitled to service in exchange for relinquishing their children, or as obstacles to the well-being of their children — parents whose rights must be terminated so that adoption planning for their children can proceed.

Any discussion of birth parents within the adoption framework does them a disservice, because it focuses on the children and because it defines the birth parents not by any indigenous characteristic but rather by the plan for their children. Adoption in this country was originally developed as a service for childless couples. For about the past 30 or 40 years, however, adoption agencies have focused their energy primarily on finding families for children who need families, rather than on locating children for families who want children. The birth parents of the children who are adopted, however, have been seen as incidental to both of these viewpoints.

Birth parents do not conform to society's conventional patterns for rearing children. Society is still grappling with what to call these "other" parents. If their children go into adoption, terms that have been tried include "natural parents" (which may suggest that adoption is unnatural), "biological parents" (which implies that the tie is physical, not affectual), and "real parents" (which denies the reality of the adoptive parents' role). In an attempt to define and respect more fully the role of the parents by birth, and to distinguish them from other parents who may be rearing those children in adoption or foster care, "birth parents" is now the preferred term. This term is ambiguous, since any parent who gives birth to a child is a "birth parent"; however, in a discussion of adoption the term does serve to distinguish such parents from the subsequent adoptive or foster parents who rear children to whom they have *not* given birth.

Services to birth parents have not been well developed because of biases against them—biases that are firmly anchored in religious convictions, community norms, and genetic misinformation. It is "sinful" to conceive out of wedlock and to fail to accept the responsibility for rearing the product of such sins, or to abuse or neglect one's child. It is "unnatural" for people not to want to parent children born to them, or to abrogate their parental responsibilities to society. Those who do so must be sick. Or perhaps the explanation for such deviant behavior lies in "bad blood" or "weak genes" that may be passed along to the next generation.

Based on our many years of experience in working with birth parents, we feel that when young and single birth parents are viewed primarily as the producers of the commodity needed by adopting families, any services that the community develops for them are directed only toward facilitating adoption planning, not toward helping them keep their children. When parents are viewed as abusive or neglectful of their children and unable to take adequate care of them, any services are directed toward saving their children from them, not toward helping them with the struggle to become adequate parents. In both instances, birth parents are denied services in their own right.

Young Unwed Parents: Myths and Realities

To handle the negative feelings that birth parents have stirred up and to provide a rationale for the plans for their children, society has created myths about birth parents that have been modified in response to the way the community viewed and served such parents. Before 1930, people generally believed that children born out of wedlock belonged to society. Children so born were innocent victims of their mothers' behavior and needed protection from them. Their mothers were sinful and had to be punished. How the mothers should atone for their sin was largely determined by their race, health, and class. If a child was white, was healthy, and held "good promise," there was likely to be a family available for adoption, and the mother's atonement came through suffering the pain of relinquishing her child for adoption. For mothers of minority children, mothers whose children were born handicapped, or others for whose children there were no potential adoptive families waiting, atonement came through the birth parents' bearing the burden of rearing their children as best they could—sometimes with the support of family or through informal kinship "adoptions," but seldom with formal, organized community support.

As social work developed as a profession and claimed adoption as a specialty within its realm, adoption became more focused on the therapeutic aspects of serving young unwed birth mothers and less punitive in its approach. Leontine Young (1954) suggested that these mothers were sick rather than sinful. In practice, at least, this was believed if they were white and middle-class. While social workers espoused therapeutic neutrality, they helped birth mothers decide to keep or release their infants according to the availability of adoptive homes. If a birth mother was white and healthy, and delivered a healthy infant who was adoptable, the social worker often presented the surrender of the child for adoption as a solution that would enable the mother to place this "tragic experience" behind her. In some instances, hospitals had rules that prohibited mothers who were going to surrender their children for adoption from even seeing them.

Unmarried fathers of children who moved into adoption fared even less well. Society has traditionally viewed pregnancy as the responsibility of the woman involved. Men who impregnated single women but who did not marry them and rear their children have been considered exploitative, irresponsible, or criminal. Until court action in 1972 *(Stanley v. Illinois)*, birth fathers who were not married to the birth mothers of their children had no legal rights with respect to the children they fathered. It is true that in pregnancies that are unplanned and occur before marriage, the women must directly confront a situation that the men may be able to deny or avoid more easily. That does not mean, however, that the birth fathers are not in pain, might not need services, or would not be responsive to intervention. Quite the contrary, there is evidence that birth fathers want services that are generally not available (Klinman, Sanders, Rosen, Longo, & Martinez, 1985; Pannor, Massarik, & Evans, 1971).

Attitudes toward pregnancy and child rearing outside of marriage have always been determined by a matrix of cultural, sociological, and economic factors; individual characteristics and needs; and family dynamics. Over the past 30 years, the impact of the "sexual revolution" has made it acceptable for more women to rear children born to them outside of marriage, and even to conceive such children deliberately with no plan of marriage. In some subcultures, such pregnancies may be more acceptable, may play an important part in a complex sociological kinship network, or may fulfill an economic purpose (Stack, 1974). In some families the pregnancies may follow a generational pattern, and in others such a pregnancy is a historical anomaly.

For the most part, service providers continue to consider an early, unplanned pregnancy outside of marriage as a concern of the pregnant woman, and to ignore the dynamics of the birth father and his need for service. When agencies do serve unmarried birth fathers, it is usually in conjunction with agency service to the birth mothers. Community stereotypes have influenced agency programs for unmarried parents. They have overlooked the developmental struggles, societal pressures, and family dynamics that contribute to young men's involvement in premature pregnancies, as well as the pain that such pregnancies can cause. Many such fathers do not have a chance to be involved in planning for their babies. Although a young man may say that if a young woman loves him she will "give him a baby," such a gift is seldom given outside of a sustained, reciprocal relationship. Usually, a young mother views a baby born to her before marriage as hers alone. Even when the father is willing to become involved in the caring or the decision making for such a child, the dynamics of the birth mother's family may limit his participation.

Behavior is multiply determined. There is no one reason why young men become fathers before they become husbands. For some adolescents, the wish to become fathers is linked to their need to establish their manhood. The act of impregnating a woman is not always enough to achieve that goal, however.

Randolph was a 17-year-old who had always been a poor student, and who dropped out of school as soon as he legally could. He was the third oldest of seven children. All but one of them were living at home with their mother, who had never married and who supported her family with public assistance. Randolph's older brother, aged 22, was incarcerated on a drug-related charge. His older sister, aged 19, was unmarried and lived at home with her 2-year-old child. Randolph had younger sisters aged 16, 15, and 13, and a brother aged 12. Although the father of the youngest child did not live in the home, he was a regular visitor and an occasional contributor to the family income.

Randolph worked at a neighborhood fast-food restaurant. He paid for his own clothes and incidental expenses, and contributed $25 a week toward the family food budget. Beverly, who worked part-time at the restaurant, was a high school senior who lived at home with her mother and her siblings. Randolph and Beverly started dating, and soon agreed that they wanted to get an apartment and live together. Before they could do that, however, Beverly became pregnant. Beverly was upset, but Randolph was pleased. He said that it just meant he would have to get a better job, so they could move out and begin living on their own before the baby came.

Neither family supported such a plan. Randolph's mother did not want him to leave home; it annoyed her that only now was he trying to get a better job. Beverly's family blamed Randolph for the pregnancy and was concerned about her finishing high school. Beverly quit her job and withdrew into her family, where Randolph was not welcome. It soon became clear to him that he was not going to have a chance to be involved either in Beverly's life now or in the decision about the baby. He had sought help in getting another job from a "Jobs for Teens" program. In talking with a counselor there shortly after the baby was born, he said, "I thought making a baby would help me feel like more of a man, but they won't even let me see my baby. They're making plans as if I had nothing to do with her. Hell, I don't feel like more of a man. I feel as if my dick had been cut off!"

Pregnancy in very young unmarried women frequently reflects the dynamics of their family systems, and the men who have impregnated them are incidental.

The Tubbs family consisted of Mr. and Mrs. Tubbs and Mrs. Tubbs's two daughters from an earlier marriage—Eve, who was

18, and Rhonda, who was 16. Within a year after Mr. and Mrs. Tubbs were married, they sought counseling. The presenting problem was Rhonda's pregnancy. In family sessions, Mr. Tubbs acknowledged the difficulty he had felt in trying to parent two teenage stepdaughters. Rhonda described how much she had looked forward to having a father in the home since her own father had deserted the family 10 years before, and how disappointed she was that Mr. Tubbs seemed not to want to play that role. As the therapy continued it became clearer that Mrs. Tubbs had covertly limited her husband's parental involvement with her daughters because of her concern that he would find them more attractive than her. Rhonda's response to her mother's fear of competition had been to become pregnant. When discussion in therapy shifted to supporting Rhonda in planning for her expected baby, Eve announced that she was also pregnant and would deliver 4 months after Rhonda.

The dynamics of the family had played a part in the onset of the pregnancies, and plans for the future could best be considered within that family system. As family roles were sorted out and family communication improved, Mrs. Tubbs, with her husband's support, could say that she was unwilling to assume responsibility for rearing either grandchild. Rhonda decided to place her child for adoption and to continue to live at home until she graduated from high school in 2 years. Eve, who would graduate from high school before she delivered, decided that she would keep her baby. Initially she hoped to go on Aid to Families with Dependent Children, but when her baby got a little older she planned to become involved in a job training program, or perhaps to go on with her education.

The family stayed in treatment through the delivery of both babies. Rhonda's placement of her child was, predictably, hard on all members of the family. Mr. and Mrs. Tubbs were able to come together as her parents, to provide her with a great deal of support, and to meet her 16-year-old developmental needs more adequately. Rhonda then became very invested in Eve's pregnancy and her planning for independence. She helped Eve locate an apartment and accompanied her when she went to public aid. Eve accepted Rhonda's help and encouraged her to visit often after the baby was born. Rhonda continued to say that she knew she had made the right decision for herself. She said she was ready to be an aunt, but not a mother. Although one cannot know the long-term impact of the decisions the Tubbs girls made, the family stabilized, and all members agreed it was functioning better when treatment terminated.

A situation with a rather different outcome involved Dorothy Vance's family. When Dorothy's two daughters were 6 and 7, she

Moving from Myths to Realities

Birth parents have not been served well, not only because of negative biases toward them, but also because service providers have focused on the children and on adoption. The necessity of planning for a child can easily divert attention from the needs of the birth parents—both the attention of the parents and of those who would offer services. Both groups tend to see the child as the appropriate object of attention or as a problem that will vanish once placement is accomplished. This serves as an obstacle to the design of services and reinforces the denial of birth parents themselves that such services are important.

Most adoptive parents, too, want to deny the importance of the other family to which their child belongs. In an effort to do this and to handle their discomfort about viewing the child's birth parents as real people, adoptive parents often construct an image of the birth parents that fits their own belief system and present this mythical construct to the child whenever he or she raises questions about the birth parent. The myths that adoptive parents construct tend to reflect one of two opposite positions, and tend to focus on the birth mother. In the extreme, these are that the birth mother was a nearly perfect young woman who on her way to or through college and a great life made one tragic mistake and became pregnant, or that she was a wanton girl who was sexually promiscuous and whose child was saved by adoption for a life much better than could have been provided within the birth environment. Agencies themselves often joined in helping construct these mythical birth parents in an effort to ease adoptive parents' pain in coping with the reality of the birth parents. Not surprisingly, the two mythical images are the ones that adopted children use as the central points in constructing their fantasies about the parents who brought them into the world and abandoned them.

Adequate service to birth parents requires viewing them as real people who are suffering real pain, and who may be able to utilize adoption as one means of resolving some of their problems. They are entitled to services, whether or not they become involved in adoption. Although a range of adequate services is often not available to birth parents, a good deal is known about how to develop and deliver them.

divorced their father; as a single parent, she reared the girls to adulthood. When her older daughter was 20, she got a good job, moved to an apartment of her own, and soon became pregnant by a man she did not want to marry. Dorothy wanted her to keep the baby and to bring it "home." The younger daughter, who was living at home, going to a community college, and working at a part-time job, also wanted her sister to keep the baby. She offered to change her schedule in order to help her mother care for the child, so that the older daughter could continue at her job. The older daughter instead elected to relinquish the child for adoption. Shortly thereafter, the younger daughter rushed into a marriage with a man she did not know well, and very soon became pregnant. Her husband abused her, and when he threatened to abuse the new baby, she divorced him and returned home to her mother with her baby. The older daughter had also entered into a marriage; although the marriage seemed to be working out, she complained to her mother that she and her husband wanted to have a child, but so far she was having no success in becoming pregnant.

Not only family systems but peer groups have influence on adolescent sexual behavior and pregnancies, sometimes in quite contradictory ways. In some cliques of adolescent girls, when one member becomes pregnant, the pregnancy seems to "inoculate" the other members and generate peer support that prevents the other girls from following suit. In other groups, quite the opposite occurs: The initial pregnancy seems "contagious" and is followed by pregnancies among several of the peer group members. In some adolescent cultures and in some families, pregnancy is viewed as a rite of passage—either a means of being accepted within the peer group or the family as an adult, or a way of establishing independence from the family as an adult.

So the clinician or the adoption worker must be cautious with any initial generalizations about the specific etiology of an unintended pregnancy, other than the fact that if the parent is considering adoption as a plan, that parent is experiencing a crisis in regard to parenting the child. As always, a careful assessment of the particular situation is the beginning of good service. The acceptance of any simple explanation of the "reason" for the pregnancy or the choice of adoption as a solution indicates the clinician's lack of understanding of the complexities involved; it will serve poorly a birth parent who is surrendering a child, whether that birth parent is being served at the point of the adoption decision or later in life.

Abusive or Neglectful Parents: Myths and Realities

Of course, clinicians also need to be cautious in generalizing about families whose rights to their children may be in jeopardy as a result of their parental failure—the families whose children come into adoption as a result of involuntary terminations of their parents' rights. Parents who have had children within their marital relationship but who then abandon, neglect, or abuse these children are even more severely discriminated against than young unmarried parents who relinquish their babies. Service to these abusing or neglectful parents has been shaped by society's attitudes toward such parents. Once again, these attitudes are determined by a host of cultural, sociological, economic, individual, and family factors.

Within the last century, our ideas of what constitutes abuse or neglect have changed markedly. In an agrarian society, the success of a family farm often depended upon having many hands to work it, and children had little social access to those outside their families. They were seen as part of a family labor pool. How they were treated was the prerogative of the parents and was generally unknown outside the family. The Industrial Revolution and the systematic utilization of children's labor in factories rather than on the family farms stirred society; the focus shifted from exploiting children to protecting them. Since then, we have struggled with where to draw the boundaries around the parents' right to manage their children without society's intervention. Because of our ambivalence about exactly where these boundaries should be drawn, society has always reacted punitively to those families that it perceives as abusing or neglecting their children.

Until fairly recently, little effort was made to help the transgressors become more adequate parents. Rather, when parents demonstrated their inadequacies in rearing their children, society responded by punishing them and "rescuing" their children. This plan to save children by taking them from their families was based on two faulty assumptions: first, that parents who abused or neglected their children were never going to be able to become good enough parents to rear them; and second, that society had the resources to adequately parent the children it rescued. Unfortunately, children were not served well by the system that rescued them, as was dramatically documented by Knitzer and Allen (1978) in a Children's Defense Fund monograph, *Children without Homes*. Because the children removed from their parents were older, were

not always white, and often suffered from earlier depriv[a] trauma, they were viewed as unadoptable. Many of the[m] consigned to being raised by social agencies in foster fam[ilies] (usually a series of foster homes) or in institutions.

Within the past 20 years, agencies have realized that ma[ny] children should never have been taken into the system in t[he first] place, and that for most of those who could not be reared [by] birth families, adoptive families could be found. These two [impor]tant changes—the emphasis on keeping children within thei[r] families, and early permanency planning for those who co[me into] care—resulted in federal legislation (the Adoption Assistan[ce and] Child Welfare Act of 1980) and the family preservation mov[ement.] The romantic myth of rescuing children gave way to an atte[mpt to] keep more of them with their birth families, and to be certa[in that] those who entered the system did so with a plan to meet their [needs.] Anger and contempt gave way to awareness and concern. [Birth] parents who mistreated or neglected their children were no [longer] seen as uncaring people who did not deserve sympathy or s[ervice.] Service providers learned that such parents could be help[ed to] manage parenting better; that many might be able to rea[r their] children if they were given appropriate help; and that if [their] children did come into adoption, these children fared better [if] the reality of their birth families was a part of their ad[optive] experience. A new family preservation movement emerge[d and] provided intensive, time-limited, in-home services to families [whose] children were at imminent risk of placement (see, e.g., C[ole &] Duva, 1990); as a result, the adoption process became more [open] and humane for all of the participants.

One of the most difficult and sensitive areas in opening u[p the] process is that of the access that it may provide adopted childr[en to] birth parents whose rights were involuntarily terminated, and [of the] access that those parents may have to the children to whom [they] gave birth. Although there is reason for concern, of course, it i[s not] true that parents who lose their children to adoption through [court] action are not in great pain, do not care about those children, [or do] not deserve services both in their own right and in efforts to m[ake] the adoption plan more successful. Because adoption creates a [new] family system, if birth parents' issues are not addressed, an[d if] service is not provided to this part of the adoption triangle, agen[cies] not only have abrogated responsibility to a group of peopl[e in] distress but also have increased the risks that the adoption plan [will] not work for the others involved.

5

Services to Birth Families

Adopted children come from birth parents who differ widely in terms of age, culture, race, religion, economic status, family systems, indigenous support, and psychological makeup. Most children are placed in adoption, however, for one of two reasons: Either their parents have voluntarily surrendered them, or have abandoned them, or their parents have had their parental rights involuntarily terminated by court action because they neglected or abused the children.

Regardless of the reason, the birth parents are involved in adoption in order to resolve a parenting crisis in their lives and all face a number of common problems as a result of losing their children to adoption. There are important differences, however, in the primary family systems in which they operate, in the developmental issues they may be facing, and in their children who come into adoption. Birth parents who voluntarily surrender their children generally relinquish them as young infants. They are usually unmarried, frequently young, and often living with their families or trying to separate from them. Because adoption has been viewed for so long as a way for infertile couples to become parents of infants, these are the birth parents who usually come to mind when people think of adoption. Parents whose rights have been terminated involuntarily by court action are generally older; they are often married and living in the families they have formed with their children. These children are of varying ages and are often considered to have special needs as a result of one or more of the following conditions: congenital deficits, age, neglectful or abusive early life histories, or the traumatic circumstances that have brought them into care.

Members of both groups of birth parents face a parenting

71

"crisis" because of their own uncertainty about their ability to rear the children to whom they have given life, or because of society's concern about the same matter. The overall therapeutic goals for the members of both groups are the same: to review the range of options available in planning for their children; to support them in making or accepting a decision about their children that allows them to feel they have been the best parents they can be; to assist them in maintaining their dignity and sense of self-worth and in managing the pain of the adoption experience, if that is to be the plan; to help them mourn the loss of their children when that is the case; and to help them integrate this experience into their lives.

Although the long-range goals are the same, the treatment is usually different for each group of clients because of their developmental needs and because the parenting crisis is defined and examined within a different family context. The services that the birth parents receive also vary according to when and where they seek help. Many young single birth parents receive no counseling or therapy. They face the crisis of their pregnancies by themselves or within their indigenous support system. Unless their decision is adoption, they may see no need for professional help; even if they decide on adoption, they may elect to work outside an agency structure. Other young single birth parents are served by child welfare or adoption agencies. These young expectant parents usually seek service at the point of the pregnancy/parenting crisis, but seldom continue to work with an agency once the decision for their children is made. In recent years, a number of these birth parents have been returning to the agencies with whom they placed their babies, to inquire about their children and to seek help with reunion. (This aspect of adoption is discussed in Chapter 11 of this volume.) Some birth parents seek and receive help from therapists who are independent of adoption agencies or programs. And finally, some birth parents who have abused or neglected their children come to therapy or to an agency as a result of a court order

For all birth parents, however, treatment consists of two phases: crisis intervention and developmental integration. The context for helping a birth parent at the initial point of contact or with concerns at any subsequent point is the parent's family system. Watson (1986) has identified six areas highlighted by a pregnancy crisis and the possibility of adoption: decision making; autonomy and control; family boundaries and membership; separation and loss; relationship to the opposite sex; and self-image. The following case illustrates how several of these themes surfaced in a case in which service was provided through an agency.

Joanne, aged 4, and her two half-brothers, Billy, aged 3, and Adrian, aged 2, came into emergency foster care because they had been abandoned by their 21-year-old mother, Anne. She had left them with a friend who agreed to keep the children overnight. When Anne did not return after 3 days, the friend called the police. The friend did not know where Anne was and reported that the children had been left alone all night in the past; the children were then taken into foster care. When Anne was located, she admitted being a heroin addict who supported herself by prostitution.

Anne's history revealed that she herself had come into foster care in Chicago at age 12 because of sexual abuse by her father. After a series of foster home placements, she ran away when she was 16 and went to New York. She began working as a prostitute and taking drugs; she lived with a pimp, Rob, and worked for him. She married him when she became pregnant with Joanne, but left him when he broke the baby's arm in a fit of rage. Her refuge with another abusive man, Arnie, was worse: She fled back to Chicago after he threatened to kill her. Alienated from her family and with no friends, she soon met Ralph and moved in with him. Ralph was also alienated from his family. Although he used drugs and was not steadily employed, he wanted "to be a man and have a family." He was delighted each time Anne got pregnant, and proudly listed himself on the birth certificates as the legal father of Billy and Adrian. He viewed himself as the father of all three children. Although sometimes abusive of Anne, he was kind to the children and never hurt them. The family was supported through Ralph's drug dealing and other criminal activity, and by Anne's prostitution.

When Ralph was sent to that state prison on a burglary conviction, Anne had trouble supporting her children and her drug habit. Her intent in leaving the children with her friend was not to abandon them, but to try to provide for them while she was working or strung out. Anne quickly became involved with a social worker in working toward a more stable life for herself and her children. She did not feel that there was any future in her relationship with Ralph, and was initially reluctant to involve him in the planning for the children. She feared he would hurt her if he knew she was leaving him and considering placing the children in adoption. She said that sometimes she though that the only reason he wanted her was to be close to them.

When she was able to see that her life was tied into the family that she, Ralph and the children had formed, she agreed to family sessions at the prison. These involved both parents and all three children. Before Ralph was paroled, however, Anne made it clear that she did not wish to continue her relationship with him. She had established an apartment on her own and had full-time employment. The children were still in foster care and had been told that their family was not going to be reunited. Both parents visited the children, but not together.

Anne entered a drug rehabilitation program. As she began to feel better about her ability to support herself legitimately, she talked of going back to school. She said that she could not be a good mother until she became a good person, and began to seriously consider relinquishing the children for adoption. Ralph was opposed to this, both because of the close relationships he had established with the children and because he hoped that through them he could get back to Anne.

Anne joined Ralph in family sessions (now without the children), but did not let him into her apartment. One night when he arrived at her apartment high on drugs and demanding to be let in, she called the police. She then moved to another apartment and did not give him the new address. She began dating another man, but quickly terminated the relationship when she realized he was yet another woman abuser. She used individual counseling sessions to explore why she always ended up with that kind of man.

Ralph was less successful in managing his life. He continued his criminal activity with drugs and thefts. He entered a drug rehabilitation program and a job training program for ex-offenders, but did not stick with either of them. The brightest part of his life was visiting with the children. Initially these visits were supervised and took place in the agency. When the foster family was comfortable with him, the visits became unsupervised and were moved to the home of the foster parents. The worker's role with both birth parents was to remind them of the impermanence of the current plan for the children, and to try to help them explore the possibility of either of them taking the children. As Anne began to function better (by now she had entered a relationship with a non-abusive older man), she was able to say in a joint session that she could relinquish the children if she were sure that they would not go to Ralph, who she felt would never be able to take care of them. This was said less with anger than with sadness.

Ralph said that he would never release the children. The worker raised the possibility of seeking an involuntary termination on the basis of his drug abuse and criminal activity. Ralph said that he could see no way he could parent the children in the near future, but that they were all he had in life. When the worker posed the possibility of his continued contact with the children even though they were adopted, his position changed. Both parents relinquished the children. Because of the children's special needs, adoptions were arranged with two different adoptive families (the two youngest children stayed together). Following their adotpion the children maintained contact with each other, and both parents maintained contact with each child, but separately. Anne did go on to school, recovered from her drug addiction, and married the man with whom she had been living. Ralph was rearrested and returned to prison. The adopted family has maintained contact with him, and the whole family has visited him there. When he is released, he will be welcome in their home.

Making Contact: Birth Parents' Involvement with Helping Professionals

Birth parents voluntarily become involved with agencies or family therapists about adoption issues in three ways. Most go either to an adoption agency or to a therapist because they are seeking help in connection with the personal crisis of a newly confirmed pregnancy, and they want help in making a plan and in sorting out their reactions. For a second group, a "problem pregnancy" occurs within a family that is already engaged in therapy, and the resolution of the difficulty becomes a part of the continuing treatment. And finally, the experience of being a birth parent long ago, or of being involved in a family where an unplanned pregnancy or an adoption was a significant issue, may press a family into treatment or affect the dynamics of one that is already in treatment.

Most young unmarried women who view pregnancy as a problem for which they need counseling and for which adoption may be a partial resolution are not already in treatment and do not view their "problem" as part of a family system. Although pregnancy generates an increased sense of family consciousness in such women and encourages them to look at their relationships with their families, actually involving a birth mother's family in planning or treatment usually proves difficult. Many of these young women are still part of their families of origin and are living with their parents. Those who are seeking adoption with their families' support are the most likely to be seen in family sessions, but it is still unusual for an entire family to be engaged. Usually only the birth mother and her mother are involved.

Sometimes young pregnant women who are unmarried and who are ambivalent about whether they wish to rear their children are reluctant to share their pregnancies with their families because of shame or the family dynamics. When the families do learn of the situation, they may join in the denial of the pregnancy crisis by avoiding agency involvement and family interviews. The visible "symptom" of a pregnancy makes it easy for a family to isolate the pregnant woman as clearly having the problem, rather than viewing her as the family symptom bearer. And, always, the built-in time frame keeps the focus on the pregnancy and the arriving child; it presses the birth mother, her family, and the therapist to focus on the issues involved in planning for the baby.

For those young birth mothers who are living apart from their families of origin, their pregnancies may be directly related to conflicts centering their separation from those families. Family interviews are often difficult for these birth mothers for both pragmatic and dynamic reasons. Some of these women have separated from their families of origin by moving to a new community — sometimes prior to becoming pregnant and at other times because of pregnancy. In either case, the families of origin may not be available for family sessions. Those who are living in the same community as their families may be very resistant to sharing their pregnancies and reinvolving the extended families, especially if the separation has been difficult and there are many unresolved issues.

Pregnancy for some young women who are on their own for the first time may be the result of an attempt to assuage loneliness. Such a woman may have turned to a new acquaintance or a long-time boyfriend. If the young pregnant woman is in her first job in a new city, she may have limited financial or social resources to aid her. If she is newly emancipated, her feelings and her view of her parents' feelings about her independence offer assessment clues. Closely related is how she expects her parents, particularly her mother, to react to her pregnancy. The woman's age, the length of time she has been on her own, and the status of her relationship with her parents are other important considerations.

Requests for therapy in regard to a crisis pregnancy also come from single, well-established career women who are in or near their 30s. Such women may have become pregnant through the accidental failure of birth control, or through an "accident" caused by unconscious motives related to a relationship or to their awareness of the biological aging process. Although the relationships of a somewhat older woman are important in helping her with the pregnancy crisis she is facing, a more critical factor may be the state of her own development. The biological clock ticks on. Her attitudes about children, with or without marriage, may have undergone changes. A very young woman may lack the resources to rear a child by herself, but this becomes a more realistic option for the established career woman. This option can be compelling if the woman views her pregnancy as her only option for having a child.

The First Phase of Treatment: Crisis Intervention

Whether their contact is voluntary or involuntary, when birth parents come into contact with an adoption agency or a therapist because of a pregnancy/parenting crisis, the appropriate response is crisis intervention service. As in other kinds of crisis intervention, there is an assumption that a person or family in trouble was functioning adequately prior to the crisis. That does not mean that the crisis may not be a cry for help, but only that the first goal of the intervention should be to re-establish the former equilibrium and satisfactory level of functioning. The focus is on the here and now and on finding ways to plan for the child or children involved.

For parents who face the threat of losing their parental rights, the return to the former state of equilibrium is often viewed as getting back children who are already in temporary foster care, or preventing the removal of children still with the parents. When such a family consists of an unmarried woman and several children, the father(s) of the children may not be a part of the family unit or may not be available for agency involvement. If the family is intact, there may be serious tensions between the parents, which they can use as a barrier to seeking help; or the parents may have formed an alliance against those who are threatening to remove their children or who view them as having problems. The wish to keep the family together, however, can be powerful leverage for engaging parents in treatment, and they may be accessible for family interviews.

For many young unmarried birth mothers, the goal of returning to the former state of equilibrium suggests avoiding the responsibility of parenting in the quickest way. If a client has not had an abortion, adoption may appear to be that way. Either abortion or adoption may reflect a denial of the impact of the pregnancy, the significance of the pregnancy for the entire family system, and the underlying problems that may have contributed to the pregnancy.

For some families in therapy, adolescents are involved in pregnancies. A daughter's behavior may have brought a family to treatment, as in the case described at the end of Chapter 3, or a family may be in therapy working on other problems when a pregnancy occurs. Most often the problem is with a pregnant daughter, but sometimes at issue is a teenage son who has impregnated a young woman. When teenage pregnancy occurs during the time that a family is already involved in family therapy, the therapist not only has an assessment at hand, but probably can deduce the meaning and function of the pregnancy within the family system. Beyond individual meanings, within the family there are two main possibilities. One is that the pregnancy calls attention to the needs of a person who is neglected; the other is that the pregnancy serves to distract the family from some other serious problem. Often the pregnancy does both, in the paradoxical way of symptoms. A therapist must tailor the response to the pregnancy to the assessment of the family, and fit this new crisis into the continuing treatment process.

For those who are not already involved in therapy, the crisis intervention follows an initial assessment of the family system and of the circumstances that generated the pregnancy and the request for service. In every case, the birth mothers in crisis must first be allowed to tell her story. Beyond the pregnancy itself, the therapist or adoption worker must pay careful attention to how the woman identifies the problem and the associated emotions. Some women arrive in shock with emotions numb; others express fear, anger, humiliation, rejection, or the inability to cope alone.

If in the course of telling her story, the pregnant woman has not volunteered information about her relationship or attitudes to the man who has impregnated her, the therapist needs to inquire. When possible, both partners in a problem pregnancy should be involved in this initial crisis resolution phase. It is important to know the man's views about sharing responsibility for the pregnancy and decisions about it, as well as his availability to the woman and to therapy. Whenever possible, the woman should be encouraged to invite him to sessions. Some men come to the first session without an invitation, eager to show their support or to make their views known; others are ready, or at least willing, to come if asked. If there is a strong relationship between the birth mother and the birth father, particularly if they are considering rearing the child or they expect to continue their relationship after they reach a decision about planning for their child, the family that they have created with their child is the family system within which service to them should be considered. If adoption is being seriously contemplated, the birth father's family of origin will be important (especially if its members wish to be the part of the extended family who will be rearing the child), and these persons should be included in the planning sessions.

Once everyone's stories have been told, the next step in treatment is to review the range of options for planning for the child. These include abortion, marriage, agency adoption, adoption by other family members, independent adoption, or the mother's rearing the child as a single parent. The therapist explores each option for its meanings related to values, emotional responses, and feasibility. If the individuals do not mention a particular option, the therapist should bring it up and provide some basic information. Frequently the birth parents want to deny the pain of the experience, and the ambivalence they feel in making any decision, by quickly seizing upon one option to the exclusion of all others.

The birth parents should be encouraged to thoroughly explore the possibility of keeping their child themselves or of arranging for the child's care within their extended families. This is not to denigrate the value of adoption, but rather to recognize its inherent limitations. As clinicians and agencies have come to understand more clearly the importance of genetic ties and of the birth bond, as they have seen the difficulty of grieving for a child lost in adoption, and as they have come to realize through experience that adoption is not a magical solution for rearing children, they have begun to place greater emphasis on programs designed to preserve birth families.

In addition to help in resolving their pregnancy/parenting crisis by planning for their children, birth parents may need a range of other services. If the birth parents are young and unmarried, these may include such things as education on responsible sexual behavior and the prevention of unintended pregnancies; adequate prenatal medical care; opportunities for continuing education; and support for carrying through on their plans for both themselves and their children, whatever decision they have made. Birth parents who are in danger of having their parental rights involuntarily terminated should be instructed in early risk detection; offered intensive family preservation services and adequate legal services to protect their rights in any litigation; provided with help to re-unify their families if children have been removed and placed in foster care; and offered the possibility of continuing service for themselves, including involvement with their children who may be going into adoption when such involvement seems in the best interests of the children and is accepted by the adoptive families.

The adoption agency need not be responsible for providing all of these services. It is, however, professionally unwise and morally

questionable for an adoption agency to make adoption placements if
it is unaware of the context within which adoption decisions are
being made by birth parents, and to assume no responsibility for the
absence of the range of services that are necessary to meet the birth
parents' needs adequately.

The Second Phase of Treatment:
Developmental Integration

Once a decision has been made about planning for their children,
birth parents can move into the second phase of treatment and focus
on the developmental integration of their experience. The impact of
the pregnancy/parenting crisis on the individuals involved will
depend on where they are in terms of their development, as well as
on the dynamic meaning of parenting with respect to their life
situation and family membership.

Often in years past, and even today, birth parents who have
chosen adoption have been cut off both from the adopting families
and from the agencies that arranged the placement. This meant that
little help was available from the adoption agencies to help them
cope with the issues of the adoption placement — such things as their
sense of loss and the feelings of abandoning their child. These are
often the issues that bring birth parents back into treatment later, as
is illustrated in the following case example (Roles, 1989, 1991).

> Phyllis Garrett was 16, 5 months pregnant, and unmarried when
> she arrived with her mother at the agency. Mrs. Garrett took
> charge of the interview, while Phyllis sat quietly with her eyes
> downcast. Mrs. Garrett was interested in locating a maternity
> home in another city to which she could send Phyllis to have her
> baby and give it up for adoption. Phyllis's father and 19-year-old
> sister had not been told of her pregnancy. Mrs. Garrett said that
> Mr. Garrett had a bad heart and it would kill him to learn of
> Phyllis's pregnancy, and that there was no need for Annette to
> know her sister's business. Phyllis did not participate in the
> interview, other than to nod or shrug her shoulders when asked a
> direct question. When all attempts to help Mrs. Garrett consider
> other options for handling the pregnancy proved futile, informa-
> tion about the out-of-state maternity home was provided.
>
> Three months later Mrs. Garrett called again. The out-of-
> state plans had not worked out, and Phyllis was now a resident of
> a local maternity home. The other family members still did not

know of the pregnancy; they thought that Phyllis was visiting relatives out of state. Mrs. Garrett said that Phyllis wanted to give her baby up for adoption, and Mrs. Garrett was calling to make placement arrangements. Phyllis was next seen in the maternity home. She was quiet, sullen, and unable to talk about her pregnancy or plans. When pressed, she said that her mother had said she could only come home if she gave the baby up for adoption and promised never to talk about it. She said that she had no other choice.

When there is a teenage pregnancy, a special condition applies. Since the adolescent is still in the family, there is a tendency for the parents to take over the decision; thus, the adolescent may be forced to marry, have an abortion, place the child for adoption, or bring the child home to its grandmother. To the extent that family dynamics permit, a therapist can use the alliance with the whole family to empower the teenager. At the least, a therapist can model concern for the young person's emotions and preferred solutions. The treatment of the whole family may be furthered by helping each member to articulate emotions and opinions in a responsible, nonpunitive manner. In this situation, Mrs. Garrett wanted Phyllis to have no part in the decision making and was blocking Phyllis's expression of her own feelings. Immediately following the birth of Phyllis's baby, surrenders were signed by Phyllis and Mrs. Garrett. Further service was offered them, but they declined and the case was closed. The baby was placed in an adoptive home within 6 weeks.

Twenty-one years later, the social worker who had taken the release saw Phyllis, now a plump middle-aged woman with the same sad expression on her face, sitting in the waiting room of the agency. She recognized the worker and asked whether the worker remembered her. The worker did, and although Phyllis had an appointment with another worker, she asked to talk to the first worker for a few moments. Phyllis asked the worker whether she remembered what she had said to Phyllis when she relinquished her baby. The worker was not sure, and asked what Phyllis remembered. Phyllis recalled that the worker had said that now the release was signed, Phyllis was free to go on with her life. She now said to the worker, "Let me tell you something: I think my life stopped the day I signed that release. Not one day has gone by that I did not think of my daughter, and not one week that I have not cried because of my decision."

The worker asked about her family and her current life. Phyllis was living with her mother; her father had died; and her sister had left the area and they didn't hear much from her. Neither her father nor her sister had ever been told of the pregnancy, nor had they ever asked. When the worker said that meant that Phyllis had only her mother to talk with about the baby, Phyllis said, "Wrong! My mother and I have never once mentioned her. That is why I am here. I want to talk about my daughter, and now that she is grown, I want to find her."

Phyllis was offered an opportunity to do some of the grief work that she had been denied 21 years earlier. She had not told her mother of her revisit to the agency and asked to be seen alone. Soon she recognized that the family system within which she was operating had been established by her daughter's birth and placement, and that it included her mother. She then asked that her mother be included in the treatment sessions.

It is in the second phase of treatment that attention is usually directed toward one or more of the six interrelated issues mentioned earlier: (1) decision making, (2) autonomy and control, (3) family boundaries and family membership, (4) separation and loss, (5) relationship with the opposite sex, and (6) self-image.

Decision Making

Young unmarried birth parents who resolve their parenting crisis by deciding to place their children for adoption make one of life's few irrevocable decisions. Such a parent usually does this during the teen years, with little prior decision-making experience and often with limited support. This major decision, of course, follows a series of other decisions along the way that are frequently not recognized as critical: the decision to engage in sexual intercourse, the decision not to use birth control, the decision not to terminate the pregnancy, the decision not to marry the birth father, and the decision not to rear the child within the family. Many factors influence a young pregnant woman in making these decisions, and many of them have been made more by default than by design. Now, however, she must make a conscious decision that will separate her from the parenting responsibilities for her child. The trauma of facing this decision, and the implications not only of the decision but of the way it is made, are enormous. An all-too-typical case illustrates this and also underscores the fact that many young women face this trauma without the support of their families or of a social agency.

After graduating from high school at 18, Agnes made her first major life decision when she left her home in a small town in Indiana. Her parents wanted her to stay at home and continue to work at the drugstore where she had held a part-time job for a couple of years. Instead, she used her "life savings" to move to Chicago and enroll in a school to become an airline attendant. She successfully completed the course but was unable to get an airline job. She did not like Chicago but was reluctant to go back home a "failure," so she got a job as a filing clerk and spent most of her free time at the airport trying to get hired. Her only friends were two other girls whom she had met in the airline school: Sue, who had been hired by an airline and now spent a lot of time away from Chicago, and Pat, who also had to take another job after the training.

Agnes had broken up with a high school boyfriend, with whom she had engaged in occasional unprotected intercourse with no expectation of pregnancy. Pat was living with a man and told Agnes that she didn't care one way or the other if she got pregnant. If she didn't, she would keep trying for an airline job; if she did, she was sure that Roger would take care of her and the baby.

Agnes met Hugh at the airport, where he worked as a luggage handler; he began driving her back to the city when he got off work, and soon they started dating. Sometimes they would go out with Pat and Roger, or go over to their apartment for the evening. They first had intercourse when they stayed overnight there. Agnes had not "given any thought to birth control" and Hugh did not have a condom. Sexual intercourse soon became a regular part of their relationship. They did not use birth control, and they never talked about long-range aspects of their relationship or about the possibility of pregnancy.

When Agnes became pregnant, her first concern was to conceal the pregnancy from her family because she viewed this as a second "failure." She confided first in Pat, who urged Agnes to carry the child to term and offered to let her stay with her and Roger before and after the delivery. When she told Hugh, he was supportive, but said that the decision about what to do was hers. Neither one of them considered marriage as a real option. Hugh said he would pay for an abortion if she wanted one. Agnes made no immediate conscious decision about the baby, but she continued working and told no one else of her pregnancy. She was concerned about her job, about her parents' finding out about her pregnancy, and about what she would do with the baby. She concealed her pregnancy until the end of the seventh month; then she quit her job, gave up her apartment, and moved in with Pat and Roger. She had resisted getting prenatal care, but did so at Pat's insistence about a month before she delivered.

Agnes and Hugh were no longer seeing each other, but he periodically called to see how she was and to ask about her plans beyond delivery. He had given her the amount of money that an abortion would have cost and offered to help out with the delivery expenses. One week before she was scheduled to deliver, she attended a group meeting for single pregnant women at a social service agency, at the urging of the nurse at the prenatal clinic. She expressed an interest in adoption, and arranged an appointment with a social worker to explore the options. Before she could keep the appointment, however, she delivered. She told the hospital social worker that she had decided to relinquish her child for adoption. She was seen in the hospital by an agency social worker, who arranged for her baby to go into foster care on the day that Agnes was to be released from the hospital. She came into the agency a week later, saying that she wished to sign release papers as soon as possible. She was planning to return to her parents' home and seek employment down there, but she was not planning to tell them of her baby. Hugh had covered the hospital bills and Pat was allowing her to stay at her apartment until the baby could be relinquished.

For families whose parental rights are being terminated by court action the decision-making process is also critical. The decision to terminate parental rights is based on abandonment, neglect, or abuse. As in the case of a young unmarried mother, a number of other decisions have formed a chain that ends with the decision to separate the child from his or her birth parents through adoption. In most instances, the decisions along the way have been made by the court or social agencies in response to actions the parents have either taken or failed to take; yet often the parents feel that they have had no part in the decision-making process.

Abandoning parents have acted out their resolution to their parenting crisis in a way that precludes service to them at the time of the abandonment. Those parents facing charges of neglect or abuse generally have a history of involvement with the courts and social agencies. They may have made attempts to provide adequate care for the children within their families at the request of the court, as part of a plan to prevent their children from coming into care or to reclaim their children from a temporary foster care plan. Increasingly, the courts are showing a reluctance to remove children from their families except as a last resort. More agencies are developing the wider range of services that these troubled families need if they are to succeed with their children.

Many birth parents are threatened by and suspicious of any intervention by either agencies or the courts, however. They often view court-mandated "help" as an intrusion into their right to make decisions about their own children. The decision to terminate parental rights, of course, is seen as the ultimate loss of decision-making power. For example, parents who are addicted to drugs and who have neglected their children may find that their children are in temporary foster care and the court is ordering the parents to get involved in a drug rehabilitation program if they want their children back. The court and the agency may view this as a great opportunity both to help the parents recover from their addiction and to assure the safety of the children. The parents, however, may feel that the decision to accept treatment has been forced on them, and may resent the intrusiveness of the agencies and the court. Depending upon where the parents are in terms of accepting and managing their addiction or in arranging alternative care for their children, the court may decide at some point to terminate their rights. The parents may feel that they have had no voice in that decision, especially if it comes at a time when they feel they are making some headway.

Autonomy and Control

Both the pregnancy and the decision to relinquish the child serve to enhance the autonomy of the young unmarried mother. Both acts establish her more as her own person and force her to accept a greater degree of adulthood. Most jurisdictions recognize the act of becoming a mother as one of "emancipation," which signals the end of minority status. Although contracts by minors are not usually binding, the agreement to relinquish a child for adoption may be accepted as a legal contract. A pregnancy carried to term makes a "girl" a legal adult, regardless of her age. The birth mother's capacity to function as an adult depends, of course, on much more than that. The degree of autonomy the birth mother will claim depends upon her age; her capacity to function as an adult in other areas of her life; her personal and familial dynamics and the meaning of the pregnancy therin; and the family's capacity to recognize and allow her to exercise her increased autonomy.

Parents whose rights are being terminated have had their sense of autonomy diminished. They view the court action as an assault on their family and feel powerless to respond.

Family Boundaries and Family Membership

Family boundaries and family membership are related both to the issues of autonomy and to family systems. We are talking here about the impact of the pregnancy and the adoption decision on the perception of the birth parents by their families, and vice versa. Sometimes, the family of a young parent feels that the birth of a child gives a young person (particularly the birth mother) adult status. For another family, the court's acceptance of the birth parent's majority status may not have much impact.

Separation and Loss

The most significant issue for all of those participating in adoption is loss. In the past, social workers who worked with young single birth mothers felt that once those young women had decided to relinquish their children for adoption, they could put the experience behind them. Workers were fond of telling such young mothers, as the worker told Phyllis Garrett in the case example given earlier, "Now you can go on with your life." As most helping professionals now know, this is impossible. The birth mother is forever bonded to the child that she has carried, delivered, and relinquished, and the normal process of mourning is impeded by the decision to place the child for adoption. Not only does the research to date indicate this (Winkler & van Keppel, 1984), but the increasing numbers of birth mothers who are returning to adoption agencies or seeking mental health services related to their pregnancies and the decision to relinquish their children demonstrate it poignantly.

In the most extensive study to date of what happened to mothers who had relinquished their children for adoption (Winkler & van Keppel, 1984), a most significant finding was that approximately one-half of the sample of 203 subjects reported an *increasing* sense of loss over periods of up to 30 years following the surrender. Loss through adoption is not the same as loss by death. A loss by death is final; one can be certain that one will not encounter the lost person in an earthly form again, and the normal mourning process can proceed. The pain of the loss subsides as the years go by. In a loss by adoption, the birth parents know that somewhere out there, the children they have relinquished still exist. The statistical odds of an accidental meeting or of being found through search are clearly greater when adopted children are grown and moving about the world than when they were relatively secure in the confines of their adopted families. The likelihood that birth parents may see their children again, either by coincidence or by design, increases with every passing year. An adoption relinquishment can never be a clean and total break that eliminates the possibility of future contact; as a result, the grief process cannot follow its natural course.

The issue of loss may be even more acute for parents whose children go into adoption as a results of parental termination. Many of these parents already feel impotent; they react to the loss not only of their children and their sense of family integrity, but also of any control over the destiny of their children.

Relationship with the Opposite Sex

It is hard to know the impact of a pregnancy and an adoption decision on the kind of future relationships young mothers may have with men. Many of them express anger toward the birth fathers at the time of pregnancy or relinquishment, because they feel that the birth fathers have not offered them support during their pregnancies or in the adoption decision. It is hard to know, however, the extent to which the absence of this support may be the result of the birth fathers' exclusion, in keeping both with the role that society has assigned them and, perhaps, with the wishes of the birth mothers or the mothers' families. Whatever the reasons, it is true that most young women who surrender their children for adoption do so by themselves, or with the support of their own mothers or other members of their families of origin. Very few do so in the company of the birth fathers, unless, of course they are married or are planning to be.

Birth mothers frequently say that their relationships with men have been seriously affected by their adoption experience, and some who feel they have been betrayed express reluctance to form a new relationship with a man. If a pregnancy and a decision to place the child for adoption serve to end the relationship between the child's birth parents, it can be assumed that the loss of the birth father compounds the birth mother's feelings of loss as a result of her decision to surrender the child for adoption. However, the long-term impact of the pregnancy and surrender on birth mothers remains unclear, and of course even less is known about their impact on birth fathers. Most women who relinquish their children for adoption do later go on to marry (Brodzinsky, 1990b, p. 301), but, this does not mean that the early pregnancy and the relationship with the birth father do not continue to have an impact on the birth mother. Her selection of a mate may itself be influenced by the earlier events; in addition, the decision to tell her husband of her earlier pregnancy, and the conscious or unconscious comparison of the husband to the birth father, may continue to affect the marital relationship.

Although it is possible that court-ordered termination could also have an impact on the birth parents' future relationships with others of the opposite sex, it is more likely that the adoption action will exacerbate problems in the existing relationship between the parents.

Self-image

An early pregnancy outside of marriage and a decision to relinquish the child for adoption present a double blow to a birth mother's self-image. Premature pregnancy may transgress religious tenets or family moral values. The birth mother may view herself as "bad" or be identified within the family system as the "bad child." A part of adolescent development is a testing of one's omnipotence. To become pregnant is a blow to the self-esteem of many young women who felt that this could never happen to them. Although family and friends may rally to their support, there is often some initial isolation, which only serves to make these women feel less secure and valued.

A birth mother is on the horns of a dilemma with respect to her relinquishment decision. She will never make the decision without ambivalence, and whatever it is, it will be received critically by at least some members of her support group. The birth mother's low self-esteem may be further lowered by those who view "giving away one's own flesh and blood" as a far more serious transgression than having a child before one is ready to be a parent.

For parents whose children are removed by the courts, the blow to self-esteem is even worse. Such parents are ruled "unfit" in courts, and some may suffer criminal trials and penalties as a result of the abuse their children have suffered. Perhaps because of people's knowledge of how hard it is to rear a child and their awareness of their own limitations in parenting, parents whose failure is publicly noted come in for a great deal of criticism and scorn.

Birth Parents in the Context of Their Family Systems

It is clear that these complex issues cannot all be resolved at the time that the adoption decision is being made, even when there is optimum therapeutic opportunity. Some recur in response to environmental pressures along the way, and some surface only as the birth parents face further developmental tasks. It is also clear that to offer clinically effective interventions to birth parents, whether at the initial point of contact or later (whatever their presenting problem), it is important to consider these six issues within the context of the family systems within which the birth parents are functioning.

As a couple or woman goes through the treatment process, the possibility may arise of inviting parents, siblings, or other significant persons to a session. If this is done, there should be a specific reason for doing so and a well-prepared plan in order to assure that such a meeting is productive. For example, a woman may wish to invite her parents to a session so that she can tell them of her pregnancy in safety, ask their reactions to various options, or both. Sometimes a sister or a friend may be invited in order to inquire about practical resources from extended family members.

An alternate to inviting significant people to sessions is to coach a woman to approach them elsewhere. Such coaching may apply to contacts with family members, friends, medical personnel, or clergy. Some women, still in shock, need encouragement to approach people not only for support, but also for information about options such as adoption or abortion.

An instance in which a therapist must deal with pregnancy/parenting issues as a crisis occurs during the treatment of a dysfunctional adult or couple. When pregnancy occurs after therapy is well underway, the therapist already has an assessment and may have been dealing with the possibilities of pregnancy. An individual woman functioning at this level may be sexually promiscuous in a search for attention and nurture. A couple, married or not, may want a child as a source of new emotional involvement. Or a dysfunctional couple may be in conflict about having a child—one partner may be insisting on a child for dependent reasons, while the other may be resisting because of the threat of replacement by the child and rejection. Once a woman is actually carrying a child, a man may threaten to leave if she has the child, or, conversely, may threaten to leave if she aborts it .

The process of working with these people in regard to their decision is the same as discussed above. The options must be considered for their implications for on each individual and the relationship between the partners in pregnancy. However, the dysfunctional nature of the dynamics means that the process must be tempered to fit what the people are able and willing to do. The neediness of these individuals is such that a well-thought-out decision is rare.

There is a final way in which a family therapist may encounter the effects of a problem pregnancy, especially when the decision was made to place a child for adoption. These effects may be uncovered years later when a family that includes the birth parent is in therapy. They may surface when a therapist senses a missing link in the family dynamics, especially in connection with the meaning of a pregnancy or a child. As the therapist explores this area, the fact that one of the parents was a birth parent who earlier surrendered a child to adoption comes to the surface. Sometimes the parents had a child together before marriage, and surrendered that child to adoption. In either situation, continuing grief about the loss of the earlier child has affected the parental relationships with subsequent children. Furthermore, anxiety may increase as one of these children approaches the age of the parent when the earlier pregnancy occurred.

When this loss is uncovered, the therapist should help the person to vent the grief and perhaps fear of exposure. Usually an earlier pregnancy that resulted in adoption is shared with a subsequent spouse, but it is less common that this information is shared with their children. Even if the adoption was known to the entire present family, the parent often has not felt permission for open grief. The pain of that loss may have been suffered silently on each anniversary of the child's birth, or perhaps even on a daily basis.

When given the opportunity by the therapist, a birth mother is likely to acknowledge her grief and pain. A birth father, however, is likely to dismiss it, probably because his part in the pregnancy has so far only received censure. A therapist should not readily accept such dismissals. Once a birth father is sure of acceptance, he too can share his grief and pain, and the clinician can help with the techniques of grief therapy.

Siblings, members of the extended family, and close friends of birth parents can also be affected by the experience in ways that may show up much later, as the following case example illustrates.

Evelyn Marvin was the youngest of three daughters. When she was 15, her oldest sister, Jean, who was 17, became pregnant. The family supported Jean in her decision to place her baby for adoption. Evelyn was the only family member who wanted Jean to keep the baby. She wanted the baby brought into the family, and offered to babysit any time Jean wanted her to. Following the placement of the baby, Evelyn's grades in school dropped temporarily, and she appeared depressed. She sometimes remarked that she wondered how the baby was doing, and on several occasions asked Jean whether she didn't miss her baby.

The next year the second sister, Karen, who was then 17, became pregnant. Karen wanted to keep her baby, and her parents reluctantly agreed to help rear it so Karen could finish school. This time Evelyn did not express an opinion about the planning, and when asked said that it was up to Karen to decide what to do. She did not offer to babysit; in fact, after the baby came into the family, she objected to assuming responsibilities for its care. She sometimes seemed to be watching the baby in a detached way, and more than once wondered out loud whether Jean's baby had developed in the same way. At the time Karen became pregnant, the mother said that she certainly didn't want Evelyn following in her sisters' footsteps and having a baby when she reached 17. Evelyn replied that she wasn't sure that she ever wanted to have a baby. Following the birth of Karen's baby, Evelyn withdrew from a 2-year relationship with her boyfriend and did not start dating any other boys. Evelyn became distant from both sisters, too.

Jean went on to college and began living with a man whom she planned to marry. They were both going on to graduate school and had decided to postpone marriage and parenting until they had completed their graduate work. Karen remained in high school and maintained her relationship with the father of her child. After she graduated, they were married and took their baby to live with them. Evelyn, who was still living at home, did not seem to react to the loss of this child. Evelyn had earlier talked of going to college, but when she finished high school she decided to take a job as a teacher's aide. She continued to live at home and to date only rarely—usually not the same man more than once or twice. She had few outside interests and spent a lot of her time watching television. She began to put on weight and pay less attention to her appearance and personal hygiene. Her parents were concerned and urged her to seek help from the therapist who had been involved with the family in regard to planning for Jean's baby. Evelyn entered therapy. The focus of the work was on her unresolved grief for Jean's child and Evelyn's arrested sexual development, which was the consequence.

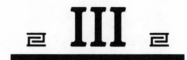

III
FORMING
AN ADOPTIVE FAMILY

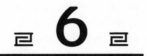

Marital Therapy
for Problems
of Infertility

Marital Dynamics and the Decision
to Have Children

A man who married during the 1950s remarked that the process was so much easier for him than for his young adult children. For him, the hard part was stammering a proposal to his girlfriend. Once she accepted, the rest was simple and understood — they would announce their engagement, marry and have children. At the same life stage, his children have much more freedom of choice, and therefore much more perplexity. Now a man and a woman must decide when they are officially "a couple"; whether to live together and/or become engaged; whether and when to marry; and whether and when to have children. Furthermore, the sequence of these decisions is also a matter of choice. For couples who marry after college and postgraduate education, the path to marriage may be quite individualized (Reitz, 1982).

On the other hand, the diverse population of the United States includes many young couples who approach marriage in a more traditional way. The particular tradition, however, may derive from one of many religious, ethnic, and socioeconomic cultures. Cultural factors not only affect marriage, but also usually prescribe norms in regard to having children. Some traditions do not consider having children a matter of choice; they simply expect that couples will have children after marriage. Whatever the culture of a marrying couple, it has been taught and mediated by each family of origin.

Particular meanings of or variations on broad cultural themes instilled by the family have a strong influence on the next generation's attitudes to marriage and children. Thus, even if individuals who are marrying come from a similar cultural background, differences in expectation instilled by each original family need to be worked out. If marriage partners come from different cultural backgrounds, the differences in learned values about marriage and children may require strenuous negotiation.

In recent decades, there have been more two-career couples who openly try nontraditional patterns of intimate relationships. They may postpone marriage, and, once married, may put off the decision about having children. Such couples, especially those who discuss their decisions at length, may be convinced that the results are their own free and personal choices. But whether or not the individuals agree with their parents' expectations, psychological energy is required to sort these matters out with a partner who also must contend with parental expectations. When parental values are disavowed to such an extent that contact between the generations is cut off, this may seem to create more freedom and availability of energy for the marriage. Ironically, however, the maintenance of such a defensive barrier against parents may bind so much psychological energy that much less is available for the marriage and any future children.

How couples go about the decision to have children varies as much as the ways in which they decide to marry. In cases where children are assumed to follow from marriage, there may be not direct discussion. References such as "When we have children . . ." convey the mutual assumption. Some spouses marry early with an agreement that children are wanted, but then plan the timing (e.g., perhaps after particular financial or career goals are met). Others may discuss at length questions and ambivalence about children. If they resolve to have children, they may work out a careful plan or schedule that addresses the misgivings. Not infrequently, one spouse wishes strongly to be a parent while the other has doubts about ability or readiness for parenting. Such spouses may proceed to have a child, with a plan that the ambivalent parent will have less responsibility for child care. This may mean that the father stays home with the child or that child care is provided by someone other than a parent.

Some spouses are not able to resolve the decision about children, because their wishes are so adamantly opposite or both are so strongly ambivalent. They may simply defer the decision indefinitely, in covert acknowledgment that they feel hopeless about reaching a mutually satisfactory resolution. In these instances, the biological clock may finally force a decision, perhaps throwing the couple into crisis. Finally, there are cases in which the decision about children is a prior condition to the decision to marry. Some individuals who live together decide to marry only after they decide to have a child. Others make the decision about children and perhaps marriage by default, when an unplanned pregnancy occurs.

When a man and a woman decide to become parents, there can be many reasons. The most common is that parenthood is a "normal" next stage of the life cycle and the means of continuity in life and generations. Most individuals have a sense of wanting children as part of their personal continuity. Some people have a strong wish to nurture the young and may choose spouses who are seen as good potential partners in parenting. A well-functioning and happy couple may wish to extend a mutual sense of well-being by opening the family circle to children.

The age-appropriate psychological theme for a marriage of young adults is competence. The issues of this theme have to do with gaining competence in the social roles of worker, spouse, and perhaps parent. Integral to this theme are the spouses' decision-making negotiations and role development as regards marriage, careers, and children.

As a result of successful negotiations and experiences of competence in these roles, the best-functioning couples move on to the theme of identity. This theme moves the outcome of young adult development into a matured sense of "who we are" in terms of values, gender identity, and plans for the next stages of life.

Some couples whose marriages are based on a theme of competence remain stuck in the issues. These individuals have usually come to marriage with damage to self-esteem in the area of social role competence. Moderate to severe anxieties in this area may stem from experiences in families of origin, which perhaps have been aggravated by difficulties at work or in dating. Some of these marriages have been proceeded by stormy, on-and-off courtships, marked by conflict centering around issues of competence as partners or employees. Spouses mired in competence-related anxieties may want to have children in order to have the opportunity to prove competence in a new role (i.e., that of parent). Others may be very reluctant to become parents because of fears of failure in still another role. A complementary pattern wherein one spouse strongly wants to prove competence as a parent and the other is very anxious about incompetence in this role can polarize a serious problem.

Couples whose marriages are based on any of the three earliest themes (nurture, behavior control, and expressivity) are already developmentally behind schedule. Such a lag relates directly to experiences in families of origin and is connected to skewed or partial emancipation from them. Such couples may see having children as a means of verifying their adulthood and completing the separation from families of origin. Thus, children may be viewed as a means of solidifying the boundary around a marriage and defending against the extended family.

When there are boundary difficulties between a marital pair and their parents, there are also often difficulties in the marriage. Thus having a child may also be an attempt to repair marital difficulties. Having a child may be meant to bring the couple together or to be an attempt at appeasement from one spouse to the other. Such solutions usually do not work out when the couple's functioning is centered around an early developmental theme. Instead, the child becomes closely allied with one parent, while the other is distanced from the dyad. Some needy adults consciously desire to become parents, or even to enter marriage, in order to have children who will be better nurturers than their own parents or spouses.

Forms of Infertility

Regardless of the reasons why children are wanted or the dynamics of a marriage, any spouses who want a child but are unable to produce one undergo severe stress and a strong sense of loss. The standard definition of "infertility" is that there has been 1 year of unprotected sexual intercourse at the appropriate monthly times without a pregnancy. The simplicity of this definition does not suggest the various forms of infertility or the range of emotional reactions experienced by individuals and couples.

Some couples never conceive, even though they may have tried for years. Whether and how soon they seek medical intervention depends on a number of factors—mainly, their reasons for wanting children and the urgency of this desire. For example, a man and woman in their early 20s may plan to start a family a year after marriage; they may try for some years before becoming concerned and going to a physician. But two-career spouses may have waited until their mid-30s when careers were well launched, before trying to conceive. They may become quite concerned if pregnancy does not occur within 3 months. In the circumstance where a couple wants a child to serve needs for basic nurture, desperation may take the pair to medical help soon and over long periods.

Regardless of a couple's level of functioning, the longer the spouses have deliberately tried to conceive and have not succeeded, the more severe the cumulative stress and grief become. Each new menstrual period brings renewed grief for an unrealized dream and

sometimes expressed through pressure on the infertile spouse to continue medical treatment or new technology beyond the spouse's physical or emotional endurance. Such pressure can be very subtle or may take the form of an ultimatum ("You do this for me or I will leave you").

Spouses' Reactions to Infertility: Grief and Stress

The profound emotions involved in frustrated wishes for a child can change the course of a marriage. In the 1980s at least 70% of couples undergoing treatment for infertility eventually have a child (Johnston, 1983). But the stress and grief of infertility can make inroads in the quality of a marriage, and these do not magically disappear when a child is born. If a marriage already has serious dysfunction before the problem of infertility arises, the marriage can worsen or dissolve even if there is a child eventually.

Writers about the effects of infertility agree that families undergo a grief process, but one with special elements. The stages of grief about infertility are usually described in similar ways (Carter & Carter, 1989; Covington, 1988). The most comprehensive discussion is that provided by Patricia Johnston (1983, pp. 9–16). Johnston says that stage 1 is the shock of confronting the fact of infertility. Stage 2 is denial, often of the sort that leads to redoubling efforts to follow a medical regimen, to changing doctors, or to becoming obsessive about the search for ways to change the outcome. In stage 3, as the data sink in, the spouses withdraw from outside contacts in order to nurse their sadness and grief together. Such withdrawal also serves to eliminate the pain of constant reminders of other people's fertility, which are all around.

In stage 4, the spouses return to looking outside themselves and the marriage, but now with anger. Often anger is projected onto medical personnel for perceived broken promises to help them have a baby. The anger also may land on relatives, friends, anyone who does have a baby, anyone who has been insensitive to the spouses' plight, and/or anyone who has pressed them about becoming parents. The experience of anger usually leads into active grieving, which comprises stage 5. The grief may have multiple facets, but whatever its form, it is necessary before the couple can move on. Stage 6 follows from grieving: It is the laying down of the dream for a biological child. As the pain of that loss is experienced, the couple may move to beginning resolution.

At this point, Johnston says, there may be three outcomes.

First, the spouses may become stuck in all the emotions and facets of grief. Second, the woman may become pregnant, but the spouses still suffer from the stress of what went before, which is now channeled into further fear of losing the pregnancy. Third, they may come though the process ready to look at alternatives for their lives: childlessness, the various forms of adoption, or the newer birth technologies.

Just as spouses must confront the specific nature of their infertility and find means to deal with it, so must they find their own means of grieving. If the grief is not recognized, or if one spouse moves through the stages in a different manner or pace than the other, there is much room for misunderstanding. Even couples whose marriages have been functioning well may regress during the grief process to old problems. When the grief of infertility compounds prior deficits of nurture, people are likely to get stuck in their emotions—the first of the possible outcomes noted by Johnston.

By contrast, if spouses are able to share their grief and accept that each may handle it differently, they may be able to ease difficult situations for each other. For example, a wife may know that her husband has difficulty controlling his temper when his father teases him about whether he knows how to make a baby; she may listen for her father-in-law to begin and then call her husband out of the room. Likewise, a man may know that his wife is having a hard time holding back tears whenever she sees a pregnant woman or an infant, so he may quietly talk to his mother about excusing his wife from a baby shower that the mother is giving for a daughter.

Infertility and its grief have some special implications for life stage and marital dynamics. It may be the first experience of being unable to master a developmental stage exactly as planned. The sense of powerlessness and loss of control over one's life can be enormous. Some persons react to these feelings by frantic attempts to regain some sense of control, sometimes eventuating in anxious or obsessive behavior. When having children was a basic reason for marrying, the blow to role competence is doubled: Not only is there a question about being able to assume the role of parent, but now there is also a question about being able to carry out the agreed-upon role as spouse. The same can apply even when children were not an explicit part of the marital agreement. Fears, guilt, and helplessness about inadequacy in the two roles of parent and spouse may interact and escalate. While reeling under such blows to sense of competence, the spouses may face decisions that further challenge the adequacy of their coping under duress. They must decide about further medical procedures and about intrusion into their personal and sexual lives; at the very least, they must determine how long they wish to schedule their sexual lives around the monthly clock.

Because dealing with infertility puts a big strain on any relationship, there is a tendency for the regulation dimension to shift toward an extreme. Under the crisis of infertility, the regulation of even a well-functioning relationship can move some distance toward an extreme. For example, a couple with open regulation and a symmetrical pattern of behavior can maintain these arrangements through the stages of infertility grief. This means that the spouses grieve openly together, talk through all the decisions, and cooperate in carrying out the decisions; they accept and are supportive of each other's emotional ups and downs. During this process, however, the symmetry can be upset if infertility-related issues begin to create differences between the spouses. One major example is that the physical infertility of just one spouse is a factual insertion of difference, which may engender very different emotions in the partners. Another possibility is that one or the other tires sooner of the treatment process or is more stressed by it, which again injects difference into their symmetrical pattern. Such disjunction can lead into a pattern of blame for not being well motivated or strong enough, creating an imbalance. Such conflict increases guilt and distance; as a result, the regulation of the relationship becomes looser.

A complementary relationship with balanced regulation may also shift toward an extreme under the duress of infertility. What usually happens to this arrangement is that the more assertive or outgoing spouse, or the one who has been the caretaker, becomes more so. This spouse assumes more responsibility for making and carrying out the decisions related to the infertility. The assertive partner may be acting out his or her own grief or guilt about not being able to fulfill a marital agreement and/or may be protecting the other from grief and guilt. Most often the arrangement serves both spouses, in that one pushes forward on decisions and the other agrees, thus permitting both to stay task-focused and to deny emotions.

The effect of this shift is that role divisions become more differentiated and predictably regulated. If the struggle to have a child continues over years, with increasing buildup of stress and emotions, the complementary pattern can become increasingly extreme and rigid. A rigid complementary arrangement in which one spouse eventually becomes symptomatic may be the permanent outcome. If a child is added at some time by birth or adoption, the rigid arrangements then may shift. The child may ally with the caretaking spouse, join with the symptomatic one, or take over the symptomatic role as the focus for both parents.

For couples whose sense of competence is loaded with anxiety, infertility can tip the balance and confirm a sense of inadequacy. Such a deep blow to self-esteem and ensuing grief may be too difficult to withstand and thus is avoided. Often such avoidance of emotion occurs though relentless, desperate pursuit of medical and/or adoption alternatives. In a symmetrical pattern, the path of desperation is pursued together. In a complementary pattern, one spouse may be relentless or even obsessive, while the other goes along. In either case, if the emotions of either spouse break through the denial (especially in the form of not wanting or being able to continue the pursuit), there is a crisis. One or both spouses may feel deeply depressed or anxious, or they may fight about whether or not to continue the pursuit. The future of the marriage may hinge on whether they can agree on what to do next.

Finally, when infertility is faced by couples who are arrested at the earliest developmental themes, situations that are already dysfunctional become more so. Whatever the dynamic arrangements, there is more conflict, distance, enmeshment, or extreme symptomatic behavior. However, since these couples generally do not have the ability to cooperate, their decisions about medical procedures, sex on a schedule, or other alternatives are marked by misunderstanding, mistakes, and conflict. Sometimes one fierce spouse drags around a passive partner to meetings and clinics. Other spouses feel hopeless and retreat to greater enmeshment, perhaps using pets as substitute children. Some who are frightened by or give up on medical procedures may switch their desperation to adoption. Since they probably do not meet agency criteria because of their psychological deficits, they may go after private adoptions. There have been instances in which the paterfamilias of the extended family uses powerful connections to arrange (and pay for) a private adoption for a couple that even the family considers dysfunctional.

The Role of Families of Origin

Although the spouses' personal and marital dynamics are the most important factors in their response to a problem of fertility, their responses are conditioned by past and present experiences in their families of origin. The contributions of original families are often overlooked in discussions of the effects of infertility on marriages; Burns (1987), however, does stress the importance of the effects of infertility on the relationship between spouses and their own parents.

When a couple contemplates children as the natural progression of life and development, this value is directly connected to families of origin. Not only was this value learned in these families, but it has the implication of giving back to parents the gift of continuity in generations. Spouses who are thwarted in this development must deal not only with their own grief and frustration, but also with the reactions of their parents and siblings.

The would-be parents have an emotionally complex task in explaining to the people who gave life to them why they cannot do the same. The complexities have to do with the nature of each person's alliance with each parent, the source of the infertility, and potent gender issues. At the broadest level, the couple's pain about the lost dream child may be mirrored by parents' disappointment about not having grandchildren. There can be four different reactions by the potential grandparents, each of which has repercussions on the relationships between each set of parents, their offspring and the spouse.

Shifts in alliances between an infertile couple and their parents can exhibit the numerous variations possible between two connected triads. Some common possibilities are provided; the imagination can fill in many more. For example, in the case of a young wife who has a conflictual relationship with her own mother but has been warmly welcomed by her husband's parents, her infertility can mean bringing grief to her husband's warm parents and further depreciation from her own mother. Another wife may be close to her own parents but not so valued by her husband's parents. Then her infertility may be openly mourned and she may be comforted by her parents, but it becomes another black mark against her with his. The situation can get even more complicated if the wife and her parents think she should not have to go through any difficult medical procedures, while the husband and his parents think that every possibility should be tried.

A would-be father may have a good relationship with his parents, but always "did things" with his dad rather than talk. Thus, to put into words to his father that he is not able to reproduce biologically, may be very difficult. This can be especially true if he knows that his taciturn father sets a premium on bloodlines and surnames. Another man may have married into a family that considers itself above his in social status. Then if he is unable to contribute to a pregnancy, his value to his wife's family may go even lower. As a result, her family may increase its pressure on her about her marital choice.

The reactions of parents to a couple's problem of infertility may lead to exaggerations of typical behavior. At the extremes, they may become intrusive by inquiring into details or may withdraw and ignore the situation. Often there is considerable concern about the question of "who is at fault." Once they have information about the physical problem, parents may unpredictably intensify or change alliances along biological or gender lines. Sometimes the potential grandparents are most concerned about having responsibility in the situation and what this means for their relationship with their son or daughter. They may worry that they somehow "caused" the problem through genetic heritage or through perceived mishandling of an illness or accident. The thwarted grandparents may also grieve for the missed opportunity to make reparations for a troubled relationship with their child.

Any potential complications between an infertile couple and their parents are exacerbated when the couple has siblings who are producing children. Then the spouses' roles in their original families have a strong effect on all the relationships involved. The number of possible variations in outcome matches the number of alliance patterns possible according to original family size. Let us consider two examples. First, the oldest and most favored of three brothers is the only one not bringing highly desired babies to the grandparents. This could lead to a shift in all the original alliances as the oldest moves down in favor. Second, the middle daughter of a large family where children were much valued has nevertheless always felt left out. If she is the only one unable to reproduce, she may experience her position as worsened. She may avoid family gatherings and even become hostile to fertile siblings with whom she previously had a warm alliance.

All the generational levels of meaning and values about children are pulled upon again at each decision point. Each time, there is a psychological impact on each individual and on the marriage, which may ripple (or thunder) through extended families and social networks. Such emotional waves can become strongly reactive when the couple decides to proceed with powerful fertility drugs or procedures such as *in vitro* fertilization or artificial insemination. Multilevel intensity is particularly evident when a couple contemplates adoption or childlessness. In any of the situations where there will not be genetic continuity, the whole extended family's values concerning children are challenged, leading to emotional reverberations across generations.

Working through Grief and Reviewing the Options

No couple that has experienced infertility is unscathed or "cured," regardless of their coping skills, their level of functioning, or the outcome. Infertile couples report that all areas of their lives are affected: the lost dream child, financial stress from medical treatment, deterioration in the health of at least one spouse, tension in sexual relations, damage to careers, challenge to family and religious values, and particularly the sheer stress of coping with it all (see Burns, 1987; Glazer & Cooper, 1988; Johnston, 1983; Mason, 1987; Mazon & Simmons, 1984; Salzer, 1991; Valentine, 1988). The attempt to regain control of one's life can lead to a high incidence of obsessive behavior, eating and substance abuse, and sexual acting out. Affairs, having a child with someone other than a spouse, divorce, and remarriage are not uncommon in the aftermath of a fertility problem.

Yet couples do work through the entire grief process, find a way to make peace with the infertility, and return to their previous level of functioning. Even then, the grief of infertility is not cured or totally removed, any more than any other major loss is completely expunged. But when spouses have faced the grief and worked through the meaning of infertility, they are more able to make a conscious choice about where to direct the generative energy that would have gone to a birth child. When choices are based on conscious grief work, emotions are less likely to go underground and subsequently to sabotage future arrangements. For example, when a couple chooses a childless life style, the spouses may decide to put more energy into careers or to try a new venture, which becomes a "brain child." Otherwise, they may become mentors to younger workers or a special uncle and aunt to young relatives. Finally, the childless couple may become stars in some volunteer service to children.

Spouses who eventually obtain a child through the biological contribution of at least one of them must still work through the infertility. As a pair they have been infertile, and this is a grief that remains for both. Furthermore, additional emotional work arises from the circumstance that only one is a biological parent. If the difference in means of becoming parents is not well addressed, suppressed emotions have strong potential for subverting future relationships between them and with the child.

The same issues apply to couples who adopt; adoption solves childlessness, not infertility. Here also, the grief of infertility must be worked through for its effect on both spouses and on their relationship. This makes it possible for a child to enter the family for his or her own sake, rather than moving into a role already established by suppressed emotions, projections, overprotection, or ready-made alliances. What complicates this decision over some other alternatives is that the wait for adoption is usually long and uncertain. Thus, the process itself may continually exacerbate the grief process, rather than helping it to resolution.

A popular myth that is sometimes still presented to couples struggling with infertility is this: "Go ahead and adopt; then you'll relax and surely get pregnant." On occasion, adoption professionals have noted apparently high rates of this phenomenon. Katz, Marshall, Romanowski, and Stewart (1985) did a study on such observations. They found that in cases where it was difficult but not impossible for a couple to have a pregnancy, stress indeed *was* a big factor. They concluded that once a couple was accepted for consideration by an adoption agency, three factors improved the possibility of pregnancy: (1) The couple had an opportunity to talk through and resolve some of the stress and grief; (2) being accepted for study provided hope and some control over their lives; (3) some women who had certain medical diagnoses and who were younger had better chances in any case.

Therapy with Infertile Couples

When an infertile couple applies for therapy, the issues of infertility are almost always part of the presenting problems. Then, like any other presenting problems, those related to infertility are assessed in relation to the couple's dynamics and life stage. A big difference, however, is that infertility does not need to be considered for the possibility of symbolizing a deeper issue; infertility *is* the deep issue.

Nevertheless, the way in which the problem is presented provides important clues to the marital dynamics, life stage, and status of the grief process. So the therapist needs to listen carefully to how the problem is described, with what affect, and by whom, while watching for nonverbal clues.

Relatively functional spouses are open about the difficulties and the emotions involved, as well as what they want from treatment, so that a contract is easily agreed upon. When there seem to be covert agendas or suppressed emotions, the therapist may need to negotiate a broader contract than the couple initially requests. Well-functioning spouses may seek help when they have just discovered the infertility; they present with shock, depression, or anxiety. Others have worked out a mutual decision about how to proceed, but want to review the process with a therapist, in order to reassure themselves and/or to arm themselves for dealing with their families of origin. Still others may present an imbalance in their relationship, because one has been worn down by the stress or there is a difference of opinion about how to proceed.

When infertility has been a further blow to already shaky senses of competence, anxiety in some form is the problem presented to a therapist. There may be obvious manifestations of anxiety or defensive behavior that attempts to bind it. Whatever their pattern of behavior, such spouses report shifts for the worse in their relationship since dealing with infertility. A couple that was already dysfunctional prior to the diagnosis of infertility presents more extreme anxiety or behavior to a therapist. Often these spouses resist any discussion of emotions, relationships, or implications of their decisions; all they want the therapist to do is to help them get a child by offering concrete or psychological help. The psychological help requested may be to teach them how to thread their way past medical personnel or adoption agencies so that they will be approved for a particular program. Some of these couples come after being turned down by a program, so they request a second opinion and then advocacy with the program.

Another reason that more dysfunctional infertile spouses present for therapy is tremendous conflict between them. The conflict may be part of their usual dynamics, or it may have erupted in regard to the infertility or at any decision point. Such conflict may be shown in open warfare, repressed into a cold united front, or suppressed behind a thin facade for presentation to the therapist. A therapist may readily assess such situations as ones in which a child is desperately wanted to hold the marriage together or to nurture the adults. In such cases, the spouses must be told that it is an essential part of the contract that they use therapy to consider where a child would fit in with them. Otherwise, the therapist is unable to help them with their goal (and then hopes that they do not somehow manage a private adoption).

Once a contract is established, the therapist can begin with the most immediate concern — usually distress or conflict about the most recent disappointment and possible next steps. The therapist must explore and develop a good understanding of how each spouse is experiencing the present circumstances. This includes the condition of infertility, status of decisions, stage of grief, and pressures from the other spouse or from families of origin. In the course of this inquiry, the spouses soon refer to past experiences, which lead into their history. The therapist needs the whole story in order to understand what has happened both before and after the awareness of infertility. The therapist may decide first to get a detailed history of the spouses' experience of infertility. Or the therapist may start with a complete history of their relationship, beginning from meeting and the decision to marry. Two factors of the early history are especially important: First, how did the decision to marry relate to each spouse's emancipation from the family of origin and expectations of the other spouse? Second, when and how did they discuss and decide about children?

Regardless of the direction of the history taking, assessment of these cases must include two aspects. On the one hand, the therapist takes the usual reading of the dimensions of the relationship, and notes in particular how the operating rules apply to coping with infertility. On the other hand, there is the unusual tracking of a particular set of values — those related to children — and what has happened in reality in the pursuit of those values. To learn about the couple's actual experiences, the therapist must inquire about and respond to not only the painful facts, but especially the associated emotions. Since the couple may have personal reasons for or social support in denying losses, the therapist must solicit details. The history of loss begins with the first consciousness of monthly disappointment. Often it is necessary to ask specifically about any delayed menstrual periods, miscarriages, or stillbirths. The therapist needs to be particularly sensitive and responsive to the ups and downs of hope.

This process of eliciting the spouses' experiences and offering empathy not only aids the grief process, but also can bring great relief. For some individuals, this is the first time they have told anyone what they feel or received any real understanding of their pain. At the same time, when spouses react to the process with relief, the therapist learns their capacity to work through the grief process and to return to improved functioning. When there is resistance to reviewing history, the couple probably is avoiding the grief process. In such cases, beginning with the factual history may ease the way into the emotions and grief. But the most vulnerable people may be so strongly defended against grief that their history cannot be opened. With them, only a limited, behavioral focus over the short term may be possible.

When reviewing history in order to enable the grief process, the therapist should be alert to whether the spouses show major differences of response. If so, the therapist should note further whether the differences are open or covert, or used in supportive or conflictual ways. In any case, conflict should be explored as to onset, association with infertility, and degree of escalation. Such exploration enables the therapist to learn whether any blaming has taken place in regard to the infertility, and/or whether any ultimata have been issued about the future of the relationship.

Regardless of whether the marital relationship has deteriorated or not under the stress of infertility, it is very important for the therapist to stay even-handed with both spouses. Often the woman is the more articulate spouse; if in addition she is the leader in a complementary relationship, her husband's grief and any different opinions may be easily overlooked. This may be further reinforced if she has gone through miscarriages or has endured more medical procedures than he has. In such a case, the man must be encouraged to articulate his grief and loss of dreams also.

> A burly truck driver had two daughters and wanted a son. When his wife had a third miscarriage, and the lost infant this time was known to be a male, she was devastated and he was very solicitous of her. Yet, when a therapist asked him how it was for him to lose a son, he cried and said that no one had asked him before.

After the history is known, the grief process and the current stage of decision-making may require various past experiences and new decisions to be reworked again and again. In each round, attention must be given to the individuals, to the marriage, and to the impact on interactions with families of origin and important others. As the focus moves from the past to the present, the therapist tries to fortify whatever features of the marriage are vulnerable. Every effort is made to strengthen mutual loyalty and attachment, so that the spouses can support each other through the stress and in facing professionals, family, and friends.

It is especially important to promote clear, direct, and self-responsible communication between spouses in regard to stress, grief, and decisions. Specific help should be offered when spouses have a difference of opinion about what to do. Differences in the meaning to each of a child by birth must be clarified, along with any blame that is transpiring. Then the therapist can walk them through all the emotional and reality-related aspects of the decisions until they reach a common position.

Whenever possible, it is preferable for spouses to affirm that their relationship is more important than the wish to be parents. Along with that, they must give up the particular child they have imagined or even expected in a beginning pregnancy. This does not mean that they must give up trying to become parents, but it does mean giving up the expectation of a biological child or one who will perfectly fit their expectations. Without the imagined child, the spouses are freer to move toward resolution of grief. Then, they are also freer to make good judgments for their future — either to decide to remain childless, or to chose an alternative means of having a child.

The final phase of treatment with infertile couples is the working through of options. In this phase, the therapist may do much educating about the choices, perhaps offering alternatives new to the couple. But the most important role is to help both spouses try out emotionally all the pros and cons of every alternative of interest to them.

Sometimes a pregnancy will occur during the grief work or while the spouses are deciding about options. They may wish to leave therapy immediately because the problem is "solved." Under such circumstances, the therapist should urge them to stay in treatment, at least occasionally during the first trimester. Often the stress of infertility is not solved during this period, but rather intensified. Whatever the therapist has previously helped the couple to do in the management of stress and grief needs strong support and reinforcement at this time.

When couples begin to consider giving up on medical treatment that might lead to conception in the usual way, they may wish to discuss the various new birth technologies and means of adoption. Although a therapist may not be an expert on the facts or procedures of any of these, important work can be done with the spouses' emotional reactions to them. Not only the individual reactions can be considered, but also the effects on the marriage of becoming parents by each method, especially those involving the biology of just one parent. Also, it is useful for the therapist to consider with them the possible reactions of their families of origin to the various means of becoming parents. A good way to tap into significant emotions is to ask each spouse who would be told about particular methods of becoming parents. They may request specific help in deciding about who and how to tell about approaches to parenthood that they know will not be well received.

When a couple contemplates obtaining a child by some means other than mutual biology, the therapist can do a further service by pointing the spouses toward the future. Often at the point of decision about birth technology or adoption, the spouses are very focused on their own wishes and urgencies to have a baby. The generic desired infant has not yet become a real person to them, or one who will grow up and someday ask about the facts of his or her birth and inheritance. The therapist can prepare parents by "humanizing" the product of their decision and asking what they would tell a child about his or her origins. They can be further helped to examine the ramifications of answering the growing child with all, some, or none of the truth.[1]

Some couples work through to their own conclusion to remain childless. But when a couple cannot find a mutually acceptable method of becoming parents, the therapist may introduce childlessness as a viable option. The therapist can surely provide evidence from experience that when a child arrives in a manner acceptable to only one parent, this bodes poorly for strong triadic alliances. (For a discussion of a childless life style, see Carter & Carter, 1989.)

Sometimes while spouses are working through the grief and decision process, the lid comes off suppressed emotions. Conflict becomes intense, leading to a decision to end the marriage. Possible reasons for this are several. Perhaps the marriage was too fragile to withstand the stress of infertility, or one or both spouses wanted a child to compensate for deficits of nurture. A child may be too desperately important to forgo for the sake of an infertile partner. A therapist can accept a divorce decision as a valid choice in such a case, but should still urge the couple to work through the grief, which now has another layer. The roles of childlessness and blame are explored as factors in the divorce decision. Since these situations are usually very heated and volatile, the therapist also needs to promote calm and the least hurtful understandings.

Case Examples of Therapy with Infertile Couples

Not only are there many forms of infertility; there is also great variation among the persons who experience it, their situations, and their outcomes. The diversity of infertility-related problems presented to a clinician may be best illustrated by case examples.

---

1. For further discussions about dealing with the grief of infertility and threading the way through options, see Glazer and Cooper (1988), Mazor and Simmons (1984), and Salzer (1991). Glazer (1990) addresses possible effects of infertility on parenting. Potential ramifications of the new reproductive technologies are also considered in Chapter 14 of this volume.

Mike and Jan, in their mid-20s looked like the all-American couple, glowing with good health and confidence. Both were the first college-educated members of large blue-collar families. They met at a softball game sponsored by the hospital where both worked, Jan as a pediatric nurse and Mike as a radiology technician. They hit it off immediately, were engaged after 6 months, and married a year after meeting. Even before they were engaged, they shared their dreams for at least four children. Both laughed as each admitted to early thoughts that the other would make a very good parent.

They planned to start their family right after marriage. When there was no pregnancy after a year, they consulted a medical specialist; although both went through a battery of tests, the results were not conclusive. Further procedures were possible but costly in money and potential pain. Mike and Jan went through every step together, thoroughly discussing alternatives and choices. Eventually they decided to stop medical treatments, to continue unprotected sex, and to apply for adoption. They preferred an infant but were open to children with special needs.

After the decision, Jan and Mike sought a therapist because they wished to review their process with an objective expert. In particular, they questioned whether they had overlooked anything in the decisions to stop medical treatment and to adopt. Furthermore, they wanted help about how to approach both sets of parents. Mike and Jan knew that all four would be thrilled by a biological grandchild. But they also knew that there would be mixed reactions to an adopted grandchild, especially if the child had a handicap.

The therapist found Mike and Jan to be a remarkable couple in two ways. First, their relationship was strong, cooperative, and mutually open. This was obvious in the way they behaved in session, but also was reflected in what they described. The second remarkable feature was that neither seemed to have a need to make a child into his or her own image or an extension of self. They also agreed that to love and nurture a child was much more important than how the child came to them.

Jan and Mike came in for four biweekly sessions, in which their process was reviewed. They had indeed covered all the facts, but readily accepted support for considerable unacknowledged stress, which they had tried to hide from each other. Each was asked to predict his or her parents' reactions and was given some general suggestions about approach. Then both were encouraged to adjust the ideas according to what they knew was most likely to ease the way with each parent. Both followed up in approaching parents and then processed the results in the next session.

Subsequently, this couple came for a few more appointments

over several-month intervals. At the last meeting, they proudly brought along 3-month-old Timmy, a bright-eyed, thriving infant. Timmy also wore an orthopedic device for a skewed foot. Jan and Mike reported that both grandmothers adored him and that the grandfathers were coming around.

In contrast, when Milly phoned for an appointment, she wept while saying that she was desperate for help in coping with unsuccessful fertility treatment. Milly did not want to bother her husband, John, because "it is not his problem." She insisted on coming in alone at first.

Milly was 38 and John 43. They had been married for 3 years and were well established in careers. Both had been married before, but neither had had children. At the time of marriage they only mentioned the possibility of children, and then as an unlikely choice. But when Milly had her 37th birthday, she suddenly decided that she wanted a child very much and at once, before time ran out. Milly confided to the therapist that it had become important to her "to give a child to John," and she believed that he wanted a son. Although she and John were devoted to each other, she thought a child would do them good. She found John to be emotionally tight and thought that a child would loosen him, and thus also benefit her.

When she did not become pregnant in 4 months, Milly went to a fertility specialist, who found several problems. After several surgeries and one regimen of drug treatment, she was about to try a stronger drug. Milly was determined to proceed, but the stress was mounting. After each treatment, her hope and anxiety went up; each time her menstrual period came, she sank into depression. Worst of all for this competent, successful woman was her first experience of total helplessness in getting something she truly wanted and went after.

Milly reported that John never initiated inquiries or suggestions about the situation; however, he did patiently listen whenever she wanted to talk. John also did whatever she requested, from taking her temperature and keeping the charts, to having sex or going to the doctor. Milly was asked to invite John to the next session.

The contrast between Milly and John was obvious, but so was their affection for each other. She was small, vivacious, and very tense; he was big, quiet, and relaxed. He agreed that he would like to have a child, but thought that it was not nearly so important to him as to Milly. John added that it bothered him to see her so upset, and that he would gladly give up on a child if that would help her to calm down. His clear statement surprised Milly and caused her to pause thoughtfully. Then her anxiety again poured out about what could happen to her, to their marriage, and to her wish to give her widowed father a grandson.

A main part of this treatment was dealing with the meanings and emotions related to children, beginning with each spouse's expectations at marriage. Milly's redecision had caused a sudden shift and thrown aspects of their relationship out of balance. At the base of this was a fundamental dimension of their relationship: John thought Milly overly expressive of emotions, while she found him underexpressive. This issue was played out against and was exaggerated by the fertility procedures. The therapist used the content of their history and the question of children as vehicles for practicing a more balanced communication process. In particular, this meant eliciting John's comments and picking up on his emotional nuances, while getting Milly to be more brief and succinct in her expression of reactions. Once the communication became more balanced and open, attention was given to Milly's sense of powerlessness in regard to producing a child (and also in eliciting John's emotions).

Eventually both spouses accepted that they could not control whether they would have a child by birth, but that they could be empowered by taking charge of decisions. Thus they reviewed possible alternatives. They concluded that Milly would undergo one more round of fertility drug treatment. If she did not conceive during that time, they would work on how to be a happy childless couple. During the last month of treatment, Milly conceived.

After initial disbelief, anxiety soared, throwing the situation into a state almost worse than that at the beginning of therapy. Milly was so afraid that the pregnancy would not last that she was distraught and demanding of John, who withdrew. Over the next 3 months, the focus was on containing anxiety by structuring behavior and discouraging emotional outpourings by Milly. It was equally important to get both spouses to vent the stress in therapy and to cooperate in behavior that eased the situation as much as possible. After the first trimester, the situation calmed somewhat, but John and Milly continued to come for support to cooperative coping. By the end of the second trimester, they were again more comfortable as a couple, but Milly was more physically uncomfortable. So they suspended treatment.

John and Milly named their healthy daughter Jill Carla — "Jill" as a combination of their names and "Carla" for Milly's father. When they brought Jill Carla for a wrap-up session with the therapist, John carried and took care of the baby while Milly beamed at them both. John was obviously expressing himself, although still in a quiet way while Milly contained her pleasure over a warm connection with both John and Jill Carla.

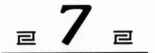

7

Affiliation and Assessment Issues of Adoptive Families

Becoming a successful adoptive family is not easy. Adoption complicates the developmental stages of family members and affects the family dynamics at each life stage. The first task of the adoption worker who helps bring an adoptive family together, and of the clinician providing service at some later point, is careful assessment. Families that add members through adoption come from the entire spectrum of family systems; they include a wide range of individual histories and needs; and they may be facing different family life stages. What they share is their desire for a child through adoption, or certain common difficulties as a result of such an adoption. It cannot be assumed that they are alike in any other ways. Even these common factors must be considered carefully with each particular family. The unique pattern of the interaction among the adoption factors, the dynamics of the family's system, and the life stage the family is facing is what distinguishes each from all others.

Assessment in Preparation for Adoption

Families wanting to adopt range along a continuum from wishing to have "adoption anonymity" to desiring "adoption notoriety." Parents who seek anonymity are infertile and are looking for a child who resembles the child they wish they could have had by birth — a young, healthy infant of good potential, who looks like them — and their fantasy is that this child will then be "theirs" in the same sense that a child born to them would have been. They have no wish to emphasize the fact that their child is adopted, but rather wish to blend into the community and be viewed and treated like any other family. At the other end of the continuum are parents who attract community attention by virtue of either the size or the unique composition of the adoptive family they have formed, or both. They seek, or at least do not shun, adoption notoriety. They adopt children whom most other people do not wish to parent. These are the parents who adopt several children of different racial and cultural backgrounds and who view themselves as a "United Nations family," or who successfully parent one or more children with severe developmental or physical difficulties. Between these extremes are parents who adopt children of all ages, backgrounds, and abilities for a variety of reasons.

The Tasks of Agencies

Agencies placing children for adoption confront two major problems in the recruitment, assessment, and preparation of parents and families for adoption: (1) There are not sufficient families for the children who are waiting, many of whom are not healthy infants; and (2) those parents who want to adopt, especially those toward the anonymity end of the continuum, are often unaware of or wish to deny the continuing complexities that adoption will bring them. Although the awareness of potential problems in adoption increases as one moves along the continuum from anonymity to notoriety, the number of parents interested in adoption decreases.

The strongest argument for agencies' handling adoptions is that there is no other way to assure that adoption is available to all children who can benefit from it and that adequate service is provided to all members of the triangle. The task of adoption agencies is to try to find parents who can successfully rear the children who are in need of permanent new families, and to be as certain as possible that newly formed adoptive families can meet the needs of all of their members. To accomplish this, agencies placing children for adoption must do six things:

1. They must be certain that the birth parents whose children will be adopted have received the services they needed.
2. They must recruit families for all of the children who wait.

3. They must help prospective adoptive parents assess their capacity for adoption, and help them understand and prepare to accept all that adoptive parenting encompasses.
4. They must assess, prepare, and place children for adoption, trying to be certain that any particular needs of a child are matched to the special strengths of the family into which that child will be placed.
5. They must help make available the range of services that adoptive families may need following the adoption, as they face developmental issues and struggle with the differences that adoption makes.
6. They must serve as the repositories of information and records that may be essential to any member of the adoption triangle in the future.

Essential to all six tasks is an agency's clear perception of adoption as a different way of putting a family together, and a commitment to helping adoptive families accept the fact that they are different from other families. Adoption changes the perspective on all of the things that parents do for their children. The adoptive parents must incorporate the adopted child into their family in a way that recognizes the difference that adoption makes, yet gives full membership to the adopted child and maintains the family as a well-functioning system for all of its members.

Four Phases of the Adoption Process

A way to conceptualize the adoption process that enables both the adoption worker arranging a placement and later clinicians who may be involved with a family to be effective is to divide the process of adoption into four sequential phases. The first phase, the "uncertainty" phase, includes everything that happens before the child comes into the adoptive family. The anxiety of the adoptive parents at this time can be captured by the question "Will we get a child?" The second phase covers the time from the new child's entry into the adoptive family until the time the adoption is consummated. During this period of time, the "apprehension" phase, the question of the adoptive parents is "Can we keep our child?" Then follows the "accommodation" phase, which continues throughout the period of the child's growing up. During this period of time the anxiety of the adoptive parents may take the form of the question "Do we *have* to keep our child?" (This question occurs in the minds of parents rearing children born to them, too, of course; however, it has quite a different meaning in adoptive families because of the more tenuous tie between the parents and the child.) The fourth phase, the "integration" phase, extends for the rest of the lives of all who are part of an adoption. Then the core issue can be characterized for the adoptive parents by the question "How is being an adoptive parent different now?"

The worker from the adoption agency will ordinarily be actively involved during the first two phases and, depending on the range of the agency's service, may be active in all four. Other clinicians ordinarily do not get involved until the third or fourth phases, when a family seeks help for a problem that has been identified. During each of these phases, the adoptive family is coping with the "regular" development tasks of its members, the family life cycle issues, and the unique issues that families formed by adoption must face.

The most important special issue faced by adoptive families is that of accepting that adoption makes a different kind of family and learning just how to handle these differences. For those families that fall toward the notoriety end of the continuum described above, it may be difficult to deny that they are different from families that develop strictly by birth. All families, however, face the question of just how much to make of the differences and what to do about them. Later we discuss how the rules within a family system shape its response to this issue.

H. David Kirk, in his seminal 1964 study of adoptive families, *Shared Fate* (see Kirk, 1984) was the first to clearly identify the acceptance of an adoption as a critical variable in its success. His survey divided adoptive families into two groups: those that acknowledged the differences made by adoption, and those that denied those differences. His conclusion was that a balance between denial and acknowledgment worked best, but that if a family were to err, it would be better to err in the direction of acknowledgment rather than denial. Our experience supports a variation of Kirk's continuum, with denial of differences at one end and *insistence* on differences at the other. Bourguignon and Watson (1987) list seven other issues that are different for the members of adoptive families and that have the potential to be troublesome: entitlement; claiming; unmatched expectations; shifts in family systems; separation, loss, and grief; bonding and attachment; and identity formation.

It is important for adoption workers to explore all of these issues in their initial contacts with families, in order to help them understand adoption better and get off to a good start, and also in order to set the stage for them in terms of identifying the context in which future problems may emerge. It is equally important for clinicians to be familiar with these issues, so that they can assess the extent to which adoption is a major component of the distress in adoptive families seeking therapy. It is also useful for therapists to note which of the four phases of the process families are in when they present (the phases are not always chronologically congruent), as well as what unfinished business the families may be carrying into this phase from earlier phases.

Agencies involved in working with families that wish to adop meet these families in their uncertainty phase. There has been some confusion among adoption agencies about their role during this phase. Traditionally, agencies have viewed themselves as representing society in terms of protecting children, and have assumed an investigatory or assessment role. The contact between an agency and the prospective adoptive parents has been called the "home study"; frequently, anxious couples have viewed this as an obstacle course with a child waiting as a reward for the successful completion. Because of the more recent focus on the placement of special needs children, and the growing understanding of the complexities of adoption, many agencies now call this period of contact the "preparation period." This term redefines the home study as a period of mutual assessment between agency and prospective family, to ascertain together whether or not adoption is a good plan. In this process, the focus is on the impact of adoption on the family system, and the background and capacities of the parents are explored in this light. As information about the family emerges, the members learn both about themselves and about adoption. In theory, the agency's power is reduced, and those families for which adoption is not a good plan will either withdraw on their own or as a result of a mutual decision-making process. In fact, however, the power to approve or disapprove a family for adoption ultimately lies with the agency.

In most jurisdictions, a license is required to adopt. The power to grant that license is vested in an adoption agency or in some legally designated representative of that agency. So the evaluative component is built into the agency's role during the uncertainty phase. Yet if the adoption is to be successful, the family and the agency must make an alliance, and it is important that the agency help the family members understand adoption and prepare for the changes that it will bring to their lives. Some agencies separate the first step of the process into two: They have an assessment period that is essentially geared toward meeting licensing standards or agency requirements, and a preparation or education period that is directed toward exploring the impact of adoption on a family and preparing the family for that event. A family systems approach helps to reconcile these two potentially contradictory components and enables them to be effectively combined.

In addition, this approach allows the first two phases of the adoption process to flow together, and reduces the anxiety of the family after the child arrives but before the court has issued the final decree. Basic to family systems theory is the fact that family systems change whenever a member is added or leaves. The first phase explores with the family members their dynamics and the way in which their system will accommodate a new adopted child. After the child is placed, the family interviews continue; the focus in the second phase is on the real impact of the arrival of the adopted child, and the ways in which the family is rearranging the system to accommodate the child and re-establish the family equilibrium.

Conducting the Family Interviews

As in conducting an interview with any family, the first task of the professional in conducting an interview with prospective adoptive parents is to join the family. It is important that the worker recognize that this family differs in two respects from those seen in treatment: *There is no presenting problem, and there is no identified patient.* To view a prospective family from a pathological frame of reference is to do it a disservice — and more importantly, perhaps to deny a child a chance for a family. This is especially true, of course, in working with families that are interested in adopting special needs children; most families are not. To focus on what is "wrong" with a family that wishes to proceed in this way is to interfere with the joining process, which has as its goal allying oneself with the goals of the clients. The alliance is centered, then, around the shared goal of the family and agency: namely, to place a child in adoption and to have that placement meet both the placed child's and the family's needs. The focus of the family sessions remains always on exploring adoption within this particular family system.

Bourguignon and Watson (1990), in *Making Placements that Work* suggest that the majority of prospective families have average qualifications for adoptive parenthood. They say that the success of an adoptive placement depends upon assessing the needs and particular strengths of each family, selecting a child whose needs match the family's strengths, and providing the initial preparation and subsequent support that the family needs to do the job.

This is not to say that all families wishing to adopt should do so.

The adoption agency does have a protective function, and it must evaluate families to be as certain as possible that no child is subjected to unnecessary risks. Bourguignon and Watson (1990, pp. 13–15) outline a number of essential traits for adoptive parenting and suggest some "red flags" indicating that adoption may be risky for a family. These warning signals include: impulse control disorders, major unresolved issues in personal history, history of a felony, extremely rigid moral or religious beliefs, significant problems in child rearing, strong needs and unrealistic expectations, history of mental illness or substance abuse, and marital difficulties.

The first phase of the adoption process,then, has as its goals *both* assessment and preparation. The task is to support parents in their quest for a child, using their anxiety to explore with them the differences that having a child by adoption makes, and assessing their motivation and capacity to fulfill the role of adoptive parents. Group meetings that answer factual questions and review agency procedures, and contact with other experienced adopted parents and with birth parents, are both useful tools in this assessment and preparation. However, the best way to proceed is with a series of family interviews that address the question of what becoming a family through adoption really means to that family. The interviews are geared toward helping the family members understand the way their family system functions; helping them come to terms with why they are adopting a child; helping them understand and come to terms with why a child becomes available for adoption; helping them accept that another family comes along with every adopted child; helping them recognize and explore the impact that any adopted child will have on their family system; and helping them "select" the kind of child whose needs most closely meet their needs and who is able to respond to their strengths.

It is important that all family members participate in these meetings, since the adoption will affect the entire family system, but not everybody needs to be on hand for every interview. Many adoption workers like to see prospective parents separately at least once, usually to gather background data and to discuss each partner's perception of the spouse. Others feel that family members' perceptions of each other emerge quickly in family sessions and that background information can be gathered as easily then. The advantage of gathering information this way is that it is garnered in relation to the family's interest in adoption and keeps the adoption process from being "owned" by any family member or subsystem. Ann Hartman (1984), in her book *Working with Adoptive Families beyond Placement*, describes the use of several techniques—such as genograms, eco-maps, family diagrams, and family sculpture — as devices to engage adoptive family in productive discussions of the family in relationship to adoption.

Sometimes parents approaching an agency to explore the possibility of adopting a child do not want to include all family members in a family interview. They may wish to exclude any children they may already have, or one of their own parents, who may be part of the household, particularly if they are going to be discussing their infertility and their sexual relationship. Workers have different ideas about working with family systems and different rules about who must attend. These are matters of worker and family discretion. The important issue is that both the worker and the family view the adoption as a family systems issue and that the entire family have some involvement.

Almost without exception, one member of a couple is much more interested in adoption than the other. Usually it is the woman who takes the lead and the man who is more reluctant. It is not a good idea to see either partner of a couple alone for the first interview. The first session should be either a family or a joint interview. Questions can be raised then about how the decision to pursue adoption was reached and what roles each family member played. One can explore whether the process the parents used to arrive at this decision was the one they ordinarily use in decision making; if so, how well the process works in this family; or, if not, what accounts for the difference here and how that is working.

Another early issue to be explored is why the parents are seeking a child through adoption. Most parents who adopt infants, and some who adopt special needs children, are prompted by infertility. A smaller group of parents are fertile but wish to adopt rather than to conceive biologically. For the first group, the acceptance of the infertility is essential in coming to grips with the meaning of the adoption. Unresolved issues related to the infertility work against the acceptance and integration of the adopted child. For the second group, the family's reason for not having children biologically needs exploration — not because such a decision is pathological, but in order for the family and the agency to understand why this family chooses to deviate from the norm.

Some additional important assessment questions include changes in the marital balance as a result of having children (if there are already children in the family), attitudes toward birth families, the nature of the family's experiences in seeking a child by adoption, the existence of a vacant family role that needs filling (such as a replacement child or one that is needed to shore up a shaky marriage), and how the family would handle being turned down for adoption.

Seven Key Issues Affecting Adoptive Families

Regardless of whether the adopted child is a healthy infant or a special needs child, the seven key issues that impact upon adoptive families, as outlined earlier, provide content for the family interviews. All of the issues need to be identified and discussed in the beginning of the first phase of the adoption process. Although the exploration at this time is primarily at the cognitive level, adopting families can begin to integrate into their own family system the reality that adoption is going to make a life-long difference.

The issues are explored in the context of each family system. During this first phase of the adoption process the emphasis is on helping the family accept the reality that a child will soon be joining the family unit through adoption and developing pragmatic ways that the affiliation can be supported. With that in mind let us review the seven issues identified earlier.

Entitlement

The first issue, entitlement, refers to the adopted parents' sense that they have both the legal and emotional right to be parents to their child. The legal right is conferred in court, the emotional right grows out of the parents' increasing comfort with their roles as mother or father to the child. Open adoption procedures in which the birth parent has some voice in the selection of the adoptive family or even hands over the child to the new family are powerful entitlement experiences. In more traditional or confidential adoptions, the worker can convey that the agency is entitling the prospective family. Workers reinforce the sense of entitlement by sanctioning the parental role of the potential adopters at every opportunity and by supporting the adoptive parents in making parental decisions before they have completed the initial phase of the process or have been licensed. They use "entitling language" early in the process, referring to the child as "your child" and to the adoption as a *fait accompli*. For example:

> Mr. and Mrs. Wilkins approached the agency feeling tentative about adoption. They had successfully raised a family of five boys, four of whom were living out of the home, and now they

wanted to explore the idea of adopting a "second family." Three of
their sons were married and two had young children. Those sons
both lived out of the area, however, so the Wilkinses had no
frequent contact with their grandchildren. Mr. Wilkins was in his
late 60s and was a retired postal worker. He had an ulcer and took
nitroglycerine for a heart irregularity. Mrs. Wilkins was 12 years
younger than her husband and in good health. The Wilkinses
indicated that they had questions about being accepted as adoptive
parents because of their age and Mr. Wilkins's health problems.
They were clear, however, about their interest and about their
capacity to parent. They were proud of their sons and felt that
their parenting experience equipped them to take on the challenge
of a "boy or two who had not had it easy in their early years and
really needed a good home." Mr. and Mrs. Wilkins were engaged
in family interviews, and their 24-year-old son, Allen, who was
still living at home, joined them at their request. As the three of
them talked about their family—both how it had functioned for
the children while they were growing up, and what its current
structure was—critical issues were discussed as they related to the
possible adoption. Among those issues were Mr. Wilkins's age and
health; Allen's plans for independence; the relationship of the
other sons to their parents now, and their investment in the
adoption plan; the way the Wilkinses currently spent their time,
and the changes that becoming parents again would mean; and the
expectations that Mr. and Mrs. Wilkins had, both for themselves
as parents and for any child they might adopt.

As the exploration continued, the worker began to focus on
how the Wilkinses thought they would be able to use the parenting
skills they had developed with their sons to parent a special needs
adopted child now, and in what ways they thought the new
experience might be different. As Mr. and Mrs. Wilkins began to
realize the complications of adoption, they began to question the
validity of their earlier parenting experience. Allen was helpful in
reinforcing their capacity and in specifically suggesting adapta-
tions of their techniques that might be necessary to cope with the
child they would get in adoption. As soon as Allen began to talk
about "the child you will get in adoption," Mr. and Mrs. Wilkins
relaxed and began to join in a real exploration of how they could
apply their knowledge and skills to the new parenting situation.
Allen validated their capacity and sanctioned their request. Immediately, the worker began using the term "when your new child
comes to you" rather than "if you were to adopt a child," to support
the entitlement process further.

Claiming

A second common adoption issue, "claiming," is the mutual process
by which an adoptive family and an adopted child come to feel that

they *belong* to each other. The process usually begins when the adopted parents find similarities between the child's appearance or behavior and their own or those of members of their families. Although there is always the danger that such physical claiming can be used by the adoptive parents to deny the differences of adoption, it is a positive first step, since it clearly conveys the message that this child belongs. During the first phase of the process, other ways of claiming should be explored. The claiming process with an infant is unilateral, since the infant cannot take conscious actions to claim the adoptive family. There are a number of ways in which the adoptive parents can stake their claim. If the infant is unnamed, they may consider giving the child a name that ties him or her to the family; if the child already has a name, they may choose to use a nickname or add an additional middle name with the same purpose in mind. Not only the adoptive parents, but the members of the child's new extended family, should claim the child. Photographs are helpful here. Pictures both of the child and of the new family unit can be sent to relatives; at every opportunity, pictures of the child with various members of the adopted parents' extended families should be taken.

With an older child the claiming process can include all of these techniques, but since the child must also claim the family, the options are expanded. The task is to draw the new child, with all that the child "owns" from earlier times, into the boundaries of the new family. Probably the most useful tool in this process is a "life book." A life book is a scrapbook that a child in placement is encouraged to keep. the child pastes photos, cutout pictures, drawings, or comments about his or her past life into such a book. For a child whose life has been disrupted, the book serves to provide a thread of continuity and provides a way for him or her to access some of the feelings about past experiences. It also is a way to bring the child's past into the new family, so that this family can lay claim to the parts of the child's life that the family and child have not spent together.

A "life book" prepared by the prospective adoptive family is also a useful device in family assessment and preparation. Like the genogram or eco-map, such a book serves as a way of helping a family focus on aspects of its own history and family dynamics that may be important to consider in terms of adoption. A life book also serves as a way of helping the family to begin to identify with some of the problems that children coming into adoption may have in terms of gaps in their family histories. If an agency allows birth parents a voice in the selection of families for the children they are relinquishing, the members of a prospective adoptive family can share their life book as one way to allow the birth parents access to more information about them. If a family is considering adopting an older child, the exchange of life books between family and child is a good first step in helping both begin to get acquainted with the other.

> Six-year-old Julie's life book was used to help in the claiming process. She had joined her new adoptive family in mid-November, following a history of early abuse by her birth parents that had brought her into foster care at age 4. She had two subsequent foster home experiences. Her adoptive mother, Mrs. Brown, would frequently have Julie sit in her lap; together they would look through Julie's life book, and Mrs. Brown would ask about the things and people in the pictures. Early in December, Mrs. Brown noted a picture of a Christmas tree, and asked Julie whether she remembered when and where that was taken. Julie talked freely about her last Christmas and the foster family with whom she was then living. Mrs. Brown commented that it appeared from the picture that the tree was set up in front of a window so that people on the outside could see it. Julie said that it was. Mrs. Brown said that they usually put their tree in the corner, but it would be possible for it to go in front of their window that looked out on the street. She wisely did not ask Julie where the tree should go, which would have forced Julie to choose between her two most recent families. Instead she wondered whether Julie remembered about any other Christmas trees in other families in which she had lived. Julie remembered none. Mrs. Brown then reflected that the Christmas tree would look good in either place in this room, and that she would talk with Mr. Brown about where they might put it. They solved the dilemma, integrated Julie's past, and laid a firm claim to the child's present and future by having two Christmas trees — one in the corner and one in the window. The following year the family made a decision to have only one tree, and Julie suggested that it go in the corner.

Unmatched Expectations

"Unmatched expectations," another adoption-related issue, refers to the fact that families and children beyond infancy enter into adoption with excitement and with high expectations. Unfortunately, the expectations of both parties are often unrealistic and have very little in common. With infants, of course, the issue is one of the parents' unfulfilled initial parenting expectations. In such a situation, the worker's role is to help the family articulate its positive expectations and begin to temper them in terms of the reality, and to provide access to support (by a visit or a phone call) during the first 24 hours of the placement.

When children being adopted are old enough to participate in the process, insensitivity to the issue of expectations is something that gets many adoptions off to a bad start. In such a case, both the adoptive parents and the older child are ambivalent about the adoption. Although both may wish for it, both have reservations. The parents are wondering whether they have done the right thing and are mindful of the enormous changes in their lives that the adoption will bring about. The child is pleased to have a permanent family in which to grow up, but is very aware that the adoption closes off forever the possibility of returning to grow up with his or her birth parents. Both sides feel that the adoption will work out "if only . . .", all too often, however, these qualifications are not shared, and both parties are disappointed or frustrated early in their new family relationship.

There is a lot of work involved in becoming an adoptive family, and it is essential that all the family members experience some early satisfactions in their relationships, so they have something upon which to build and can put their fantasies aside. Those early satisfactions should be structured into the placement, which means that discussion and planning are a part of the work in the first phase. Family members can be asked to list some specifics that would make the first day with the new child seem great for them — a pleasant dinner; playing with the neighbor children; bedtime without tears and with a request for a story; being called "Mom" or "Dad"; questions about the school or neighborhood; or the like. The importance and reality of these expectations should be discussed in the family interviews before the placement. Shortly before moving into a new placement, the child can also be asked to list what would make the first day great for him or her. Such a list can help identify common ground with the adoptive family if theres is some, and can also serve to help defuse the child's unrealistic expectations and provide suggestions to the adoptive family for getting things off to a good start. For instance, an adoptive mother may say that it would be great to fix her favorite meal and to have the child enjoy it as much as the other family members always have. That does not sound too unrealistic — unless the meal is one that the child has never eaten before or the child's characteristic response to stress is nausea. Or a child may want more than anything else to have a room of his or her own and to have a little privacy to sort out the events of the day, but the new family may be planning a get-together so that all of the local members of the extended family can welcome the new member.

Another simple technique is to have both the adopted family and the child make a list of some of their favorite things (recreational activity, TV program, time of day, smell, etc.). When there is agreement, a sharing of the favorite activity or stimulus can be built into the first day. If there is no common ground, the negotiating process of trying to decide on something that the family can share that will provide pleasure for all serves as a way to reduce the chance of both sides' missing each other.

Shifts in Family Systems

The addition or subtraction of a member is a critical change point in the life of any family that always requires an adjustment in the family system (Watzlawick, Beavin, & Jackson, 1967). Such shifts in family systems are not limited to adoptive families, but when a member is added through adoption, a number of unique factors are likely to create anxiety. An adoptive family is more vulnerable to these shifts, because the tie between the adopted child and the family is more tentative. The nature of the prior experiences will shape the process of negotiation between parents and child for the place and role of the child in the family. An adopted infant has a very special status. This child usually represents something in terms of the infertility of the parents, and is the "prize" at the end of what may have been a long and arduous journey. Agencies used to play right into the fantasy expectation that the parents may have had for such a child by talking of the "chosen child." Even though this terminology is no longer encouraged, both the child and the new family may sense the special role the child has been given.

An older child coming into an adoptive family brings into the new family systems roles that have been assigned and practiced in other families. This presents several potential problems: This role may already belong to another member of the new family system; it may be a role that is not syntonic in the family system of the new family; or it may be a role the child has practiced in a prior dysfunctional family as a means of protection or control—one that is inappropriate in a functional family system. If the adoptive family members are aware of their own dynamics as a system and of the role(s) that the child has played in earlier families, the integration of the child into the new family will be much easier, of course.

A fairly common example of this is the preteen girl who has suffered sexual abuse in a past placement and joins a new family. Within the prior family system, parental attention, pleasurable intimacy, and perhaps survival have depended upon her sexualized relationship with the adult male in the household. She will practice what she has learned, and can be expected to sexualize her responses to her new father and to act in inappropriate ways. A family that is not anticipating this and is not prepared to help this child find a new role within its system will focus on correcting her "seductive" behavior in ways that place an unrealistic burden on her, and this pattern of interaction may soon lead to her rejection as a child who cannot fit into the family.

To return to its prior equilibrium, any system tends to cast off what it perceives as foreign. Changes in the family system that are demanded by the incorporation of a new child may cause existing members to ally themselves against the new child, and (consciously or unconsciously) to conspire to reject that child. When the new member is a birth child, the strength of the birth bond and the sanctions of society usually work to hold the child within the system until the system can make the necessary adjustments. The adopted child is viewed, correctly, as more "foreign" than a child born into the system, and is therefore initially more vulnerable to being rejected.

Separation, Loss, and Grief

No issue is more universal to all families, nor more important to adoptive families, than that of loss. "Loss" is the affectual state one experiences when something of significance is withdrawn. The participants in adoption are immersed in loss issues. The infertile adoptive parents have lost their fantasy of a biological child, and may have lost a specific child (or potential child), through death or miscarriage. They have in addition lost the image of themselves as adults with healthy reproductive systems; status among their peers; a sense of adequacy in following through on their life plans; roles or status within their families of origins; and a sense of control over the events of their lives.

The birth parents have lost a child born to them; self-esteem through their sense of failure as parents; and a measure of control over their own lives and futures. The child has lost birth parents — a source of fundamental grief, no matter what the circumstances or the degree of awareness of the impact of that loss. For the older child this is an immediate issue; for the infant it will become so with the awareness of the adoption. Whatever the time of awareness, the level of comfort within the adoptive family, or the facts and explanation of the adoption, adopted children struggle with why their birth parents gave them up. Since all the members of the adoption triangle have experienced loss as a prior condition to participating in the adoption, loss serves as the foundation of adoption.

Separation and loss are universal human experiences. As children grow up, they learn ways of handling their feelings about being temporarily separated from important others, as well as their feelings about permanently losing such others. Losses are always painful. People get through the pain of a loss by enduring it through the process called "grief." This process has been conceptualized in various ways, which are usually based on a model developed by Kübler-Ross (1969) for loss through death. Bourguignon and Watson (1987) suggest a five-step model: denial, guilt, anger, sadness, and acceptance. The process takes time, is seldom orderly, and is difficult for a person to get through alone. Even when the person has effectively mourned a loss, there is always a residue that hurts again as he or she copes with subsequent losses. Adoptive family members need to explore their own losses, the ways in which they have handled these, and the strength of their residual grief. This is important both because a loss of a child that the parents did not have by birth underlies their wish to adopt, and because by definition any child joining a family by adoption has suffered the loss of a birth family and possibly other significant families. It is important that adoptive family members not be stuck somewhere in the process of their own grief if they are to help the child who brings the pain of his or her own losses into the family. Denial is the most common place to get stuck. Because parents do not like to see children hurting, they sometimes join them at the denial stage and fail to give them the chance to learn how to cope with the pain of loss. They tell children, "Don't worry about the past," or "Everything will be all right now," rather than quietly accepting their pain—and, by sharing, easing it a little for them. It is, of course, always possible for adoptive parents to be stuck at the guilt, anger, or sadness stages. This limits them in helping their adoptive children move through their grief process.

Adoptive parents who can share with their adopted children their own sense of sadness that they were not able to be the children's birth parents help the children express their own sadness about the loss of their birth parents. This acknowledged shared loss helps form a powerful affectual tie between children and their adoptive parents.

Bonding and Attachment

Bonding and attachment are significant issues in adoption. As Watson (1989–1990) has pointed out elsewhere, they are not the same thing. "Bonding" in this context refers to the birth bond — the complex physiological and psychological tie between a mother and the child she is carrying that begins at conception, culminates at the child's birth, and exists from then on. Birth mothers and the infants to whom they have given birth have no control over whether they bond to each other or not. The bonding is a function of the relationship they have had in the uterus and of the birth experience they have shared.

"Attachment" is the psychological process that enables people to make connections and to have emotional significance for each other. Unlike birth bonding, attachment is a learned process that is very much influenced by the behavior of the people involved. Attachment is ordinarily learned through the nurturing interaction between parent and child during the first 3 years of life. If that nurturing has been inadequate, intermittent, or traumatically interrupted, a child may suffer from an attachment disorder.

By definition, then, children are "bonded" to their birth mothers and learn how to become "attached" as a result of their early childhood experiences with nurturing caretakers. Parents who adopt infants have an opportunity to help their children learn how to make attachments; parents who adopt children over the age of 3, by contrast, frequently have to help these children overcome their attachment disorders. This means teaching these older children how to become attached to others by providing them with the consistent nurturing they missed, in ways that symbolically relate to their early years but that do not infantilize the children. Over a period of time people who are attached to each other — such as parents and their adopted children, or marital partners — develop a situational bond to each other as a result of shared experiences and affection. This bond, however, will not replace the adopted child's birth bond with the birth mother. The strength of this birth bond is one of the factors that draws adopted persons into searches.

During the first phase of the adoption process, bonding and attachment should be explored cognitively in terms of the meaning of the words, and affectually in terms of the experiences of the members of the adoptive family and their reaction to the concept of the adopted child's birth bond to the other mother. All of the children placed in adoption come with a birth bond to their birth mothers. Those who are not placed in adoption shortly after birth may come with an attachment disorder as a result of inadequate or interrupted parenting during the first 3 years of life, when attachment is learned.

The members of an adopting family need to assess their own attachment capacity. If a prospective adoptive parent has an attachment disorder, this does not mean that the parents should not adopt. It probably suggests that they should not adopt an infant (how would that child learn how to become attached?) or an older child who has had poor early attachment experiences and needs to learn how to attach in the adoptive home. But there are children with attachment disorders who will not overcome them and who need to learn how to function comfortably in the world with such a liability. Well-functioning adults with attachment disorders can be good teachers. An awareness of attachment issues and careful "matching" can lead to effective placements. Needless to say, the process of assessing the attachment capacity of children awaiting adoption is critical.

Identity Formation

Identity formation is always more complicated for adopted children. "Identity" is the sense that one is a "self" with identifiable boundaries. Since one only draws boundaries around something of value, self-worth lies at the core of identity. One's identity begins with genes and family history, is nurtured during childhood in the context of a family in which one is a valued member, and is consciously shaped during adolescence. Identity formation is harder for adopted children, because they may not have complete or accurate information about their genes and birth family history; because they may not feel full membership in their adoptive family; and because as they establish their "boundaries," they must cope with the ultimate attack on self-worth—"abandonment" by their birth families.

In the discussion of the adopted child's identity during the early phases of the adoption process, the agency will have an opportunity to identify and enlarge the prospective adoptive family's sense of its own identity. What does becoming an adoptive family do to that identity? Will the prospective parents ever identify themselves as "adoptive parents"? When? How will they help their adopted child learn the facts about the birth family? And how will they help incorporate the pieces of that child's identity that were in place before the child joined their family?

Much of the work on a child's identity will have to take place after the adoption has been consummated. Indeed, all seven of the issues discussed will continue to need attention as the adoptive family moves through its own life stages. Not all the problems in an adoptive family can be attributed to the adoption. The success of therapeutic intervention with an adoptive family seeking help after an adoption often depends upon the clinician's ability to be sensitive to the differences that adoption makes, without losing sight of normal developmental problems or the current life stage and dynamics of a particular family.

Assessment after Adoption Has Taken Place

In assessing an adoptive family that is seeking treatment at some point after the adoption has been consummated, the therapist should review the adoption experience, with an ear tuned particularly to unfinished business from the earlier phases of the process. The questions that were asked in the initial assessment should be asked again: "Why did you decide to adopt? What was the process of deciding to adopt? Who led the way? How did adoption change your marriage and family? What has been the nature of your involvement with the birth parents of your child?"

Exploring earlier experiences of the children are equally important, not only in terms of the personality or unmet developmental needs they bring with them, but also in terms of their family systems experience and the roles they may have already learned to play. Birth information, health history, nature and number of prior caretakers, and specific trauma suffered are all of great significance. The child's view of self at the point of adoption is also critical. How the child interprets what that child has experienced influences the child's behavior. If children view themselves as people who cannot be tolerated by caretakers or as the cause of the misfortune in their own lives, they may externalize their concerns and become screaming infants or acting out children, or, as is more often the case with children placed in adoption very young, they may internalize their feeling and become passive, withdrawn, and depressed.

Critical to the assessment of a family at this point is learning how the family members have handled the differences that adoption has made to them. What rules have been put in place around the adoption? If we accept Kirk's (1984) formulation that the acceptance or denial of the differences of adoption is a critical factor in adoptive family systems, there is a wide range of possible family rules. At the positive end of the range is the family rule that adoption is different but good; and that it can be openly discussed by all as needed. Most families, however, have more complex rules that specifically define when and with whom questions about adoption can be discussed. Often the rules concerning discussion of adoption will parallel other operating rules in the family about what is permissible behavior and content with whom. For example, the mother may be so fragile that no one in the family is supposed to say anything that might upset her. If the mother looks even a little dismayed when the subject of adoption is mentioned, very soon it will not be mentioned in her presence.

Another example of how open discussion of adoption within a family is limited by the functioning of the family system can be seen in the type of "two-child family" that is frequently seen by family therapists. In this type of family, one child is the "good child," and the other is the "bad child" with the problems. The child cast in the role of the "bad child" seems to break the operating rules of the family but in fact is successfully drawing the anxiety onto himself or herself. The "good child," too, carries a burden, but one that is less obvious. This child must continually please and conform to the family rules in order to maintain the role, thus giving up a great amount of autonomy and individuality. If the children are adopted, a role division in regard to adoption also can be expected. The "bad child" will bring up all sorts of questions and concerns about adoption, which the parents will find objectionable, like much of the child's other behavior. The "good child" will maintain a pleasing role by denying any curiosity or discomfort about adoption.

At the other end of the range of possible family rules about the differences adoption makes are two negative outcomes. One is based on the excessive denial of differences, and the other on the excessive emphasis on acceptance of them. An extreme form of denial is apparent in the statement that adoptive parents sometimes make: "I love this child just the same as one I might have given birth to." Such a statement reflects rigid regulation of the family system and promises trouble if ever the beloved child wishes to raise questions about the adoption. Another kind of denial is the open family secret, in which everyone knows about the adoption, but it is not to be talked about. Therapists are familiar with the harm that open secrets can do. They tend to foster harmful fantasies that do not get corrected, and they can lead to problems based on false assumptions.

Too much emphasis on the differences can be troublesome, too. (Brodzinsky, 1990a, p. 20, calls this the "insistence of differences.") When the differences adoption makes and information about birth parents are discussed openly and frequently, it may establish for the adopted child a sense of occupying an alien position within the family. This can also happen when the family makes too much of the child's adoption outside the family. The family that needs to introduce their child as "our adopted child," or that responds too quickly to community questions about a child's adoption, courts trouble.

> One mother who had adopted a child whose appearance was quite different from hers or her husband's felt, correctly, that it could be harmful to discuss the child's adoption with casual acquaintances. Whenever someone commented that the child didn't really look like either parent, her standard reply was "No, he doesn't, does he?"

In summary, when adoption is a condition of a family's life, the following questions should be added to the standard assessment that the family therapist makes: How did the therapist learn of the adoption (as part of the initial presentation, later, by questioning, through behavioral manifestations or problem elaboration, etc.)? How are the presenting problems and the adoption related? What are the family rules concerning the adoption, and how do they match other operating rules of the family? And what is the interaction among the family system dynamics of a particular family, its life stages, and adoption? The following case illustrates this last area of assessment.

> Mr. and Mrs. Lawton, in their early 50s, applied for family treatment because of concern for their youngest child, Mary, who had just begun high school. Mary was a very attractive girl who was receiving a great deal of attention from boys, including some who were much older. She was enjoying this attention. She had not come right home after school several times, had secretly slipped out in the early evenings to meet boys, and on one occasion had gone for a long ride with a boy after dark.
> Mr. and Mrs. Lawton had four children. Their 28-year-old daughter and 26-year-old son, both birth children, were successfully independent and living outside the home. When this son entered high school, Mrs. Lawton felt at loose ends and began to care for foster children. In the next several years several children moved through foster care in the Lawton home, and they adopted two of them. At the time of the treatment, Ted was 15 and Mary 14.
> Mr. and Mrs. Lawton, Ted, and Mary came willingly to the first session. All were able to discuss their views of Mary's behavior and to discuss their reactions to it and to the fact that they were a family by adoption. Ted had begun at the same high school the year before; he minimized the difficulties that Mary was having, and said that everything would work out fine. Mary and her father tended to agree with Ted, leaving only the mother

to verbalize strong concerns. Nevertheless, some very practical agreements were worked out in regard to curfews and their violation. All four left pleased about this beginning.

By the next session Mr. and Mrs. Lawton had not only implemented the agreements of the prior week, but had also worked out some additional plans that seemed to be helping the situation. In this meeting , the mother made a number of references to the need for the father to be more involved in discipline. Because of the strength of these remarks, the parents were invited to the third session by themselves.

In this meeting, Mrs. Lawton eagerly presented a list of examples in which Mr. Lawton had either not supported her or had outright ignored her wishes. Mr. Lawton was not unaware of her concerns, but said that although he tried he could not please her, and dismissed the situation as his wife's problem. Both maintained a pleasant manner with each other, but seemed distant and angry. The mother added that she and Mary had always been very close, but now she was afraid that she might lose Mary. She might run away with a boy, become pregnant, or otherwise alienate herself. Although there was some concern that Mary's identification with her birth mother might be triggering her behavior, this did not seem to be the source of the parental anxiety.

Assessment of this family indicated that life stage issues were the most significant in producing the presenting problem. The marital relationship always had a pattern wherein the wife voiced wishes and concerns while the husband tended to soothe and minimize. When there were children to raise, the pattern posed no serious problem in the family. The decision to take foster children and Mary's adoption had probably served to keep the pattern operating. Now developmental changes were influencing and exaggerating the marital pattern of interaction. Mary's budding sexuality and independence resulted in her mother's feeling more alone and aware of the distance from her husband. The mother's sense of the loss of Mary caused her to want more from her husband. He was feeling increasingly helpless about pleasing her. Both of them were aware of the growing gulf of anger between them. Although Mary's adoption was certainly a critical factor in the dynamics of the family, the current crisis was related more to the developmental issues of Mary and the life stage of her parents.

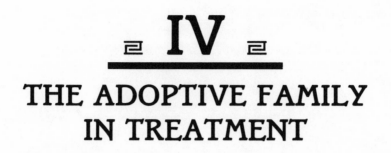

IV

THE ADOPTIVE FAMILY IN TREATMENT

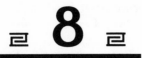

8

Therapy for Adoptive Families with Young Children

Adoptive families come for help with any of the issues that bring any other family. At intake, an adoptive family may be indistinguishable from any other, with a presenting problem grounded in anxiety resulting from a traumatic event, family dynamics, and/or life stage transitions. A therapist makes an assessment as usual and proceeds with whatever method of family therapy that is appropriate, *but with a difference*: The therapist remains alert to any features of adoption, loss, separation, or attachment that may exaggerate the situation. With this under-standing, the therapist looks for opportunities to open these issues and to make the connection between adoption and the problems experienced by the family. Once the connections are opened, they can be normalized and accepted.

But for many adoptive families who come for help, adoption *is* the central issue. In cases where the issues relate to placement, attachment, or family reorganization around an infant or older child, the fact of adoption may be the most important. In other families, adoption has become the central issue because of the family's attribution of problems to the adoption. When adoption is a major part of a family's concern, some special strategies apply. Whatever the level of functioning of the family, these strategies are best used after the original presenting problem has improved. In addition, family members should be able to talk back and forth about each person's feelings and should be open to healing. The timing may be right for more functional families after a few weeks; for more dysfunctional families, several months may be needed (see also, Kral & Schaffer, 1988; LePere, 1988; Linsay & Montserrat,

1989; Melina, 1986; Schaffer & Kral, 1988; Schaffer & Lindstrom, 1989; Talen & Lehr, 1984; Tansey, 1988).

Interventions Focused on the Fact of Adoption

The most obvious adoption-focused intervention is to open for discussion the meanings of adoption for each family member. In this process, it is reassuring to parents to teach what is normal behavior for a child's age; then, ways in which adoption issues fit in differently at each stage can be elaborated. The questions most frequently raised by adoptive parents are when and how to discuss adoption with a child. Working from the premise that adoption is a *process*, not a single event, a therapist helps parents to tailor responses to the age and interests of the child. Parents are shown how to find out just what the child is asking, especially the emotions underlying the words; then they are helped to address specifically what is at issue for the child, but not more than the child has asked. It is especially important for a therapist to prepare parents to recycle the discussion at each subsequent stage of development. The need to recycle this discussion can be connected to the handling of other ultimate issues with a child, such as independence–dependence, sexuality, and death.

Children tend to ask these sensitive questions at the most inopportune times, such as when a bag full of groceries has just burst. Therapists can support parents in making judgments about when to put off questions while making sure to return to them at another time. If a child never questions adoption, parents can be encouraged to make openings through casual remarks that tell the child that the topic is permissible. The therapist reinforces the process not only through direct education, but also by modeling the manner of talking to parents and children in session.

Another way in which a therapist can help a family with issues specific to adoption is to legitimize the process of "claiming." "Claiming," as described in Chapter 7, is the normal process by which all children and parents identify with each other and thus reinforce their attachment. A special stage in claiming occurs when the child discovers gender and connects himself or herself with the parent of the same gender. Usually there is a spontaneous, continuous process of claiming, with episodes occurring at any time, begun by child or parent, and involving any members of the family. Claiming usually occurs in connection with very ordinary subjects, such as who has blue eyes, has curly hair, likes the color red, hates broccoli, or can tell jokes.

Adoptive parents sometimes express concern that a child who is as fully aware of adoption as his or her age permits may claim physical similarities to parents, as well as social ones. This concern can take an extreme form: The parents may label the behavior as "pretending" or "lying." They may ask whether to correct such ideas immediately for the sake of "truth," or at least openness, about adoption. A therapist can help parents distinguish the facts and emotions of adoption from normal claiming, which aids attachment. If adoption is always mentioned whenever a child makes a claim of attachment, this can have the negative effect of reinforcing the idea that there is something different and wrong about adoption. A therapist can aid attachment by encouraging parents to enjoy moments of claiming, while leaving the harder issues of adoption for another time. Such a moment occurred when a small girl (adopted) announced that she could draw well just like her big brother (adopted), and that they both took after their daddy, who showed them!

A positive conclusion of therapy for adoptive families is a ceremony embodying the circumstances that have brought them into treatment, as well as the changes made. Whatever the form of the ceremony, its purpose is to recognize the circumstances and issues of family membership. The process of family building and the emotions associated with each addition are reviewed; the ceremony concludes with affirmation of family attachments.

Ann Hartman (1984) describes the use of the family membership story. She has the members of a family tell in detail the story of their coming together, beginning with the parents' meeting and courtship. They go on, describing their decision to marry, have children, and to adopt. As the chronology proceeds to the addition of children, each child's story is told. Whatever is known about the birth of that child and his or her life prior to this family is repeated, and the arrival in the home is described. Each person who was in the home prior to the child tells the details of first contacts, impressions, and emotions. The family story is unfolded right up to the need for therapy and through the changes that have occurred. Finally, a symbolic ritual may be created to epitomize the whole process. The ritual may become a regular part of family life, as well as the closing of family therapy.

> In tracing their whole story, the members of one family realized that they were special because each of them had been born in a different country: the parents in Germany and Canada, respectively; the daughter in Mexico; and the son, in the United States. They already knew that chocolate cake with chocolate frosting was everyone's favorite dessert. Their closing ceremony, symbolizing family unity, was the production of a chocolate cake. The cake was baked by the mother, iced by the children, and decorated by

the father into equal sectors marked by small national flags of their countries of origin. The family enthusiastically voted to repeat this ceremony on certain designated family days.

A related intervention is a "time-line genogram." Essentially, this is telling the story of family building on paper, often large sheets. Each parent's family of origin is diagrammed, with descriptions and stories of all the persons. What is known about each adopted child's family of origin is also diagrammed. When all sheets are brought together, the representations of the current family are put in the central position, with a strong boundary line drawn around them. All the families of origin are also shown, in connection, but outside the boundary. This kind of genogram, which the family can take home, may become the symbol of family unity.

Some families may create a family motto and/or family crest that captures the renewed sense of family. Other families may choose ceremonial days, to be observed as a means to honor family inclusion. For some families, this means deciding on appropriate celebrations for birthdays and/or days of joining the family.

Another means of affirming life histories is to review together any existing "life books." "Life books," as described in Chapter 7, are often provided for children who have been in foster care prior to adoption; they may include statistics of birth and development, as well as photographs of birth parents and any subsequent caretakers. An adoptive family also already may have "life books," in the form of photograph albums or scrapbooks. Then, all together, the members of an adoptive family can create a life book that honors their joining as a family. Items from their first days, such as photographs, announcements, and cards of congratulations, can be included and then updated regularly. Photographs and letters from prior families may be included.

A child who wishes to make a life book but has no documentation of prior life experience can be helped to supply the story. For any details that are known, such as city or hospital of birth, pictures can be obtained. When there is little information, children may wish to create their own. Children may draw, photograph, or select pictures that represent whatever facts are accessible.

One 10-year-old girl knew only that she had been left in a particular church shortly after birth. Her parents helped her to obtain photos of the church and its surroundings. She used these, along with pictures cut from magazines, to create her story, including how her birth parents looked and what had happened to them. Whether or not her fantasies came anywhere near the facts seemed unimportant. What was important was that she found a way to address her concerns within the supportive relationships of her adoptive family. Thereby, her identity within both of her families was anchored.

Sometimes a child wants to do or redo a life book in a new way.

For example, one day an 11-year-old boy took all the photos out of his life book and rearranged them in nonchronological groupings, interspersed with his own drawings. His explanation indicated that the new order had much meaning to him, even though the significance was not apparent to others.

Other kinds of rituals may be used in the treatment of adoptive families. Evan Imber-Black (Imber-Black, Roberts, & Whiting, 1988) gives five themes for use of rituals in family therapy: membership, healing, identity, belief expression and negotiation, and celebration. Specific needs of a particular adoptive family in any of those areas may require the design of a ritual tailored to the situation. A therapist draws on understanding of the family's dynamics to suggest a meaningful ritual. If the family agrees to cooperate, engaging all members in the creative process ensures a potent outcome. Sometimes families spontaneously create their own rituals of membership and healing.

An example comes from a family of three daughters aged 10, 11, and 12, where the middle girl was adopted. As the oldest approached puberty, questions of female anatomy, sex, birth, and adoption were rampant in the family. The 11-year-old was quite distressed that she too had not grown inside the mother and openly wished that she had.

The girl herself devised a ritual, which was carried out with the full cooperation of the whole family. First, the mother was placed on the floor, fully covered with a blanket. The adopted daughter joined the mother under the blanket and then emerged from the foot end, to be received with rejoicing by the rest of the family and placed in the mother's arms.

Interventions for Difficulties with a First Child

Beyond the generic approach to treatment of adoptive families, specific constellations of dynamics related to adoption are frequently presented to clinicians. The first of these has to do with life stage difficulty in adding a first child. Even when the child is a much-wanted and eagerly awaited infant, whether by birth or adoption, the spouses must reorganize their lives to make room. Whatever the prior form of the marital relationship, the new role as parents can put much strain on a marriage. An infant coming to a couple responds to the partners' expectations and anxieties as expressed in the quality of care offered. The infant's reactions, in turn, affect parental expectations and future actions. Thus, even newborns actively negotiate with their caretakers and help to shape the relationship between them.

Most parents acknowledge that their inexperience adds to anxiety in the care of a first infant. For adoptive parents, this anxiety adds to whatever emotional loading they have already undergone to become parents. Some say that the adoption process makes them feel under such general scrutiny that they must be perfect to prove their worthiness to become parents. Any first-time parents may experience difficulties in regard to attachment, and more such parents are seeking help from clinicians. Unfortunately, it may be harder for adoptive parents to seek help, out of fear that they will be criticized as unworthy parents.

When adoptive parents do seek help with nurturing their first infant, the therapist first listens to what factors are presented as contributing to the difficulty. Do they focus on not knowing what to do (inexperience)? Do they focus on the baby and how he or she does or does not respond (worries about adoption)? Do they talk about how this experience is not turning out at all as expected (role strain)? Does one spouse focus on how the other does or does not take care of the baby (marital adjustment)? As soon as possible, the therapist gives a concrete, educative suggestion directed to relief of the most pressing concern. This not only serves to reduce anxiety, but also acts as an intervention addressed to the simplest level. The result of the first intervention provides good assessment information about the nature of the problem and the couple's dynamics.

When the problem is that new parents are having difficulty integrating an infant into their lives, intervention at the educative and behavioral levels may be enough. If deeper marital or individual issues underlie conflicts related to being parents, behavioral interventions probably will not work; even if they do, the conflict will move to some other issue, perhaps child care. When there are deeper sources of distress, all the experiences surrounding the adoption are explored. The therapist begins with the circumstances

daughters. Coming home from school in midafternoon, these girls continually vied to hold the baby, well into the evening. Donald was apparently screaming for the level of comfort to which he had become accustomed!

With this information, both Margaret and Jonathan radically readjusted their attitudes. They cooperated on a new schedule of care, whereby each held Donald for shorter periods earlier in the day. When Jonathan left for work, Margaret held Donald for long periods, which were gradually shortened.

Most families whose alliances polarize severely are not so fortunate as to have an early intervention; instead, the alliances become entrenched and continue in the same form indefinitely. Many times such families come to a therapist much later, after the child is attending school and the problem has become more public.

Interventions for Families with Overweight Children

The problem of an overweight child may be presented for treatment at any time, during the child's infancy or later. Parents may come because of their own concern, because of a medical recommendation, or because of a school referral. Since food is not merely a physical necessity, but also is symbolic of and is associated with nurturing relationships, it may take on prime meaning in an adoptive family.

Overfeeding an infant may be a means for inexperienced parents to prove themselves capable, to solve anxieties about attachment, or to reinforce an alliance with the child. Although an infant can indicate grief through food refusal, a baby can also demand large quantities of food in order to compensate for loss and to feel securely filled, even stuffed. When such an infant is permitted unrestricted quantities of food, particularly sweets, the stage may be set for an overweight child.

Even when the pattern is not set immediately after placement, several types of family dynamics can induce a child's weight gain at any point. Harkaway (1987) has identified five types of families who come for therapy about an overweight child. Although she does not refer to adoptive families per se, several of the dynamic pictures are relevant.

In one kind of situation, the parents are united in concern about the child's weight and seek treatment voluntarily. Their concern may focus on the adoptive parent's dilemma: How much of the child's weight problem is due to genes and how much to food management in the family? Often, the more anxious the parents are, the more likely they are to attribute the problem to genes. A therapist must point out that regardless of a possible genetic contribution, appropriate food management is necessary. Suggestions are made about alternative means of managing food and fostering attachment. Then the therapist addresses worries about being good parents to a child who does not share their genes. Parents may be encouraged to seek medical consultation or further information about the child's genetic legacies.

The situation is more serious when parents with a mutual concern for an overweight child have formed a "united front." This dynamic avoids conflict in the relationship and/or about the issues of infertility and adoption. Thus, the mutual investment in the child's intake of "our nurture" becomes the focal third point needed to maintain the united front.

Another type of dynamic involving an overweight child occurs when parents are not united but are in conflict, possibly polarized. Here the best prognosis is for a situation in which the child's weight gain has been recent and sudden. The prognosis is still better when parents themselves have recognized the problem, even though they may be sharply divided about its cause and management. The usual dynamic underlying such conflict between adoptive parents is that at least one has experienced a difficult loss. Increased anger between spouses serves as a substitute for or as a distraction from the new grief. If the stricken parent has a tendency to self-soothe through ingesting food or other substances, this is likely to become part of the escalated marital conflict. An adopted child, then, out of an alliance with one parent or to distract from the conflict, is in a position to take on the symptom-bearing role through overeating and weight gain. Then the quarrel can be continued over the child, thus distancing the issues from the marriage. At the same time, the family is kept intensely connected during a time of new loss.

Less promising for treatment is the case in which parents have been in conflict about an overweight child for a long time, perhaps from the time of adoption. These differences may reflect major differences in the parents' motivation to adopt, along with other dissatisfactions in the marriage. After the infant arrives, the more motivated parent may reinforce an alliance through feeding the child, perhaps exclusively. Thus the other parent is distanced and has fresh fuel for the conflict. These dynamics can be exaggerated if weight has already been a source of conflict, such as when a lean spouse attacks an overweight spouse about appearance and lack of sexual attractiveness. If the overweight parent was the one who promoted the adoption, the child has probably been drawn into an alliance with the overweight parent through eating, and thus has gained a symptom-bearing role. Then the overweight child and parent are allied in "proving" to the lean parent how intractable the problem is.

Beyond early issues of attachment and nurture, each pattern involving an overweight child can emerge at any later developmental stage. This most easily happens when the child's development reaches the issues of the psychological theme of the marriage. A common example occurs when a 2-year-old's demands for autonomy in regard to food connect with parental issues in regard to behavior control. A similar situation applies when a child becomes more emotionally expressive with parents who have problems with expressivity. (Certainly adoptive parents have reasons to be familiar with grief and depression.) Such parents may provide the child with food instead of modeling appropriate expression of emotions, and food may thus become the child's habitual consolation when hurt or sad, or a reward for getting over temper tantrums.

In a final type of situation, the problem of an overweight child is little amenable to change, regardless of age or stage at the time of referral for therapy. In this instance, the entire family is overweight and weight is not considered a problem. In a family where being overweight is a sign of being loved and part of the family, an adopted child is soon inducted into family membership through overeating. The only recourse a therapist may have is to appeal to the family members' value about nurturing, while raising anxiety that their main means of nurture may harm the child. McVoy (1987), observes, "When a parent brings a child for treatment of obesity, for example, usually the greater the disparity between degree of obesity and degree of parental concern, the greater the likelihood that the 'obesity' is a symptom of other family stresses" (p. 74). He also states that the greater the degree of overweight, the more time treatment will take, and the more difficult and more subject to sabotage it will be.

To address the problem of an overweight child, both Harkaway (1987) and McVoy (1987) emphasize family therapy along with nutritional/medical attention. Both also suggest that a careful assessment is needed of the history and function of the problem in the family. Central to the assessment of overweight in an adoptive family is the relationship of the problem to adoption.

When a child is preadolescent, the parents must be willing to change their own behavior before any weight loss program for the child is undertaken. Therefore, the initial phase of treatment should focus upon behavioral change in food and exercise management for the entire family. Early interventions include specific directions to parents. An overinvolved mother can be asked to switch her focus onto studying nutrition and to make smaller meals that are both nutritious and attractive. An underinvolved father may take charge of limiting snacks and/or going swimming with the child. Families where neither the degree of overweight nor the dynamic need for it is severe may experience sufficient weight loss as a result of these changes. Some respond well to the initial family focus, thereby indicating readiness to engage in a more definitive weight loss program for the child. Other families resist the initial family focus by protest and/or sabotage.

When an initial family focus does not alleviate the problem, the therapist continues to arrange modest behavioral change. At the same time, therapy delves into the family operating rules concerning weight and adoption. In this process, families who can tolerate change (albeit slowly), distinguish themselves from those who can not, for the latter depart.

The following example typifies an adoptive family in which the child's weight was the concern that brought them to treatment.

Maya's parents sought help for her because, at age 10, she weighed 150 pounds. Their older child (Maya's half-sister by birth), Teka, aged $11\frac{1}{2}$, was slender, as were both parents. The girls had been adopted together when Maya was 1 year of age; at that time, both parents were just over 40. Both had come to the city from farm families as young adults, and both held poorly paid office jobs. They had met and married in their middle 30s. Because of health problems that precluded pregnancy, limited finances, and severe disapproval from her own mother, the wife had been very reluctant to adopt. The husband was enthusiastic about wanting to be a father; he finally persuaded his wife that she could quit her job and that he would provide all the child care when he was home.

To this couple came Maya and Teka. Their birth mother, said to be a beautiful, slender woman, apparently had a series of live-in lovers. When Teka was born, she went to live with her maternal grandmother; however, when Maya was born $1\frac{1}{2}$ years later, the grandmother refused further responsibility. So Maya remained with her mother, being fed and cleaned erratically, nor getting medical attention for frequent colds. Finally she was removed by the court, and, without protest from the mother, her rights to both girls were terminated.

Both parents remembered fondly the early days of place-ment. The little girls happily responded to supplies of good food, clean clothes, comfortable beds, and ample toys. But the parents also remembered that right from the start, Maya always accepted all offered food and generally asked for more. Soon a pattern developed that continued to the time of therapy. The mother, whose stamina was not great, found it easier to be permissive with the children during the day. This meant that Maya's steady requests for milk and cookies were granted. When the father came home and assumed child care, his attempts to get Maya to eat a normal meal were met with lack of interest. If he denied further requests for milk or cookies, Maya howled and clung to the mother. Generally, the father gave in rather than become the "bad guy."

By the time Maya was 2, she was strikingly chubby and her weight continued, to increase. The mother's permissiveness con-tinued along with sporadic efforts by the father to institute various diet plans. The family came to therapy after a pediatrician told them that Maya's health was suffering.

The early phase of treatment revolved around making small changes in each parent's role in Maya's food intake. The mother agreed to limit after-school snacks to anything but sweets. The father would let Maya have a dessert after dinner only if she ate normal portions of the other food. Teka was to go bike-riding with Maya at least every other day. This initial plan was difficult to establish. Often the mother gave in to Maya's begging for ice cream and cookies. Later the father would criticize the mother, who cried, and gave in even sooner the next day.

Finally, the parental conflict was addressed in sessions without the girls. The origins of the conflict were traced to the decision about adoption and the hostility of the in-laws. Once the parents aired their grievances and clarified the two sides of their emotions about marriage and parenthood, they made a commit-ment to working together. Not surprisingly, when it was no longer effective to plead for sweets or stir up parental guilt over her "deprivation," Maya lost weight steadily.

Interventions for School-Related Problems

Most families who seek therapy because of concerns for a child do so after the child begins school. Whatever the family dynamics, with or without adoption, early difficulties and solutions usually are contained within the relative privacy of the home. With a child's attendance at school, the family's organization is challenged in two ways. First, change is required in the family arrangements in order to free the child to enter school and to participate in learning and in peer relationships. Second, relationships in the family are now exposed to the outside world through the child as family representative. Thus, as a child enters the outside world of school, the family is opened to outside scrutiny, and in turn to the impact of ideas from the outside.

An adoptive family's struggles with the issues of attachment and adoption are likely to be underscored with the child's entrance into school. The family rules in regard to discussing adoption are often confronted right at registration. There may be further challenges as a child deals with peers or adults at school about adoption. Whether or not a child feels free to report such school experiences at home is also determined by the family rules.

Attitudes of school personnel toward adoption may also be quite obvious to parents in conferences about a child's learning or behavior. Although judgments of blame may land on any parents for a child's problems, adoptive parents are more vulnerable as targets of school personnel as well as of their own fears. They may meekly submit or engage in continuing conflict with school authorities.

Any time school personnel refer a child and family to a therapist, the circumstances of the referral and the parents' view of it should be explored. Questions about the perspective of the school include the following: Was the referral made casually during a first phone call about problems or after many conferences with parents? Does it focus on learning difficulties, behavior, or both? Is an ultimatum involved? Is the child viewed with affection or as some sort of monster of short stature? Is adoption mentioned in the referral? Points for a therapist to notice about the parents' perspective on a school referral include the following: Do they disagree and see it as evidence of an abusive or inept school? Do they understand the reasons but minimize or resist them? Are they relieved that their distress about the child has been recognized by others? And, again is adoption mentioned?

How soon and with what connotation adoption is mentioned, either by the referring school personnel or by parents, is significant. When anyone mentions adoption early or with intensity, it is likely that it figures in the problem. In any case, the issue related to adoption may be located in the family, in the school, or in the interaction between them.

When school problems of a preadolescent child are presented, it is preferable for a therapist to see the parents alone first, without the child. This step serves to reinforce the responsibilities of the adults, to provide a forum for their views and solutions, and to involve them immediately in the change process. In the initial exploration of incidents of the problem, the therapist looks for any mention of adoption. When there is an opening, the therapist explores whether adoption is used as an explanation of the school problem. At the same time, the therapist learns how the family rule pertaining to adoption compares to the family's other operating rules.

As soon as possible, the therapist makes a hypothesis about the primary nature of the problem: an individual learning difficulty of the child; a behavioral problem serving a systemic function at home, at school, or both; an adoption-based issue; or an interactional problem between parents and school. Whatever the hypothesis, some initial plan of action should be offered in the first session. Often this plan includes getting more information, especially through contact with the school. Most important is to learn about the teachers' and others' experience with the child and parents and to gain a sense of cooperation. If there are aversive attitudes toward the child, adoption, or the parents, the therapist must be in a position to be an advocate.

The need for an accurate assessment of an adopted child's school problems is as essential as it is difficult. The complex interaction of genetics, aptitudes, family dynamics, adoption, and school dynamics poses a challenge for diagnosis. If medical or psychological testing have not already been done, they may be suggested to aid diagnosis.

Learning disabilities of all forms and degrees of severity are reported at higher rates for children who have been adopted than for others (see Deutsch et al., 1982; Dorris, 1989; Nelson, 1985). To date, there is no hard evidence for why this is, but there are some strong possibilities from both the biological and social spheres. In the biological sphere, there may be a genetic, inherited factor. Another biological component may result from the condition of the birth mother during pregnancy: Perhaps the birth mother was so young that her body was not fully ready for pregnancy, or perhaps her prenatal medical care or even nutrition was inadequate. Of increasing concern is whether a birth mother abused alcohol or drugs during her pregnancy. All the effects of varying degrees of substance abuse on a developing fetus are not known, but it has become tragically clear that substantial abuse of alcohol or drugs by a pregnant woman can have dire effects on the child. Among these, learning disabilities are a strong possibility, although sometimes they are not easily identified until a child begins school or even later.

In the social sphere, there are also several possibilities. In a moderately closed family system, the rules may not permit openness of feeling about most things, including feelings about adoption and birth parents. A child may respond to such closed regulation by suppression of interest and feeling about his or her origins. Thereby a pocket of repression is created in the personality, or any existing tendency toward a introverted and/or depressed stance is reinforced. In either case, energy is required to keep such emotional dams in place. The dams restrict the energy available to learning, and may also limit openness to inquiry in general.

Another aspect of the adoptive situation may affect school performance. Adoptive parents have no way to temper their expectations for an adopted child through comparison to their own and their families' educational history. Fears about the unknown elements of the child's genetic inheritance may combine with the extra need of adoptive parents to prove themselves. If the child has some sort of learning disability, frustration about lack of information or misdiagnosis can escalate the anxieties. This combination of factors can feed a negative spiral of reactions and pressure on the child's school performance.

After making a contract, a therapist may educate parents and school personnel about coping with learning disorders, adoption, or family situations. Also, behavioral interventions may be suggested, such as a study program and/or behavior control program based on rewards. No matter what the therapist offers the parents or the school separately, often continuing mediation between them is needed.

More functional families that are able to respond to intervention at the level of education, behavior, or advocacy show fairly prompt improvement in the presenting problem and anxiety level. This is the clue to move into the area of emotion and meaning related to school performance. The therapist addresses how the school problem fits into the family's general operating rules and alliances. If the connection to adoption is not already part of the discussion, the therapist points it out.

Negative interaction spirals centered around a child's school performance can become most severe in family systems that have the theme of competence. The vulnerabilities of the adoptive situation are likely to exacerbate parents' anxieties in regard to competent role performance. Then a child's difficulty in school is an additional assault on the parents' self-esteem and pushes the organization of the family toward a greater extreme of regulation.

In a family that exhibits more rigid organization, the child and the school performance are likely to become the focus of family anxiety. Thus the child's symptom-bearing role for the system is created, and this can become so extremely entrenched as to be unmovable. In a family that exhibits more random regulation, by contrast, the child's school problems may be ignored or avoided. In such circumstances, the child's education and position in the family may drift unattended unless school personnel demand intervention. At either extreme, the outcome for the child can become severe, leading to psychosomatic symptoms, behavior problems in school or community, depression, illiteracy, or eventually dropping out of school.

An example follows wherein a child's school performance became the means for his adoptive parents to bind grief.

A phone call from a mother began as follows: "I want you to see my adopted son, Joey, who is failing all fourth-grade subjects but math even though he is bright." She would only attend the first session with her husband if Joey came too. In the initial session, Joey's solemn expression and reluctance to speak mirrored his accountant father. The mother, in turn, was fidgety and opened the session by speed-speaking about Joey.

Joey's grades had been average until they deteriorated over the last 2 years. His teacher was concerned that Joey was very quiet, seemed lost in daydreams, and had no friends. The mother proceeded through a litany of all the school had not done, while she was doing so much. Further exploration revealed that every day after school, the mother and Joey worked at homework together until the father came home. Then while the mother prepared dinner, the father did math homework with Joey, often covertly playing number games. After dinner, the mother and Joey again sat at homework until just before Joey's bedtime.

The mother conveyed an attitude that Joey was an ungrateful, stubborn child who gave no joy. An inquiry about expectations uncovered the information that these parents had once had a child who did fulfill their lives. The story emerged that the parents married late after working together for years in routine jobs. After 6 years of marriage, they had a child by birth, named Jimmy. At age 8, Jimmy died of leukemia. Prior to his illness, Jimmy was said to have been a bright, vivacious child who was their shining light. After Jimmy died, the mother spent months in Jimmy's room weeping and refusing to leave the house.

Some months later, the pastor of their church approached them about Joey, then 17 months old. Joey's young mother had been trying to work and raise him alone, but in despair she had come to the pastor, saying she could not go on. Once the adoptive parents were persuaded, the transfer took place soon. A tearful young mother handed Joey over and ran, as a screaming Joey tried to follow.

Apparently, the adoptive mother flung herself into Joey's care. Joey responded obediently, but rarely spoke or smiled. The mother began to compare Joey unfavorably to her fond memories of Jimmy. Because of her guilt and need for distraction, the mother always resolved to try harder. Although the father was relieved that his wife was functioning again, Joey responded with passive resistance and more depression. By the time he entered school, a very rigid pattern was in place. Symbolic of the dynamics was that the mother spent the long hours with Joey at a table above which hung a large, lighted oil painting of Jimmy.

The first behavioral intervention was that the mother should relieve herself of responsibility and give it to the father, who would supervise only 2 hours of homework each evening. For every evening that family members successfully did their own tasks, each accumulated points toward a reward from a previously agreed-upon list. All parts of this plan were carefully worked out and written down on paper. Weeks went by before the plan got a fair trial; the mother often found a pretext to interfere with or change it. The father claimed to have hope in the plan, but would not stand up to the mother. The plan finally started to work, when the mother resumed some church activities given up when Jimmy died.

Shortly thereafter, Joey received a report card on which his grades had inched up to D's and two C's. His teacher noted that he had begun to smile in class. The mother, however, complained that there was no real change, that therapy was not helping, and that she was forced to take back the supervision of Joey's homework. The father and Joey looked upset, but would say nothing. The therapist tried to touch the underlying grief, but was met with indignant protests that the family had only come about Joey's school problems. The mother concluded that she needed to find a different school for Joey and left therapy.

Interventions for Problems Related to Secrecy about Adoption

Another configuration of adoptive family dynamics that frequently comes to the attention of therapists is presented as some personal problem of an adopted child. However, the fact of the adoption does not emerge until much later in the treatment, and then only incidentally. On first consideration, it could seem that the adoption is not a prominent factor in family dynamics. More likely this is a clue that the adoption is a somewhat hidden factor on the order of a secret.

Family therapists are well aware of the negative effects of secrets in families, even when these are not "secrets" in the most literal sense. Often family "secrets" center on known, painful items that are not to be talked about or are just avoided. In an adoptive family where the pain of losses and/or the difference of adoption is denied, the adoption may be protected by a rule of nondiscussion. (For the only reference found in family therapy literature to the effects of secrecy about adoption, see Boszormenyi-Nagy & Spark, 1984.)

In earlier days, denial and secrecy about the fact of adoption was often more complete. Florence Fisher (1973), in her classic autobiographical account of her search for her birth parents, tells poignantly (p. 29) about coming across her adoption papers when she was 7 years old. Finally, in the way of a child who assumes personal responsibility, she could explain to herself her mother's tension and her father's coldness. Even today, there are still stories of adults who uncover their adoption for the first time by accident.

Either kind of adoption "secret" has the effect of isolating family members. Emotions and assumed meanings about adoption and the secrecy can be neither shared nor clarified. Barriers created by an adoption secret may add to depression and sense of detachment for any family member, but the negative impact on the adopted child's identity development can be particularly severe. Betty Jean Lifton (1975) describes this process in *Twice Born: Memoirs of an Adopted Daughter*. She reports how her mother told her of the adoption when she was aged 7 and at home in bed, ill. Betty Jean was told not to tell anyone that she knew, not even her father, because he wanted her to believe that he was her birth father. Lifton goes on to describe how her internal identification was permanently changed, leading to continual fantasies about being someone different, a changeling, and somehow an unacceptable person.

When a family with a "secret" adoption comes for treatment, the degree of rigid regulation is most significant for outcome. In the course of nudging the operating rules that affect the problem presented as the adoptee's, a therapist notes nonverbal tension. By commenting on such clues, the therapist moves into emotions that are likely to open the "secret" of adoption. When secrets concerning adoption are acknowledged sooner and with less probing, this suggests more flexibility in the organization's regulation. But adoption secrets may be mentioned only long after the family knows the therapist well, and then still with resistance to discussion. Such indication of closed regulation and protection against strong underlying emotions must be approached carefully.

For families with adoption secrets, acknowledgment of the adoption is already a big step. Since the secret has some protective function, assumptions and fears about breaking the rule of silence must be aired. *Before* the actual discussion of adoption, a therapist must elicit each person's concern about what will happen if the adoption is openly talked about. Often the fear is that someone will be badly hurt. This may be dissipated promptly by other family members. In other cases, fears are confirmed but still can be modified. Most often each person's hidden worries and fears receive a mixed response. Relief, acceptance, and understanding counterbalance hurt, anger, and pain, stemming once again from the fact of a nonbiological relationship.

After fears have been dissipated, the secrets are opened. In this important process, ambivalences are clarified and relationships re-examined. The therapist continues to support the process of openness at a pace the family can tolerate, and emphasizes the acceptance and normality of all the mixed emotions. These families benefit from any measure of increased openness they can achieve.

Depending on the degree of closed regulation, a therapist may need to use varying amounts of pressure to point out two paradoxes. One is that the secret, which was meant to protect the family, instead has hurt the members' relationships by keeping so much of themselves hidden. The other is that the rule of silence has only worked *because* they *are* attached as a family. Such attachment can best be reinforced by sharing of emotions, even pain that may never entirely go away.

For a final consolidation of the therapy experience, a ritual or some other means of telling the family story is recommended. Whatever rite is selected, it should include the reasons why the adoption was "secret" and how the secret contributed to the problem. Most especially, the ritual should strongly reinforce the increased openness in a way that will help to maintain it.

Interventions for Problems Attributed to a Child's Inheritance

Yet another kind of adoptive family comes to treatment emphasizing that an *adopted* child's behavior is the problem. In these cases, both the adoption and its relationship to the problem behavior are central. Reports of episodes of the problem reinforce the implication of adoption as the cause and explanation. The underlying assumption, sometimes openly articulated, is that the behavior results from bad genetic or moral inheritance. Families in this group are dedicated to the belief that nature is absolutely stronger than nurture, even when a child joined the family shortly after birth.

The problems of these families often begin with tensions in the marriage, so that a third person is needed for the role of distracter. The greater the psychological needs of parents, the more their desperation for a child is likely to escalate. When a child arrives by either adoption or birth, the child is inducted into the vacant role (i.e., distractor and potential symptom bearer).

In such situations, parents explain the behavioral outcome in terms of some feature of the child to which special meaning has been attributed — for example, "Jimmy was colicky and *stubborn* about eating from the beginning," or "Sally cried in a *temper* the day we brought her home." An adoption provides a readily available explanation that "bad" behavior is caused by the unknown genes. When a child has racial characteristics different from those of the parents, the genetic explanation and associated fantasies are even more easily reinforced.

A family that seeks therapy because of an adopted child's "inherited" behavior may have any type of organization. One with more open regulation may respond to education regarding the troublesome behavior. Most importantly, the family members need help to distinguish between the realities and their anxieties and attributions of meaning. Finally, their anxieties based on expectation are connected to their reactions to the child's behavior, but are now differentiated as two valid emotional responses that need not merge.

One extreme family form in this group is a rigid, united-front marriage in which the adopted child is labeled as a "bad seed." In this form, the marriage is said to be fine, but actually is covered by a veneer of pleasantness in order to avoid conflict. Any child can be inducted into the needed third-person role, but when the child is adopted, the explanation becomes that of the "bad seed." The behavioral interventions with which a therapist generally begins are unlikely to be effective here. Beliefs used to explain the child's behavior may also be used to rate the situation as outside the parents' ability to change. As another way to protect their facade and underlying emotions, these parents often request treatment only for the child.

When initial behavioral interventions are met with resistance, sabotage, or complaints of being ineffective, the focus must move onto the beliefs. A therapist must often draw on maximum creativity to find a means of questioning the beliefs that the family can hear; such means may include education about child or system development, knowledge of belief systems, or use of metaphor. Most likely to be effective is an approach that connects with the parents' underlying hurt and permits them some way to feel better.

When it seems impossible to get at a belief about a "bad seed," another way is to go around it. This approach is to tell the parents that no matter what the child's inheritance may be, they must take responsibility for managing current behavior in their family. In a fairly closed arrangement, parental anxiety or guilt may need to be escalated by predicting a dire outcome if the parents do not take responsibility for making changes.

However the rigid arrangements and beliefs are addressed, the therapist watches for any signs of disagreement between the parents. Taking care not to pounce, the therapist carefully encourages any little differences of opinion. If a full-blown argument breaks out between parents who have a united front, the therapist may observe it with pleasure but *no* intervention. When the argument subsides (which usually happens quickly because of their fear of differing), the therapist must support each one for the courage to speak up. The emergence of disagreement between parents is crucial to release a child from the role of "bad seed." Thus conflicts are at first nurtured, then opened to discussion, and finally form the basis for a new cooperative plan for change. Differences in their experiences of and attitudes toward losses of the past and present, infertility, and adoption must be discussed. Finally, attention should be given to the anxieties that have led to suppression of differences.

As differences are aired, there is less need to attribute negative characteristics to the child's inheritance. Thus, in the process of changing the handling of projected emotions, the connection can be made to beliefs about the child. Sometimes a tragic piece of the child's inheritance is known and has contributed to the "bad seed" fears. Such information may have been suppressed by both parents or may have created a difference of opinion about how to handle it with the child.

The child may be excused from sessions wherein parents are working out differences, but may return at intervals for a review of the child's changing role. Whatever the prior plan, the child should be included in the final sessions. The family members need to review together what brought them to treatment and how they now understand the interaction of suppression of emotions, fears about adoption, and behavior. The parents are reinforced by the therapist in every way possible for maintaining their relationship with openness, tolerance of differences, and cooperative parenting.

Here is an example of a family with an adopted symptom bearer, in which the regulation was moderately open and amenable to change.

> Seven-year-old Jeremy was brought to therapy by his parents, who requested individual treatment for his nightly bedwetting. In an initial parent conference, the parents quickly pointed out that Jeremy was adopted at 8 months of age and always had been "uncooperative" about eating, sleeping, bathing, and diaper changing. Since they had waited a long time and were very eager for a child, they were sure that his bedwetting was just another sign of his innate obstinate personality.
>
> In discussing the problem, it was clear that the parents knew all the strategies for dealing with bedwetting, and that what to try next was a major topic of conversation. They described their relationship as pleasant and themselves as mild-mannered people. Except when discussing their frustration about the bedwetting, they referred to Jeremy in admiring tones as "strong-willed."
>
> Initially, the parents were asked to discuss their opinions of all the methods in detail. The first chink in their togetherness was a difference about whether or not Jeremy should have to launder his own sheets. From there, more differences in regard to handling Jeremy came to light. The next stage of treatment went into the meanings of the attributes of "stubborn," "strong-willed," and "mild-mannered." As a result of this discussion, the parents realized that they did not risk open argument with Jeremy or with each other. Early in their marriage, they had had "cold wars" that could last a week. Once Jeremy arrived, they consciously agreed to stop that way of fighting.
>
> The members of this family moved fairly quickly into the area of their patterns of interaction and attribution of meaning. With new understanding, they were emboldened to risk conflict with each other. By the time each parent could be openly angry with Jeremy about the problem of wet sheets, he could yell back, but the bedwetting stopped!

Interventions for Problems with Child Behavior Control

In still another common approach to therapy, adoptive parents present the picture of an adorable but uncontrollable child. In one type of presentation, parents say that they are so happy to have a child that they do not (or cannot bear to) discipline consistently. In another version, the parents say that the child is disobedient but charming and that they are often outmanuevered. In a third variation, a child is considered wonderful at home, but people outside the family complain about the child's behavior.

The dynamic underlying such presentations by adoptive parents may be one of several. The most favorable prognosis is for a marriage that has continued to function well despite the struggle to have a child. The parents' delight in having a child at last has led to indulgence and the creation of a little "prince" or "princess."

Another possible dynamic, somewhat more serious, is that a parental sense of entitlement has not occurred. A fully developed sense of entitlement allows parents to hold their ground when their authority is countered by the use of adoption as a weapon. For example, "You wouldn't be so mean to me if I wasn't adopted" can be answered with "You *will* clean up your room now; we can talk about adoption later if you want." Without a sense of entitlement, parents may provide fine physical care and much affection but do not set limits on behavior. Without consistent limits, a child feels insecure and may escalate misbehavior in attempts to invite limits. When parents do not respond as needed, behavior problems may become routine or may worsen.

A third dynamic has the worst prognosis. In this situation, discipline is an issue for the adults themselves and thus for their child or children, regardless of how they have obtained them. The family may have a theme of competence and may be too loosely organized or underorganized. The pervasive characterological and family structural problems make the treatment of this group the most difficult.

Regardless of their dynamics, families with children whose behavior is not well controlled have a common need: to put the parents in charge and to set appropriate limits for the children. The key in each such case is that the therapist models and teaches parents how to establish structure and pass it on to the child.

First, the parents identify one *small*, specific area in which change is desired and that they can control. It does not work to start with the wishful or general goals sometimes offered by parents — for example, "She should go to bed on her own when first asked" or "He should be respectful to his mother." After the parents choose the first step, the therapist helps them work out an agreement about who will do what in managing the plan. All contingencies are considered, along with the consequences for noncompliance. Such a plan is reviewed at the end of session, so that each family member

knows exactly what it is. If the family has a severe problem with structure, it is helpful to write the details of the plan on paper. Sometimes additional reinforcement can be provided by having each person sign the page (with the therapist signing as witness) and giving each person a copy.

In the next session, the outcome is reviewed. If the plan has worked, each person's contribution to the success is talked about and praised. If the plan has not worked, the details of what did happen are reviewed. A plan that was too difficult must be revised to provide a greater chance of success. If parents consider the plan manageable, they are encouraged to try again; they can be supported by a discussion of pitfalls and how to avoid them.

When the first small plan becomes effective, another small plan is added. Then the whole process of review proceeds again with both plans. When each new plan becomes successful, another is added, thus incrementally building up the structure of the family.

In the case of totally indulged 8-year-old Susie, the parents were in their mid-40s and married for 12 years before they adopted. These affluent parents were ecstatic with their little "princess," who was in fact blonde and beautiful. No matter what Susie asked for or how she behaved, her parents found a way to make it positive. By the time of referral, the parents recognized that they had lost control; they knew that the situation was not good, but felt helpless to change it. A pattern they had identified was that if one parent told Susie to do something she did not want to do, she turned to the other in some cute way. The second parent would laugh and let her off.

Although the parents vowed to do whatever was necessary to change the pattern, their plans were disrupted by Susie's wiles. At home and often in session, Susie could get her parents to laugh and back down. Finally, the parents committed themselves to change the nightly dinnertime fuss about what and where Susie would eat. Against permission, she bounded between the table and the television, not responding to urging to sit at the table. When she did come, she did something amusing.

The modest initial plan was that Susie had to sit with her parents at the dinner table for 15 minutes continually. She could choose how much to put on her plate, but had to taste (no matter how tiny the portion) each item on the table. Anything she put on her plate had to be eaten. If any part of this was not done, Susie would have no dessert or snack that evening. The parents were to support each other against separate appeals from Susie. As Susie continually made jokes about the plan, it was clear that the parents were in for a royal testing.

For 3 weeks, Susie won the battle more than half of the time. The turning point began when the mother became annoyed, no longer finding Susie's lack of cooperation so cute. The mother also began to speak sharply to her husband when he did not back her as agreed. Finally, one evening Susie piled mashed potatoes on her plate, and refused all else, then said she didn't want the potatoes either and ran off to the TV. The father said firmly, "Susie, you come back here or I'll smack your behind." After a while Susie danced back in and said, "Daddy, look at this!"

Daddy did not smile. Instead, he took hold of her arm, slapped her behind, and sat her firmly in her chair, saying, "Now eat, but you still get no dessert or snack." Susie smiled at the mother, who unsmilingly said, "That's right." Susie began to wail loudly, but obviously was watching her parents through her hands. When there was no response, she tried to slip off her chair. The father stopped her. For another 5 minutes, Susie searched from face to face for a sign of relenting. Finally she sighed and said, "Oh, well, cold mashed potatoes aren't so bad," and ate.

These parents went on to complete a program of behavioral and structural changes for their household. They affirmed that their love for Susie did not require them to permit their home to be run by an 8-year-old. As they regained control, Susie settled into a more cooperative mode. After that, the parents came in as a couple for a while to discuss how their waiting and longing for a child had led to the creation of a "princess."

Interventions for Parent–Child "Mismatch" Problems

A set of dynamics presented for treatment by some adoptive families differs drastically from the one just discussed. In this situation, the long-desired and long-awaited child by adoption does not match well with parental hopes and expectations. The basis for the sensed lack of match may be attachment issues or unexpected differences in temperament, physical appearance, or aptitude. The perceived lack of fit may also derive from known racial differences, physical handicaps, or illnesses that are harder to cope with than anticipated. Or a profound sense of mismatch may result from the discovery of a disabling handicap or illness well after adoption. The shock of learning that a child's physical or mental abilities may be severely limited can cause disruption even in a biological relation-

ship; thus shock added to the fragility of an adoptive relationship can lead to the relationship's becoming emotionally distant.

This dynamic is also different from than the one discussed earlier wherein a child is needed to fill a vacant role in pre-existing family dynamics. Here, regardless of dynamics, the child was adopted with high hopes and positive expectations. Often the trouble begins when a child leaves early infancy and begins to be a more independent personality, thereby highlighting differences from the parent. Uneasiness about the sense of match may emerge as the child receives more exposure outside the home, when reactions of others impinge on the family's ways of coping. Finally, school or medical personnel may make diagnoses that bring differences into unavoidable clarity.

At any of these points, the sense of mismatch can impinge upon the parental dream. At best, a sensed lack of match may cause uneasiness, which affects family relationships. If parents differ in their reactions to the child, or if they are not able to share their mixed emotions , this can create barriers in the marital interaction. Such marital tension in turn may skew parent–child relationships. Parents often feel very guilty about any feelings of disappointment with an adopted child; nevertheless, such ambivalent feelings color interactions with the child, especially when they are suppressed. Even when the ambivalence is only expressed through metacommunication, the fine-tuned antennae of a child pick it up. As this process goes on, it leads to various degrees of emotional disconnection between parent and child, as a defense against further rejection.

A child too can feel the unease of a lack of match, although he or she may have no words for it until the age of reasoning.

> For example, an adopted woman with dark hair, dark eyes, and olive complexion said that she always felt different from her calm, blonde, blue-eyed family. She also felt the need to suppress a tendency to be vivacious, as well as questions about her ethnicity. She was quite sure that her sense of difference, which could not be discussed, caused her to be less close with her parents than she wished. However, the learned guardedness did fit the family tone.

Although racial differences between parent and child are obviously known, their very visibility can cause unexpected strain. Wherever the family members go, they may be subjected to stares and comments from strangers. Even more hurt can come in dealing with reactions from extended families. Coping with other people's reactions may interfere with a family's own style, pace, and readiness to deal with the issues.

Adoptive parents can also experience unexpectedly strong emotions when they realize that a child has no aptitude for the activity central to the family, such as music or athletics.

> For example, one young man, Bill, was placed as an infant with a family whose father was a high school coach. The life of the family was oriented to sports, whereas Bill was a klutz who loved to draw. His father tried to hide his disappointment, but Bill sensed it keenly. When the whole family prepared to go to the father's games, there was always tension about whether Bill had to go along unhappily or whether special arrangements would be made. Fortunately, Bill knew the the members of his family loved him; for the most part, they took his lack of interest in sports with good humor. Nonetheless, his self-esteem did suffer, putting Bill in a prime position to become symptom bearer should something cause family anxiety to rise.

A diagnosis of a debilitating disease or an unknown physical problem such as deafness is especially shocking to adoptive parents. Because they often have relatively little information about the child's genetic background and the birth family's medical history, the diagnosis may come without warning. The shock is compounded and can add another layer of grief to the load begun by infertility. Whatever the family style of handling bad news, the new layer of grief is likely to exaggerate the modes of coping. Similarly, even when the handicap or disease was known prior to adoption, the full impact of physical care, health-related crises, or medical regimen may not have been. Fatigue and stress may wear down coping abilities. Families whose coping abilities are not so strong to begin with, may attempt to suppress these reactions; as a result, they may experience depression or hostile interactions. In such an exacerbated situation, relationships between parents and child and/or spouses will worsen, and the child becomes a prime candidate for symptom development.

A family that comes for help with problems based on a sense of mismatch usually offer something about the relationships in the family. If a family comes to a therapist early after identifying the discomfort, when there still is positive motivation to work out the relationships, much can be done. At the other extreme, the relationships may already be cold and distant, and the child may have been labeled as undesirable or rejected. In such cases, the therapist may only be able to arbitrate a peaceful coexistence or separation. Regardless of the level of dysfunction, it is important to get into grief work as soon as the family can and will tolerate it.

First, the reality basis of the sense of mismatch must be identified and acknowledged, whether it is based on differences in appearance, race, temperament, or aptitude, or on a child's physical handicap or disease. Then the origins of the discomfort are fully explored. These include the circumstances of adoption, the information available at that time, and the history of anxieties surrounding the particular feature. During this exploration, anxieties about the unknown and the uncomfortable are accepted as reality factors and are labeled as elements of the grief of not being biologically related. Each member must be given the opportunity to express, and validation for expressing, differing individual responses. For family members who have struggled secretly or guiltily with their reactions, the openness of discussion and acceptance can go far in bringing relief.

The next stage of treatment, which may take various forms, focuses upon bringing out ambivalence. Families that are early in the process of identifying their unease, may find the negative side of emotions more painful to admit. Families who are far along in the process of detachment may have more difficulty expressing any positive side to their emotions. Nevertheless, the therapist must persist in eliciting both sides of their feelings. As the therapist accepts the emotions family members find easiest to vent, usually the other side then comes forth, perhaps when directly solicited.

There may be a division of roles among family members, such that one or more are strongly positive while one or more others are vociferously negative. The therapist can use such unilateral expressions to point out that two differing reactions are possible, while expressing regret that individuals are experiencing only one side. As any family member acknowledges a mixture of emotions, each of the others is encouraged to follow. More functional families move into this process readily, even if with considerable pain. Soon members clarify responses among themselves and validate each other's reactions. Comments such as "I didn't know you felt that way," or "I feel the same way," or "Now I finally understand what that was all about," are positive signs.

The final stage of treatment for problems of mismatch involves evaluation of the state of the relationships, the potential for reinvestment, and the possibility of change. In a more functional family, the family members and the theapist can appraise the situation together. Each person's resolution of the sense of mismatch, as well as his or her motivation to improve relationships, must be considered.

First, *what has been* is compared to *what is wanted*; this is followed by planning specific changes. Together, the family members can consider alternative attitudes and behaviors. They may be able to exchange possibilities from among their different repertoires, or they may need suggestions for new ideas or different behaviors from the therapist. The therapist must take care that the realities of the source of mismatch are not dismissed, but are taken into account within whatever solutions the family agrees on. For example, a musician mother can be encouraged not to deny her dismay at her child's off-key singing, but instead to find other ways to share her love of music with the child. Or family members may acknowledge together the fear that wells up for all when a child with cystic fibrosis gets a cold; at the same time, they may reaffirm their commitment and find ways to share the distress.

When a more functional family with issues of mismatch is finishing treatment, some kind of ritual is desirable. Whatever is selected by the family, the ceremony should include the ingredient of mismatch, the underlying grief, and the specific connection to adoption for all individuals. Finally, the reaffirmation of relationships should conclude in a celebration of the relationships that includes an appreciation of individual differences.

Families in which the sense of mismatch has become entrenched or is part of more dysfunctional dynamics do not go through this process so easily. In these cases, it is difficult to get very far in exploring the underlying issues or eliciting mixed emotions. Such a family is more likely to be focused on the negative feelings, the difficulties experienced, and/or rejection of the child. Along with the negativity, roles and relationships may be rigidly fixed with little motivation for change. In an extreme case, by the time a therapist concludes that the relationships cannot or will not be repaired, the family withdraws from treatment.

In one dynamic picture based on mismatch, the relationships of the family are regulated in a bland, distant, predictable way. On the surface the family seems to function quite well, but there is a sort of pseudoattachment or sense of going through the motions. The underlying dynamic may be established by parents who are depressed or who have learned to stay emotionally detached. An adoptee in such a system learns not to make emotional waves and may obtain a sort of "guest" status. Although such a child has obviously joined the system and may be well treated, here the mismatch is between a child's need for emotional attachment and the inability of the parents to relate in a nurturing way. Discussions of the parent–child relationship resemble reports about united-front marriages, wherein everything is said to be "just fine." Queries about what "fine" means get responses that are vague or thin.

Many such emotionally bland families just go along quietly, without drawing any attention that would bring about a referral to a therapist. If such a family does come for treatment, it is because the passivity has been noticed — for example, through lack of achievement, withdrawal, or depression in the child. Blandness may be regulated either by predictable, emotionally distant interactions or by unpredictable behavior that keeps family members out of proximity to one another and therefore not interacting. Regardless of what must be done to counteract features of regulation, the emphasis is such a case is on eliciting of emotions; any emotional liveliness must be fostered and praised. If necessary, the therapist tries to raise anxiety by pointing out what is not normal or risky about the situation. Finally, the stage of appraisal of the relationships is most important for an emotionally bland family. The family members may not want to change, or may not be able to change, their tepid expressivity. In this case, a therapist may send them on their way with the prediction that the arrangement could blow up when the adopted child reaches adolescence.

When an adoptive family comes for help with a rupture already impending, a therapist must use a crisis intervention mode at once. This means bypassing the stages of exploration and dealing with ambivalence, and going right to an assessment of the state of the relationships. When they cannot be repaired, the therapist openly acknowledges the need for or inevitability of separation. While acknowledging the crisis, a therapist urges that separation be handled in the most optimal way for everyone. Planning, instead of impulsive decision making, is encouraged. Then the therapist guides the family members through the decision, offering his or her knowledge of options that may suit their needs. Any positive aspects that can be marshaled are incorporated into the plan of separation, such as a visiting program and financial support. (Separation between spouses who are adoptive parents is discussed further in Chapter 13.)

Interventions for Families Adopting Older Children

The adoptive placement of older children is quite different from the placement of infants, and usually more difficult. Since the newborn's entire family experience is supplied by the adoptive family, the child is much more likely to occupy a role designed within the family. The older child, even one who is only a few months or years old, comes with some sort of prior family experience. Furthermore, the older a child is at the time of adoption, the more likely it is that some part of the prior family experience was traumatic. Perhaps a child lived with a birth mother who was not able to continue caring for him or her, but the separation was agonizing. Or a child may have been legally removed from a neglectful and/or abusive birth family. Or, because of legal or medical complications, a child may have spent time in one or more foster homes.

Three factors provide a guide to how severely a child has been traumatized prior to adoptive placement: age, severity of neglect or abuse, and the number of prior homes. Extreme combinations of these factors produce more damage to a child's attachment abilities, and thus more difficulties can be expected in the adoptive home (see also Rosenthal, 1990; Sandmaier, 1988).

The effect of multiple changes in the early years is painstakingly described by Katrina Maxtone-Graham (1983) in her autobiographical account of reclaiming the first $3\frac{1}{2}$ years of her life. At the age of 38, after 14 years of psychiatric care for depression, phobic behavior, and low self-esteem, she embarked on her search. Gradually, she ferreted out that she had been born to a teenage mother who wanted to keep her baby, originally named Judith, but was not permitted to bring her home. For 2 months they lived together in a maternity center. Then the baby lived in two foster homes for a year, with regular visits from her young mother.

Then, without notice, Judith was moved to another home where there was a loving, maternal foster mother, who described her as "such a good little girl." Meanwhile, her 19-year-old birth mother realized that Judith was confused about who was her mother. Also, she was told that the tot would be moved yet again "because the family was becoming too attached." In the face of these factors, her birth mother painfully signed adoption papers so that Judith could have a permanent home.

Judith was next placed in an adoptive home wherein there was a mother described as "not warm" and "mechanical." For the first few days, Judith slept a great deal and would not eat, and when she did, she threw up. (Maxtone-Graham notes that this pattern continued into her adult life; when depressed, she slept a lot and did not eat.) A short time later, Judith was described as "stubborn," as " negativistic," and as "having severe tantrums twice a day." At the end of 5 months, the little girl was returned to the agency.

After a month in still another home, Judith moved at age $3\frac{1}{2}$ to a permanent home, where she became Katrina. Here the tantrums were put to an end: "The too-hard-to-handle, spunky terror was replaced by the quiet, ever-so-well-behaved child of my recollections. Judith and her fiery independent spirit were gone; in her place was Katrina, the silent observer" (1983, p. 20). Maxtone-Graham's story poignantly portrays how psychological suffering follows from loss of loving relationships and multiple placements. Equally clear is how a toddler's personality can be subverted by depression and then maintained in passive form by a rigidly regulated adoptive family.

Many children available for adoption after infancy have suffered not only psychological trauma, but also other types. They may have lacked adequate food and shelter, and/or may have been abused physically or sexually. Their care may have been very inconsistent, at the whims of substance-abusing, mentally ill, promiscuous, and/or poverty-stricken parents. Such children are considered to have "special needs," and their adoptions (permanency planning) are generally handled by social agencies, public or private. Optimally, the adoptive placement of older children should be handled with special therapeutic consideration all through the process. This may be done by agency social workers, with therapist services added at any point (see also, Elbow, 1986).

When prospective parents are selected (sometimes as foster parents who have the option to adopt [Derdeyn, 1990]), it is optimal for both parents to be involved and positively motivated for placement. Although a strong marriage is the best underpinning for joint parenting of any child, it is essential in the care of an abused or deprived child. In single-parent adoptions, a strong support system is also needed. If the parent does not already have such support, the agency should be prepared to supply it.

Deprived and abused children are known to repeat previously learned patterns of behavior in a new home. Therefore, consideration should be given to how a potential new family is organized to deal with the particular areas of difficulty. For example, a family that is tense about open expressions of anger probably should not take in a child who was physically abused during parental rages. A family that is particularly squeamish about sexual matters probably should not take in a child who has been sexually abused. A family that is fairly closed in the regulation of order and cleanliness probably should not take in a child who has not had adequate food or toilet training.

Once a family has been selected for a child, the parents should be fully informed about the child's experiences and probable difficulties in attachment. The assumption sometimes held by agencies that withholding information protects a placement is always wrong. In fact, withholding information does the opposite: It worsens the inevitable difficulties by adding dismay about the unexpected and about being misled.

Potential parents for older children are sometimes subjected to the practice of "stretching," as decried by Barth and Berry (1988). In this situation, child welfare workers have encouraged prospective parents to "stretch" the parameters of the kind of children they will accept. Then they are urged to take a particular child they would not have considered previously. Whether because of "stretching" or by accident, if an older child is placed in a family where the psychological issues are the same as the child's, the situation can deteriorate rapidly. Therapeutic crisis intervention is needed at once. There must be maximum effort to bolster structure, to offer support, and to evaluate whether the situation can work at all.

Prospective parents should also be prepared for the predictable stages of placement and relationship development: honeymoon, testing, and building of trust. They need to know the irony that when the child begins to trust, things can get rough. The initial honeymoon stage is based on best behavior all around, which aids in getting acquainted and bridges unfamiliarity. When a child begins to trust and to feel at home, consistency, commitment, and trustworthiness are thoroughly tested. Not only does a child need to find out that this family responds better than previous ones; the child also needs to live through the reworking of his or her own behavior repertoire.

Even after everyone survives the worst of the testing phase, the family will live with the child's wounds for some time. As the trust and the relationships grow stronger, all the issues are likely to require reworking at each stage of development. Usually the severely deprived older child is engaged in working out early psychological stages, which are probably discrepant with his or her physical or mental age. Social workers (Clemmons, Gora, Moline, Mulryan, & Sanders, 1989) have suggested that the adoptive parents of a deprived older child think of the child's emotional development as beginning with placement. Such an attitude can offset feelings about inappropriate behavior and can guide responses when there is a discrepancy between a child's emotional needs and size or age. Thus a child of 10 who begins to trust may need to cuddle like an infant, or a child of 8 may like to play the chase-and-hide games of a 2-year-old; in each case, the child is literally doing developmental work that was missed.

Because of the importance of food for real and symbolic nurture, such problems as binge eating, hoarding, or guarding food frequently arise. Sometimes the problems are in "digesting" nurture, and are manifested in stomach complaints or vomiting. There can be similar issues related to elimination; these can stem from lack of training or from psychological dreprivation. Problems may be manifested in atypical ways as well. The behavioral expression of the emotional trauma may be at one of two extremes: Family rules may be violated beyond what the parents could have imagined; at the other extreme, the child's behavior may be secretive, guarded, frightened, or withdrawn.

At any stage of placement or in the development of a traumatized child, adoptive parents usually need a great deal of therapeutic help. Even with preparation, the daily living with behavior (e.g., tantrums, hiding feces or food, clinging) may be more difficult than expected. There must be repeated reassurance that what is going on is a result of the child's deprivation and not of "badness," either in the child or in the parents' abilities. Parents may need education about the child's behavior and concrete suggestions for management; progress must be monitored and supported. Other services may also be necessary, such as therapeutic schools, physical activity programs, or respite care. Whole-family therapy is advisable but may not be effective during the most difficult periods. There must be ample opportunity in separate sessions for parents to ventilate and to have the support of the therapist as individuals, as well as for their teamwork. Often the child needs individual therapy in addition, in order to rework specific traumas.

The adoptive placements of older children with the most impaired ability to attach are the adoptions most likely to be disrupted. Often a psychiatric hospitalization for such a child is indicated. Although it is preferable for the adoptive parents to stay as involved as possible, sometimes a child reverts to being a ward of the state. Subsequently, an experience in group care may be indicated, where relationships can be less intense than in a family setting.

Sometimes older children are adopted as sibships. An evaluation of the three factors by which to gauge trauma must now be multiplied by the number of children. An additional factor for careful assessment is the nature of each child's relationship to the others. Any positive, nurturing, secure aspects of the children's relationships at first should be fostered. Even when an older child may have too much responsibility for its age, such security arrangements should not be disrupted too soon.

Once the children have settled into the new home, age-appropriate differentiation can be encouraged. Differentiation of siblings adopted together is perhaps the most difficult, as well as the most necessary, responsibility of their caretakers. Differences in trauma, age, gender, developmental stage, and the way each sibling deals with placement require a special response to each child. Siblings may initially contend for resources or may become rivalrous during the testing phase of the placement process. All the children must find out for certain whether each child is a fully accepted and permanent member of the family. Beyond that, each child must find his or her own role and position in the family alliances.

> In one such situation, parents adopted five children, aged 6 to 15, from one family. The children had been living in a one-room rural shack with their parents, three younger siblings, two dogs, and some chickens; there was no electricity, no indoor plumbing, and not enough food. The adoptive father said that they required huge amounts of services of all kinds from the community and often he felt that they were operating a therapeutic nursery. But the rewards came from seeing the younger children begin to settle in and to thrive. He was not so sure how it would work out for the older ones.

Another kind of family in which the issues of attachment and sibling relationships can be very complex is the adoptive family that also has children by birth. A finding of the Delaware Family Study (Hoopes, 1982) was that families who had children both by birth and by adoption were at greatest risk of difficulties. Although caution is needed because of the relatively small sample, the finding does suggest greater emotional complexities in such families. When this type of family comes for treatment, extra precautions must be taken to assess *the family's* experience and to avoid assumptions. The role of each child must be assessed in the family alliances, regardless of the means of entering the family. Sometimes a family of this type has tried so hard to make the adopted child secure that the birth child or children suffer by comparison. Alternately, the adopted child may be the most readily available candidate for symptom bearer, should the role be needed.

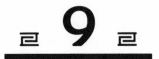

Therapy
for Adoptive Families
with Adolescents
and Young Adults

Adolescents and Midlife Parents: Basic Issues

The upheaval of the adolescent passage from childhood to adulthood is well known to anyone who has been through it. The stresses are even more emphatically known to any parent whose midlife issues have reverberated to those of an adolescent offspring. Whatever the personal experience, family therapists know that families with adolescent children and midlife parents seek help at higher rates than families with members at other ages.

Despite the emergence in recent decades of theory about stages of adulthood and families as systems, adolescence often still eclipses other stages in a family. In the systemic view taken here, the life stage transition of adolescents *parallels* and *mirrors* the midlife stage transition of parents. The adolescent is passing into adulthood and is dealing with the questions of "What will I be and do as an adult?" The parent at midlife is passing to the latter half of life with the questions of: "How did I do with my youthful goals, and now what will I do (better or worse) with the rest of my life?" (See also Ackerman, 1980.)

The adolescent does indeed undergo a great deal of change, and often has nearly convulsive ambivalence about all aspects thereof. The ambivalence of the adolescent passage can intensify

parents' review of their own youthful decisions and goals for
personal relationships and occupation; in addition, parents may be
barraged by echoes or resurrections of their own adolescent issues.
All parents instill in their children particular meanings and beliefs
about what it means to be an adult, in terms of productivity, family
relationships, gender, and sexuality. Much of the teaching is
existential; much of the learning is by observation. The real test of
these lessons comes when it is time for the young people to move
into the ranks of adults.

Each generation deals with its own questions while attempting
to influence or challenge the other. As the generations jockey back
and forth through this life stage, the arrangement of relationships
that comprises the family system is changed. In order for both
generations to make a successful transition, the central issues that
must be renegotiated are (1) physical growth and sexuality, (2)
autonomy, and (3) identity.

Physical changes in both generations can mean that all family
members are confronting new aspects of their own sexuality. As
adolescent hormones surge, promoting capacity for and interest in
sexual activity, parents may experience hormonal changes that
decrease sexual desire and ability. There may be general confusion,
at the same time that family members try to influence shifts in
values and operating rules about sexuality. All members of a family
may question their attractiveness to the opposite gender. Within the
family, a parent and an adolescent of the opposite sex may test their
attractiveness on each other and even provide reassuring validation.
At the same time, such interactions can be threatening and can
create the need for distance.

Second only to sexuality in the potential for conflict is the issue
of autonomy. A young person faces the question of whether it is
possible to leave the dependency of childhood to become an adult
who is self-directed and productive. Many teenagers vacillate
between insistence on self-determination and dependency-seeking
behavior. Finding a balance is difficult enough when adults have
modeled autonomous behavior. But when parents have shown
spotty self-direction or are dependent on their children, adolescents
may only know pseudoautonomy, as shown in the role of parental
children.

The question for parents is whether they can or will turn over
any control to the young people (i.e., who will now make the rules
for whom?). More functional parents not only have modeled
autonomous behavior but also have gradually adjusted the operating rules, providing more participation and autonomy for teen-

agers. In less functional families, changes are resisted, gained through fighting, or obtained by default.

The adolescent's struggles with sexuality and autonomy are a necessary part of the process of forming an identity as an adult. "Identity" is defined here as a sense of who one is as an adult. This includes values, beliefs, sense of gender, and expectations of self in relationships and for productivity. In order to establish an adult identity, the adolescent must sort out whether to retain parental values and beliefs, and if so, which ones. This sorting occurs through vigorous testing of parental values and is best carried out when parents are able to hold their ground and still maintain basic good will to their offspring. However, at the same time that adolescents are testing values, midlife parents may also be undergoing shifts in identity and personal values. Often at this life stage, the intellectualized, instrumental male begins to develop his emotional, relational repertory. The nurturant female begins to develop her intellectual and instrumental competence. At midlife, both genders tend to move toward wholeness.

Parents' issues can by accentuated by the launching of children, because of the obvious change in parental function and the return to being a couple alone. The groundwork laid by more functional families enables them to navigate the multiple passages successfully. In more randomly organized families, all members may vacillate rather unpredictably in their demands for closeness and distance, while the young people simply drift out of the family. Families with closed regulation resist any change; they may become even more rigidly organized, or may explode. Regardless of the type of family organization, the complex interactive processes of this life stage nearly always engender anxiety. Since all family members have their own struggles and do not move at the same pace, conflict tends to increase and may escalate to crisis proportions. The outcome may be some type of symptom production, a return to previous arrangements, or the extrusion of a member.

The Issues as Experienced in Adoptive Families

Every issue of adolescence and midlife has additional meanings for a family in which a teen has been adopted, even in infancy. Most obvious is that once again the meaning of adoption must be reworked in this life stage. The young person's identity issues are compounded by fresh confrontation with his or her dual heritage. If the birth heritage is not known and/or cannot be openly addressed because of the family operating rules, the suppression of questions and emotions can be a prime contributor to symptom development. On the parental side, midlife review and dealing with a teenager can reopen youthful dreams to have children by birth, grief about infertility, and qualms about adoption. Doubts about attachments can be exaggerated by an adolescent's bids for autonomy, separateness, and eventual departure. The actual departure of an adoptee amplifies the loss experiences of each family member.

The basic issue for all adoptive families is that the process of reorganizing dependency arrangements again forces confrontation with the lack of birth bond. Regardless of the level of functioning, all adoptive families are taxed in reworking the meanings of adoption at this life stage. On the positive side, the need to rearrange relationships, although stressful in the short run, can lead to a better resolution; hidden meanings and protective rules in regard to adoption can be opened and redone. However, when the issues of adoption have not been faced before, a family is more vulnerable to upheaval. This may come about because the adopted adolescent may finally be willing or able to break the family rules of operation against talking or even knowing about the adoption. The adolescent's behavior may be an extension of the prior family role, or may be new behavior as a way of testing the possibility of change.

A mild form of testing in regard to adoption is the raising of questions about adoption, birth, and search. Severe testing may be expressed by the wish to search for the mythological, "perfect" birth parents, because the adoptive parents are so "bad." Other tests come through behavior that acts out the hidden feelings, such as law breaking or running away.

Families with closed regulation meet the emergence of adoption issues at this life stage with hostility, threats, and attempts at suppression. Both generations are vulnerable to symptoms resulting from internalization of emotions, whether these take the form of depression or of acting out. Particularly when an adopted adolescent is depressed, this may mirror depression in a parent, usually the mother. In the extreme, a family vacillates between returning to the previous state of relationships or extruding a member, most often the adoptee. By contrast, the underorganized family may become more wildly unpredictable about the meaning of adoption, attitudes toward each other, or even the whereabouts of family members. The continued loosening of the organization may proceed at intense levels of anxiety, or the family may just quietly drift apart. In one extreme situation, eventually the adopted adolescent and each adoptive parent all returned to their own families of origin.

Each specific issue of this life stage has powerful ramifications for the adoptive family; this is especially true of issues related to the gender and sexual development of the teenage adoptee. The complexities of opposite-gender parent–child attraction can be aggravated by fears or fantasies that the incest barrier will not be strong enough within the adoptive family (Easson, 1973). Indeed, in cases where there have been problems of attachment and/or regulation (either problems specific to adoption or problems of the system in general), the incest barrier may be weakened. Even when there is no actual incestuous activity, fantasies and fears can be powerful. Thus the adoptive family may need to create even more than the usual distance between the adopted teenager and the parent of the opposite gender.

There are several ways in which a family can increase this distance. Conflict may intensify directly between the teen and the parent of the opposite gender, or the parent of the same gender may feel threatened and may foster hostility between the teen and the opposite-gender parent. Still another possibility is that the adolescent develops a strong interest in finding (or, if already known, increasing involvement with) his or her birth parents, as a means of neutralizing the sexual tension in the family. Adoptive parents may also focus on the birth parents with relief as a means of neutralizing their own anxieties. On the other hand, adoptive parents may focus hostility on the birth parents or on interest in them. This serves to keep conflict alive, thus providing a barrier between parents and teenager.

A twist for the adoptive family in regard to adolescent sexuality is that the younger generation is apparently able to reproduce while the parents are not. In the adoption literature, this seems to be primarily an issue of females, both mothers and daughters (see Schaffer & Lindstrom, 1990; Schechter & Bertocci, 1990). Why this is the case is questionable. Perhaps the orientation to females results from the childbearing ability of women, since physical, psychological, and social aspects are obvious.

More probably, however, the dearth of information about males derives from stereotypes about males. One stereotype results from the still-existing "double standard," which encourages young men to be as sexually active as possible without responsibility for the outcome. Another bias is that males do not have or will not express emotions about their sexuality or potential fatherhood. More effort should be made to ask birth fathers, adoptive fathers, and male adoptees about what biological versus adoptive fathering means to them. No doubt much could be learned, as in the case of Randolph, described in Chapter 4.

Adoptive parents may react to the apparent fertility of a

daughter in a number of ways, but inevitably their own grief about infertility is reopened. (Again, little is known about how adoptive parents react to the fertility of a son.) If only one parent was infertile and/or there was any conflict between parents about the infertility or adoption, conflict may increase between parents. Often such conflict is not directly expressed in regard to the issues between them, but instead focuses on the daughter, particularly on her sexuality and its management.

The adopted daughter who has passed puberty, for her part, has a loyalty conflict overlaying her identity issues: Does she identify with the woman who raised her but did not give birth to her? Or does she identify with the woman who gave birth to her but could not raise her? If the mother and daughter (and the father, as well) have not been able to discuss openly their mutual grief about the nonbiological connection and the questions of loyalty, the worries and fantasies go underground.

Several outcomes are possible. Parental fears about a daughter's sexuality may be expressed through a great deal of attention to her physical development, health care, attractiveness, and attention from boys and men. Another possibility is that parents may induce a daughter to engage in sexual activity by promoting their expectations in reverse, emphasizing the dangers against which she must be protected.

On the other hand, the adopted daughter who becomes sexually active, promiscuous, and/or pregnant may have several agendas. She may have a symptom-bearing role for her family, whereby family anxieties are focused on her. Or the daughter may be trying to produce a baby for her infertile parents. A third possibility is that she may be identifying with the only or most salient aspect known about her birth mother. When a single female adoptee has a baby, her decisions about her child's care reflect the reworking of her own issues about adoption and possibly reparation.

Perhaps the most powerful impact of adoption at this life stage is on the identity development of the adolescent. The fact of having two sets of parents becomes a major complication in the sorting of values. Here again, the literature almost entirely offers examples of adopted girls. Often these girls are described as cooperative family members and good students until early adolescence. Then, in a sudden reversal, they develop a disrespectful attitude toward parents and engage in unacceptable behavior. Often the behavior is designed to be noticed (e.g., breaking curfew, failing in school, changing friends, or engaging flagrant substance abuse and/or sexual activity). When the female adoptee approaches the age at which her mother gave birth, she may identify with the birth mother or at least decide to try out the mother's imagined life style. Thus, the female adoptee changes her behavior in the direction of the imagined behavior of the birth mother, often toward more rebellious and sexual activity. Simultaneously, the young woman is giving a major test to the values of the adoptive parents, as well as to the strength of the adoptive attachment.

There are few case examples of adopted boys whose behavior seems to change so radically just at the time of puberty. However, there are clues that the adopted male adolescent may begin a pattern of dating wherein there are numerous short-term contacts. It is as though the male adoptee is searching and never finding the perfect, long-lost love object.

The outcome for both sexes has to do with fantasies about birth parents. In a case where the adoptee knows little about the birth family, and operating rules have discouraged discussion, fantasy has filled in the blanks. The adolescent adoptee may privately have spun a whole life scenario for the birth mother, in which the birth father may or may not have much place. Some adoptees create scenarios of birth parents as special people — heroes or royalty who were somehow tricked or forced into placing their children. Adolescent identity issues can reinforce such fantasies and feed an urgent need to search as a hoped-for solution. Indeed, some adoptees have had so bad an experience in their adoptive families that the need to search *is* based on the wish to find a better family. Their desperation goes well beyond the normative wish to know.

> Eighteen-year-old Jane spoke emphatically about a lifelong need to search for her birth parents; by now, this was almost the only thing she could think about. It had nothing to do with her adoptive parents, she knew, because they had provided her a good life. Yet, as she spoke about them, her emotional tone was flat. The contrast in passion when she talked about wanting to know her birth parents was very noticeable, as was her pain.

As more adoptees grow up with some degree of openness about their adoption — whether through facts, letters from birth parents, or personal contact — fantasies should not be so hidden or powerful. Yet the need to sort out one's identity when there are two sets of parents remains a very complex task. Some young people cope by fixing exclusively on one family or the other, or by vacillating between the two. Many times, the struggle in regard to identity issues centers on the adolescent's name: Will the adoptee keep the given name or surname provided by the adoptive family, take either from the birth family, or select an altogether new one? Florence Fisher (1973), the first adoptee to write her search story, kept the first name given by her adoptive parents but took her birth father's surname.

> One adopted adolescent male, who had been named Marco by his birth mother, complained at length to his parents about being forced to have a name he did not want. When they finally thought to ask what name he wanted, he said he wanted to be called Dave after his adoptive father, and did not want to change the surname at all! By contrast, a teenage girl decided that neither the first name given by her birth mother (Eva) nor that given by the adoptive family (Karen) suited her at all. Henceforth, she decreed, she would be known as Rondi!

Another aspect of normal adolescence that is powerful for adoptive families is the move away from dependence toward autonomy. All members of the adoptive family may fear that emancipation means another abandonment. For the adoptee, who has already lost one set of parents, emancipation may seem to threaten the loss of a second set. Some adoptees develop symptoms that prevent their leaving home, or at least delay it. There may be failure to graduate from high school, an eating disorder, or a phobia. Adoptive parents who are faced with a child's preparation to leave may experience renewed misgivings, expressed by the way in which do or do not relinquish parental authority. The family's conflict in regard to authority usually centers around the question of who now makes the rules for the adolescent's behavior. The adoptive family has the added possibility of fighting about attitudes and arrangements regarding birth parents.

General Considerations in Therapy

When an adoptive family with midlife parents and adolescent adoptee applies for treatment, the interaction of family dynamics, symptoms, adoption, and life stage tends to be at maximum intensity. Often the presenting problem is some extreme form of behavior, and there is an element of real or impending crisis. Usually the problem — either in a teenager's behavior or in parent--teen relationships — is directly related to life stage. Often the family is aware of the importance of adoption and mentions it immediately. When risks are high, a crisis intervention must be used. The first goal must be to ensure the physical safety and well-being of all members. This means engineering a very structured truce within the home (or, if necessary, with a member temporarily outside the home). Once there is safety, then the objective is to lower anxiety, so that family members are more available to engage in working with the problem.

When there is no major crisis, therapy can proceed along the general guidelines, with consideration of the specific approaches described at the beginning of Chapter 8. But in any case where the symptom bearer is an adopted adolescent, exploration of the problem and the dynamics around it must take the life stage into consideration. That is, the onset of the symptom should be specifically investigated in regard to the onset of puberty. In addition, any changes in family relationships before and after the onset of puberty and the problem should be queried in detail. Any other changes, such as in regard to health, occupation, and the extended family, should be asked about as well. Family members who are very focused on the behavior of an adolescent may be successfully distracted from other sources of anxiety. They may be no longer be consciously aware of any other possible sources for, or of any connection of these sources to, the symptoms.

Often, along with making a structured plan of intervention, the therapist needs to teach what is normative for this life stage. This can be done through imparting expert knowledge or through telling stories from experience to illustrate common issues. Most important is that the therapist *must stay balanced and support both sides.* For example, the therapist could say, "Of course, you parents must put down some consequences for Marcy for staying out all night. But it is just as natural that Marcy, now that she is 15, wants more say and more privileges than she had at 13." Then the therapist can try to negotiate the terms of both consequences and privileges.

Interventions Focused on the Fact of Adoption

Since the fact of adoption has probably been known from the outset, exploration of issues related to the adoption can be woven into initial discussions. In contrast to the approach with a younger family, in which the pace of the family must be carefully followed, here the therapist must take responsibility to push the process and make the connections to adoption. As soon as the anxiety level about the presenting situation permits, the therapist takes advantage of the normal upheaval of relationships (and defenses) at this stage to promote change. Not only may the situation require firm management, but this may be the last chance for the family as a whole to make a better resolution.

When a therapist makes connections to adoption that may not be consciously known to a family, this must be done with ample support. When there is resistance to seeing these connections, a therapist needs to persist or to find other ways to make the points. A good alternative is to locate a member of the family who has emotion about the adoption and whose voice cannot be ignored.

In particular, if the issue is not introduced by someone in the family, the therapist must bring up the fact of two sets of parents. Even when the adoptee denies any interest, a therapist teaches that it is normal for everyone, including an adoptee, to want to know about his or her origins. This gives permission to any family member who is able or becomes able to acknowledge feelings on the matter. If a family can do no more than listen to the therapist's comments, at least the subject has been introduced for future reference.

When a therapist discusses the fact of two sets of parents, several points should be made. First, the fact of two sets of parents is a real aspect of present life, not just a musty statistic, long since stowed away. Second, the fact of two sets of parents is a complexity not just for the adoptee, but for every member of the family. Finally, the adoptee's interest in birth parents is normal; it is not *necessarily* a comment on the quality of life in the adoptive family (although it may be).

In this process, the therapist must attend to the parents also, giving them opportunity to express their ambivalence about the other set of parents. Adoptive parents may try to put the birth parents out of mind, but inevitably they have thoughts or fantasies about them. Permission and legitimization from a therapist can bring great relief in opening these hidden but active concerns. Adoptive parents may grieve for the birth parents' loss, or may worry that a child will be hurt if more is known about birth circumstances. Often, they also have fears for their own parental status and relationship with the young person who is preparing to leave and who may find the original parents. Conversely, there may be concern about getting too close, if feelings about birth parents no longer provide distance.

A therapist really cannot overemphasize the point that mutual openness and sharing about these matters dissipate barriers and strengthen relationships in the family. As painful as such discussions can be, the experience of learning about and supporting each other through the process promotes improved, more nearly adult-level relationships. In fact, the process of discussion about meanings of adoption may be the prototype for the process of emancipation.

Instead of a specially designed ritual at the end of treatment with adoptive families at the launching stage, changes related to preparation and planning for the young adult to leave can be reinforced. The adoptee may be headed for college, the armed services, or a home of his or her own. Here the ritual has to do with the family' members' way of saying goodbye, the kind of contact they expect during separation, and the ways in which future reunions will take place. Parallels between the way the family members prepare to launch a young person and the way they prepare to leave therapy can be used to consolidate a positive process (see also Lax & Lussardi, 1988).

For some families, a mutually created plan to search for birth parents can take the place of a ritual. The parents of an early adolescent may do the search work in consultation with the adoptee. Even when an adolescent adoptee is able to instigate and carry on the search, parental support may validate the adoptee's sense of autonomy and identity. At the same time, the parents have reaffirmed their parental position, but from a new basis — as enablers to a budding adult.

Concurrently with this phase of family therapy, it is often useful for parents' to have couple sessions and for the teenager to enter group therapy with other adolescents. When available, group therapy with other adopted adolescents is optimal. Such a treatment plan parallels the preparation for separation of living arrangements in the family (Schmidt & Liebowitz, 1969).

Interventions for Families with Eating-Disordered Adolescents

Beyond the general approach to therapy with families of adopted adolescents, there are special considerations for the treatment of particular symptoms. These constellations of dynamics follow from those discussed in relation to adoptive families with young children. But with the additional leavening of adolescent and midlife changes, the anxiety levels of these families are generally high when they apply for treatment.

When an adoptive family brings an obese adolescent for treatment, the duration and degree of the overweight is the central question to assess. If the adoptee's weight was within normal parameters until puberty, the next question is how the weight gain relates to life stage and preparation for launching. Often the young person has taken on the family's issues about separation, either through rebellious overeating or through creating a physical situation that could prevent the pain of separation.

Terry (1987) points out that eating can regulate the closeness and distance in relationships and the changes impending with a life stage. This dynamic may occur when an adolescent adopted daughter is very closely allied with her mother, to the exclusion of the father and all other relationships. If permissive feeding was a strong part of establishing the mother–daughter alliance, there is likely to be mutual cueing about food in times of stress. The message can be that overeating and weight gain constitute an acceptable way to stay anchored at home and avoid the pain of separation and independence.

Another form of this dynamic occurs when the strongest alliance is that between an adopted adolescent and the parent of the opposite gender; more often, this particular dynamic applies to a mother–son alliance. A "good" adolescent adopted son may suddenly gains a lot of weight by eating many burgers and fries away from home. This may be a declaration of independence from his mother's food/nurture and control. A literal wall—one of fat—creates distance between them, with the additional benefit of decreasing the possibility that the mother will find the son's sexual development attractive.

In contrast to sudden weight gain, an adolescent's obesity may be a long-standing problem, perhaps since placement. The weight can function as a wall of protection against feelings of inner void and outer lack of fulfillment in family relationships. When the obesity of an adolescent is of long duration, the important assessment question is whether there is any motivation for change *within the family*. If at least the teenager and/or the parents have some concern about the teen's health or suffering in the peer group, change is more of a possiblility.

In dealing with families of obese teenagers, the general procedures for beginning therapy must be reversed. Instead of behavioral interventions, the first steps must be to learn all about food habits and their meaning to *each family member*. If even one authoritative member of the immediate or extended family system also is obese, considers obesity acceptable, or considers weight loss unacceptable, the potential for sabotage is great. As soon as the review of food habits has led to an understanding of the dynamics, the therapist should openly connect the function of food to the issues of adoption. If the family resists, an often effective approach is to inquire about the parents' experience with food and with emancipation from their own families of origin. Related factors are the grandparents' attitudes about the parental marriage and especially about the adoption. Frequently, problems between parents and an obese teenager have some parallel in the issues between parents and grandparents. Sometimes, change must occur between grandparents and parents before a family is able to deal with the obesity of a adolescent.

Once a family examines the meanings of food and connections to adoption, intervention focused on the behavior can begin. McVoy (1987) says that since obese teens tend to have a devalued self-image, it is essential for the teen to take charge of plans for his or her own body. At the same time, parents whose overinvolvement has helped to perpetuate the problem must be kept appropriately busy elsewhere. McVoy also suggests that group therapy is very helpful for overweight adolescents, but the focus needs to be on nutrition, not weight loss. Peer support for the struggle over food habits, as well as for positive changes in appearance, is most valuable. Young people in a group can help one another spot and avoid parental sabotage.

When an eating disorder first appears in adolescence, the most common form is bulimia nervosa (Roberto, 1987; Terry 1987). The disorder may begin during high school years or just after the start of college. The typical picture is that of a daughter who has been oriented to her mother's needs. The "good adoptee" daughter who has been allied with her mother, in a family whose operating rules preclude open conflict, fits the protocol for bulimia very well. (Bulimia seems to be almost entirely a female symptom; we know of no cases in which an adopted male has had this symptom.) When a daughter is still at home, there is usually a direct correlation between the degree of suppressed conflict and the frequency of the daughter's secret bingeing and purging. If bulimia begins after a daughter has left home, the symptom may be used directly in the service of separation issues. It may become the young woman's own "secret property," separate from her family. The bulimic girl's "secret" may become a reason to avoid going home. Conversely, it can become the reason for frequent trips home or for a permanent return.

By the time families of bulimic daughters seek treatment, the bulimia has been discovered and has brought them. In the assessment, the therapist needs to take notice of alliance patterns, themes related to competence and autonomy, and operating rules about conflict. These families tend to have awareness of the suppressed conflict.

The dynamic picture is likely to include a mother who is oriented to the care of her own mother. The father either is a "good son" or is cut off from his family of origin. The inability to produce a child by birth has further injured the mother and father's sense of competence in the parental role. The adopted daughter has been inducted into an alliance with the mother, oriented to making the mother feel competent as a mother, in the same way that the mother has tried to do for the grandmother. At the same time the daughter experiences pressure to achieve in the world—to make her parents proud, and thus again to verify their competence as parents. Thus, any attempts by the daughter to emancipate herself are highly threatening. The daughter is caught in the bind of double messages: "Don't go away or stop feeding the parental self-esteem," but "Go out into the world and achieve what we have not, so that we can be proud."

In the first phase of treatment, the family dynamics centering around the daughter must be emphasized. The expectations and double messages must be addressed in particular, along with the daughter's normal need for increased autonomy. Each family member is encouraged to develop self-management skills, perhaps through training in improved communication, fair fighting, or assertiveness. Furthermore, the daughter is put in charge of her bulimic behavior. She is helped to work out a management plan, and is encouraged to choose alternative activities that she can control and from which she can gain feelings of competence. Her parents are urged to consider their own needs and wishes in a way parallel to the daughter. They must be shown their self-defeating behavior in regard to the bulimia and helped to give it up. Each parent is encouraged to pursue alternative, gratifying experiences that bolster the sense of competence, especially former sources of gratification as a couple. Each parent, particularly the mother, may need to examine the relationship to his or her own mother and the way in which that has affected the current situation.

Michelle was the beautiful 16-year-old adoptive daughter of Ed and Doris, farmers who looked much older than their roughly 50 years. The parents worked very hard to scratch a living out of a small vegetable farm, in the community where they had grown up and married late. A year after their marriage they had a son, Keith. When Keith was 15, a girl on a neighboring farm became pregnant and later gave birth to Michelle. Doris, who had just experienced the death of her mother, insisted on adopting Michelle. There was a hint that Doris suspected that Keith was Michelle's father. Apparently no one knew for sure, and the subject was not open for discussion.

Michelle, always a pretty and charming child, was kept in dresses and curled hair. Although she stayed near her mother, she was taught only "feminine tasks"; she was not allowed to engage in physical labor, as Doris did. Once Michelle began school, the message was that average grades were acceptable, but that being on stage in school concerts or plays was highly desirable. Just prior to the referral, Michelle had been selected as the school homecoming queen, much to the family's satisfaction. She was also in a position to have a lead in the school musical and to be a class officer. Recently there had been family discussions about whether Michelle should go to college. Doris favored a junior college at a nearby small city, so that Michelle could live at home and "keep the costs down."

The family requested treatment for Michelle right after a family joke was answered. Everyone liked to tease Michelle about how she could stay so pretty and slender, when she ate such quantities of her mother's good baking. Recently, Doris had become suspicious about odors in the bathroom, so she had followed Michelle to listen at the door just after Doris had seen her carry off most of a pie. When confronted, Michelle admitted that she had begun to binge and purge shortly after beginning high school. By the time she became homecoming queen, she was purging at least once a day. She claimed that it helped her get through the pressures of public appearances.

This family was not accustomed to talking about personal matters. The members' very willingness to come for family meetings indicated their degree of concern and affection for Michelle. Because of their verbal reticence, the therapist actively discussed bulimia, adolescence, and the loyalty issues of growing up adopted. Initially, the family members said little, but their faces were responsive when the therapist succeeded in reaching them. Noticing a facial reaction, the therapist asked each person to put the reaction into words. Finally, the family members began to talk more about themselves in relation to the others and to Michelle's bulimia. Every verbal and emotional expression was encouraged. The pressures on Michelle were validated, as were her attempts to cope, while her choice was labeled unfortunate. The mother, especially, was given credit for how hard she tried to make life easier for Michelle than for herself.

Although no one in this family became voluble, each person did learn to assert his or her own position and to negotiate with the others. A sizable part of their negotiations involved checking out assumptions about nonverbal responses with each other. In fact, they used the same phrases the therapist had modeled initially. By the time their communications had improved outside of sessions, the bulimia had stopped. Michelle was successfully dealing with her own urges to eat and purge.

Anorexia nervosa, or self-starvation, is the most serious of the eating disorders because it can reach life-threatening proportions (Moley, 1987). Again, this symptom is primarily experienced by adolescent females, who perceive themselves as fat despite diminishing body weight. Commonly, the problem originates with an episode of extreme dieting. This sets a precedent for distorted body image, physiological and psychological changes, and a pitched war with parents.

In a family with an anorectic daughter, conflict is generally severe but covert, and centers around the psychological theme of behavior control. All members are very skilled at power struggles, as evidenced in the match between the parental efforts to persuade the daughter to eat and the daughter's efforts in refusal. Furthermore, the starving daughter has found a way to be extremely rebellious while apparently complying with social and perhaps familial norms for thinness. The theme and the escalation can be taken to the ultimate question of who has literal control of the daughter's life.

When an anorectic daughter is adopted, the behavior control issues were probably part of the marriage from the beginning, well prior to the decision to adopt. At this point the inability to control one's own or one's partner's body in order to produce a child was a dreadful frustration. Some of these parents pursued adoption aggressively in a desperate attempt to have some control over the situation, but then got into power struggles with adoption workers. Once the child was adopted, the control issues were further fought out between parents and/or with the infant over basic functions, such as feeding and sleeping. If the control struggle did not immediately involve the infant, it began when the child gained more autonomy and mobility. By the time an adoptee raised in such a situation reaches adolescence, a daughter may seize on self starvation, whereas a son may engage in uncontrolled misbehavior.

Invariably, the parents of an anorectic daughter seek help, while the daughter does not admit a problem. If she is in an advanced physical state of starvation, she may not be able to think or talk clearly, and therefore is not very accessible. Moley (1987) comments that in severely escalated situations, parents may be just as "addicted" to self-defeating attempts to change the daughter as the daughter is to the physical experience of starvation. He also points out that there are two approaches to resolve such an escalated, life-threatening conflict: One is to empower the parents until the daughter surrenders her symptom, which is the structured approach of Minuchin. The other approach, which Moley espouses, is to operate from a neutral position and to use diplomacy with all family members. The conflict is reframed for parents and daughter as follows: Unwittingly, the daughter has harmed herself while helping her family keep conflict at distance. A related issue is that of how the alliance and control patterns shifted when the daughter was adopted or at any other developmental point in the family's life.

Interventions for School-Related Problems of Adolescents

Whenever a request for family therapy is introduced as related to a junior or senior in high school, a therapist can be fairly certain that impending change and separation are central issues. Two kinds of such requests are directly involved with school behavior. One is that an adolescent who has been doing well enough in school is now failing at least one class, breaking rules in school, or cutting classes. The second is that a teenager who has always done poorly in school — academically, behaviorally, or both — now is doing worse, perhaps threatening to flunk or drop out. Either situation may be exquisitely orchestrated by a senior about to be ineligible to graduate because of missing one credit (often in a course nearly impossible to fail, such as gym). There seems to be a higher proportion of males with pre-graduation problems, in contrast to the eating disorders. Perhaps our society conditions young males to express problems through instrumental and performance areas. In contrast, young females may be conditioned to express problems in areas concerned with nurture.

When the adolescent is also adopted, the therapist can be quite sure that normal individuation issues are causing an extra measure of upheaval in the family organization. The focus of the treatment must be on the nature of the family members' attachments through adoption and the meaning of adoption to each family member. Not only must each person's experience of adoption be reviewed; what each expects when emancipation takes place must also be determined.

When school problems are of more recent onset, the adoptive

family probably functioned relatively well until it snagged on this life stage. There may need to be an immediate, reality-based intervention, such as a plan to get the youth reinstated in school or to help him or her make up work in order to graduate. Beyond that, a therapist can move quickly to focus on the upheaval in relationships. An educative, insight-oriented approach generally produces rapid relief.

When school problems have a long history, the adopted high school student may be carrying out a family role right up to the boundary of childhood. If the young person can avoid graduation from high school, perhaps the passage to emancipation can also be avoided . Often such a family has been in an uproar for some time, but the members still blame it on the adolescent or on adoption. Long-term school problems require persistence and work in small behavioral increments before there is substantial change in the symptoms. The first agenda must be to calm the situation in any way possible. Often an appeal to self-interest is the most effective means to encourage a change in behavior. Then a careful study of how the parents and the adolescent cue each other to maintain the problem is useful. Insight is not sought, nor are the connections to adoption and attachment issues.

Families that are able to go on to work on their relationships generally manage to help the young go on to some useful activity. However, this does not always mean that high school is completed or that a youth leaves home. Others, at the first signs of change, abruptly launch the young person from home or the family from treatment.

> Rick, of Hispanic origins, had been adopted as an infant by non-Hispanic parents. His school difficulties began with learning to read. This was a major concern to his mother, a high achiever in school and work, whereas the father minimized the problem as common to males, including himself.
>
> When Rick turned 16, he announced at his birthday dinner that he wished to be called Ricardo. He planned to quit school and go to Mexico to work on a ranch. Rick had always loved horses and was good with them. Moreover, what little was known about his origins was that he was born on a Mexican ranch to a teenage kitchen worker. Later, in therapy, it emerged that Rick had the fantasy that his father was the rich ranch owner. He felt that this man would be glad to reclaim a son who was excellent with horses, if not school work.
>
> Rick's birthday announcement brought on a near anxiety attack in the mother, who dragged a reluctant son and father to

therapy. Once Ricardo was persuaded not to act on his plans immediately, but to reconsider in therapy what brought him to this, the mother calmed down. Then the father had to be persuaded that Ricardo's wish to leave had serious implications. Ricardo hesitantly told about great distress over his school performance and fears of displeasing his mother, which came as a total revelation to her. Similarly, her feeling that her efforts to help him had been rejected, right down to the name she had chosen, was a new idea to Ricardo. For his part, the father was stunned to realize that his minimizing the problem made Ricardo feel deserted, so that he fantasized a father who would really value him.

Despite this family's ability to discuss their emotions, the treatment process was bumpy. Whenever Ricardo was angry with either parent, he absented himself from school for a day or more, until there was a phone call from school to parents. Then the mother's anxiety again shot up, based on the fear that Rick had or would run away to Mexico; the father again minimized the importance of the situation, saying that Rick would not elope after his promise. Eventually, however, this plan was negotiated: The name would be Ricardo. He would attend high school and get passing grades until he graduated. For every week that he attended all of his classes and did the homework, he could spend one whole day of the weekend with horses. For their next vacation, the family would travel to Mexico together to visit the area where Ricardo was born and to see what more could be learned. Furthermore, all three began dealing more directly with each other: Ricardo put things into words, his father took him more seriously, and his mother listened more calmly.

Interventions for Problems Related to Secrecy about Adoption

In a family where adoption has been kept secret or shrouded under a veil of silence, the cover is likely to come off during the adoptee's adolescence. Normal adolescent identity struggles, enhanced by those of adoption, supply the pressure that forces the emergence. The adoption may emerge because one or both parents have finally decided, sometimes after considerable conflict, that they must tell the young adult before he or she begins a new family. In other instances, the adoptee's suspicions have led to questioning parents or other relatives or to searching the home for documents. Relatives or family friends may have blurted out some remark about the teenager's behavior, such as "What can you expect, considering where Jason came from?" Occasionally the fact emerges after a parent dies and the adoptee finds documents when sorting estate papers. Unfortunately, even late in the 20th century, there are still adults learning for the *first* time of their adoption as infants.

The upset resulting from a young person's discovering his or her adoption at so late a date may bring a family for help. If the discovery coincides with a death or other loss in the family, the upset may assume crisis proportions. The first step is to invite the adoptee to vent his or her reactions (especially grief and distrust), and to ask questions. Other family members are encouraged to listen first and tolerate the adoptee's outpouring. Then the others are given an opportunity to explain the circumstances, reasons, emotions, and possible differences about keeping the secret. While hearing these exchanges, a therapist considers the secrecy about the adoption in comparison to clues about the family's organization and operating rules. For example, a father may say that he always wanted to tell about the adoption, but he deferred to the mother's wish not to tell because they all try to save her from pain. Then the adoptee may express anger that the father always gives in or may agree that the family must protect the mother.

Major attention must be given to the sense of trust between adoptee and parents, and to the degree which it may be shaken. Sometimes an adoptee's feelings of betrayal are offset by relief at finally being able to account for and discuss feelings of dissonance. The initial upheaval must be well vented, with some recovery, before the grief of not having a biological connection can be addressed.

The sense of loss for the adoptee may be profound—a loss of life itself, in the sense of the identity and birth bond previously integrated into the self. Anger is often a strong element in such grief, especially when the adoptee feels betrayed and wonders what else about the family cannot be trusted. Therapy should stay focused on the grief as long as necessary to obtain some resolution.

When there has been a code of not talking about adoption, an adolescent may open the discussion in various ways. An adoptee who has responded through passive acceptance may be driven further into fantasy and/or depression. Other adopted adolescents respond by acting out suppressed feelings, often through some form of running or questing behavior. The adolescent may or may not be consciously aware of the connection between the behavior and his or her hidden origins. Another possibility is that the previously "good adoptee" switches into testing the family operating rules vigorously, especially the rule of silence about origins. The "bad adoptee" whose role it is to test the rules may intensify demands to know more, to see the adoption papers, or to search. Open testing may include insults to the parents' abilities as parents.

Any of these adolescent responses to a rule of silence about adoption may become the problem that a family presents for treatment. Where the adoptee has taken a vigorous verbal stand about the right to know, to talk, and to break secrecy, the therapist should have no difficulty making the assessment. Assessing the problem is more difficult when the adoptee has retreated to fantasy, depression, or unconscious acting out of suppressed emotions. If a therapist notes generally limited communication in the family, this is a clue to the probability of suppressed emotions about adoption as well.

For such a family, the very act of seeing a therapist together to discuss family matters is already a step toward change. If the family members can openly discuss their presenting concern, this is a good sign that they may be able to continue the process. Approaching the presenting symptom through the pattern of interaction clarifies the rules of silence in the family. Perhaps even more important is what the family fears will happen if the rule is changed. Once it is clear that there is a veil over the adoption, the therapist may directly address the circumstances and issues of adoption as quickly as the family can tolerate.

> Joshua, at 15, was a short, slender boy whose serious look was accentuated by dark-rimmed glasses. His parents by adoption were very proud of his intellectual ability and scholarly interests. Their household operated with order and routine: In the evenings the parents sat together, reading and listening to classical music, while Joshua studied in his room.
>
> The family calm was exploded when the parents were called in by the high school principal. Joshua, it seemed had been approaching girls during lunch periods, saying seriously that he was taking a survey. He wanted to know what a girl would find sufficiently attractive in a boy for her engage in sex. Also, he wanted to know whether she would use birth control and what she would do if she became pregnant. Joshua had persisted in his "survey," despite some girls' getting angry and reporting him, while others laughed and called him a "pervert." When the principal talked to Joshua, he politely insisted that he was doing serious research. Concerned that Joshua was becoming socially isolated and perhaps emotionally disturbed, she referred the family for therapy.
>
> The bewildered and mortified parents brought Joshua to the first interview. They had not been able to make themselves

question Joshua, nor could they imagine any explanation for the situation. Joshua solemnly and articulately filled in the silence by explaining at length the nature and rationale of his research. With a small smile, he added that all the adults seemed unnecessarily alarmed. (The fact of adoption had not been mentioned so far.)

Finding it difficult to create an opening, the therapist asked about Joshua's decision to do this research. He was acknowledged for his resourceful approach, even though his methods distressed others. The parents were encouraged to be even more concerned about the meaning of Joshua's behavior. Eventually, the therapist commented that Joshua might have trouble "researching his questions," especially about male development, sex, and what girls find attractive, within the family. Then the fact of his adoption was told.

Just before Joshua began grade school, the parents had given him a brief explanation of his adoption, and added that he was very much wanted. The parents already knew that Joshua was very bright, so when he seemed to understand and never asked more questions, they assumed that all was well. However, when he was asked the right questions, Joshua could indeed report that he had major concerns. He was worried about why he was not growing and developing more male characteristics. Also, he wondered from whom he came and whether that had anything to do with not growing. Already, he had done much book research (in the evenings) into growth patterns, genetics, sex, and adoption. This research led him to conclude that he was genetically doomed to being a small, scholarly sissy all his life. His fears led to his ingenious but unconscious means of getting his worries into the open. At the same time, he was trying to relate to girls and gaining some sense of power from their negative reactions.

Even after Joshua's concerns were known and accepted by his parents, it was not easy for them to talk about the issues but they kept trying. Things finally began to loosen up when the father told Joshua that he too, was concerned about the son's slow growth pattern, and could remember having had similar worries as a teen. The father offered to take Joshua to a doctor, and the offer was gratefully accepted. The opening of communication became complete when the mother said that she could not bear to think of Joshua's birth mother, much less talk about her. Thinking about the birth mother's loss reminded her of the grief of her own four miscarriages. The mother had struggled with her pain and concluded that the living Joshua was the most important. She told Joshua all she knew, and offered to "do research" on what else might be available from the adoption agency.

Interventions for Problems Related to an Adoptee's Role in the Family

When a child is adopted as an infant to fill a vacant role in the family, by adolescence the child is well entrenched in that role. In such cases, the adolescent is brought to therapy identified as "the problem." Depending on the type of regulation of the family organization and the psychological reasons for the adoption, the situation may or may not be amenable to change.

In instances where a well-functioning spouses have adopted to "solve their grief," that dynamic does not necessarily become problematic. The child still may be the focus of the family, as the major source of pleasure and distractor from sorrow. But the importance of the adoptee's role leads to increased anxiety for all when the threat of emancipation and changed relationships loom. In response to the family's anxiety, a teenager is likely to intensify the role of distractor, escalating behavior that has served the purpose before. Furthermore, the behavior is exquisitely designed to fly against some important family value, thereby guaranteeing parental attention and distraction from separation anxiety. The problem behavior also seems to show that the young person is irresponsible or immature, and thus not ready to leave home. For example, a policeman's son may be caught riding with friends in a stolen car; a minister's daughter may get drunk in public; a teacher's child may be suspended from school.

In a more functional family, where the adoptee's special role has only become problematic in adolescence, therapy can follow a typical path. As soon as the presenting problem has been changed, the focus shifts to issues of loss inherent in launching and adoption. If the family theme is expressivity, the members may never have expressed their grief about the lack of birth bond. Thus they are unprepared for, and perhaps unaware of, the double impact of loss when they are no longer in a daily relationship.

A more dysfunctional situation occurs when parents have adopted a child to fill the role of distractor from marital difficulties. By the time the child reaches adolescence, this dynamic has evolved into a moderately to severely problematic arrangement of a "united-front" marriage with a misbehaving teenager. In these cases, the initial focus must stay on the parental response to the adolescent's behavior. Although there is apparent agreement between the parents about setting limits on the teen's behavior, often one or both has subtle ways of not cooperating, which perpetuate the problem. The resulting message of "We can't do anything to stop you" is the cue to the young person that there really is no wish for the behavior to stop.

Two approaches may be useful with the united-front dynamic. One is to find out in great detail how much time and energy is expended by parents on the youth. Then the therapist can wonder what would happen or what else would be possible if the parents were not so invested in the adolescent.

At the same time, the therapist can admire the teenager's ability to keep the parents' attention on himself or herself, and thus to distract them from any other possible worries. Often there is some slight nonverbal recognition from the teen to tell the therapist that this is the right track. This approach can be held or amplified until a family member announces readiness for change.

The second approach is to watch for any possible cracks in the parental unity during initial discussion of the presenting problem. When even the smallest disagreements are observed, they are fostered, but indirectly. Calling direct attention to a budding disagreement may drive it back behind the facade. The two approaches may be used in combination.

At the beginning of treatment, the pivotal question is whether or not there is any flexibility in the united front. If the arrangements show potential for change, no matter how slowly, then it is possible to go beyond adjustment of the pattern of behavior. When a therapist deals with these marital issues, it is appropriate for the adolescent to be excused from sessions. If the teenager can join peer group therapy, the path of therapy runs parallel to and supports the emancipation process. When there is negligible flexibility in the united-front arrangement, however, families tend to withdraw from treatment soon. In their typical way of projecting blame, they may complain that the therapist is incompetent. The pattern then is maintained, while the family members try, and leave, many human service programs and therapists. Such patterns may be lifelong, changing only when someone dies or is incarcerated in a mental hospital or prison.

The most dismal prognosis applies to adolescents adopted in infancy to fill the role of nurturer for one or two, very needy parents. By this life stage, this type of dysfunctional family is characterized by blurred boundaries and role reversals. Usually there is a combination of enmeshed and distanced relationships, wherein the adolescent adoptee is the partial caretaker of at least one parent. Such a dysfunctional system is threatened by any change, particularly any moves toward individuation by the adoptee, and the members work to avoid it. Under such circumstances, the young person may give up on individuation and then develop psychotic symptoms, making it impossible to leave. An alternative outcome is a sudden rejection and extrusion, leading to a complete cutoff of relationships. This may be instigated by the adolescent's running away or by an involuntary institutional placement. When parents eject the adoptee, they may go to the extent of seeking dissolution of the adoption.

When an adolescent who as been adopted to fill a needed role, begins to individuate from a loosely organized, dysfunctional family, generalized anxiety causes the system to fluctuate frantically. The fluctuation moves between parental attempts to restrain the adolescent's independence and attitudes of disregard or unconcern. If these families get to therapy at all, they are seen by counselors at social institutions, such as hospitals or courts.

The specific problematic behavior of whatever family members can be induced to attend meetings must be the major focus initially, and perhaps for a long time. It may not ever be possible to address life stage or adoption issues among family members. The adopted adolescent raised in this type of dysfunctional family should be offered individual treatment as soon as possible. Therein, appropriate self-responsibility can be supported, and the adoption and the adoptee's role in the family can be addressed. (For further discussion of the treatment and hospitalization of disturbed adopted adolescents, see Fullerton, Goodrich, & Berman, 1986; Goodrich, Fullerton, Yates, & Berman, 1990; Grotevant, McRoy, 1990; and Grotevant, McRoy, & Jenkins, 1988; Pierce, personal communication; Powers, 1984).

Interventions for Problems with Adolescent Behavior Control

The adopted child who has not been given adequate limits can become totally out of control during adolescence. In this instance, the normal testing of family values translates to a scream for needed limits (see also Schmidt, 1968). An adoptive family may come to therapy with an adolescent who seems out of control to them, but the problem is still amenable to change. Usually in such cases, the family organization has functioned fairly well until this life stage. Then the adolescent's need to test has strained the family's ability to cope, thereby raising anxiety and conflict to new levels. With such a family, therapy proceeds in a typical way, beginning with an initial focus on the problems related to limits. From there the background of adoption, in view of the life stage, is discussed.

Long-standing, severe difficulty with setting limits may result from parental characterological deficits in regard to behavior control. Such parents may react by increasing ineffective responses, such as being inconsistent, canceling each other out, or giving up in helplessness; thereupon an escalation can develop to the point of risk to life, limb, or membership in the family. As the adoptee escalates out of control, parents often shop for a therapist who will somehow take control. Here, the key factor is whether or not the parents can be persuaded that *they* must take charge. Often these parents are not able to get the teenager to sessions. It is not crucial for the teen to be there initially, because the outcome depends on whether or not the parents are motivated to change. Usually the initial meetings are a struggle between parents and therapist about who should take charge of the adolescent. Parents may offer a litany of complaints intended to persuade the therapist that there is nothing the parents can do. They seem to believe that somewhere there are magical words that if discovered and said just right, will turn the teen instantly into a rule-abiding citizen.

A therapist must use any means at hand to heighten the parental sense of responsibility, whether by educating, warning about the future, or appealing to wishes to be good parents. The therapist offers much support, while pointing out that the teenager *will not* voluntarily make the desired changes and the therapist *cannot* do it. Once the parents agree that they must take charge, one very small behavioral item is selected as the starting place. Great care must be taken with this initial item for change, because the outcome is critical for what will follow. When a particular limit is selected for the adolescent, all possible terms, contingencies, and loopholes must be considered. This includes the exact nature of the limit and how it is to be applied, the advantage of compliance, and the consequences of noncompliance. Especially important is the identification of each parent's vulnerability to backing down, plus a plan for how the parents will signal for and get reinforcement from each other. Working out such terms in regard to even a very modest limit can be very difficult, but diagnostic of how much real change is possible.

The difficulty in making an initial plan is mirrored by difficulty in carrying it out. If the therapist sees that there is genuine motivation to change, but entrenched patterns that resist change, prescriptions from various strategic or Ericksonian approaches may be considered (Schaffer & Lindstrom, 1990; Whiting, 1988). In such approaches a directive or ritual is set up, which forces change in entrenched behavior patterns and/or beliefs, without engaging conscious awareness of the purpose of the intervention.

These families introduce the fact of adoption early, often as an explanation of the problem; however, if they do not, the therapist must focus upon it earlier than is typical. Because the issues of adoption and of behavior control are deeply entwined in these families, they are basic to the resistance to change. Thus they need to be addressed as soon as they surface as blocks to motivation, to negotiating an initial plan, or to carrying out a plan.

With these families, the therapist's use of self is more critical than ever. A therapist must be actively in charge of sessions, firm about following up on agreements, and clear in acknowledgment of compliance or noncompliance. Thus, the therapist models the handling of limits with parents, in a process parallel to that being encouraged between parents and teenager.

Families with out-of-control adolescents usually stay in treatment briefly or settle in for the long haul. Among the parents who stay very briefly are those who cannot or will not agree that it is their responsibility to set limits, so they depart. Others work until they begin to experience success in getting the desired changes, and then they withdraw. If parents with control problems can get past the initial hurdles, they often need a long time to work on the patterns of interaction.

> Max and Olga, a couple in their late 50s, applied for help, saying they had come about their "beautiful adopted daughter, Joy." The problem was that Joy, now 18, had left home and, they thought, was bunking with various of her streetwise friends, mostly male. The parents were quite sure there was heavy drinking and feared drug use. Parents reported a long history of problems with Joy, and an equally long list of resources from which they had sought help for her. This report was punctuated with references to Joy's beauty, popularity, and physical maturation at 11.
>
> Max, a dapper, trim man, was considerably smaller than Olga, who was tall and heavy. Both of them were refugees who had come from eastern Europe alone as young adults, and then met at gatherings of their ethnic group in a U.S. city. Loneliness caused them to latch onto each other and to hope for a replacement family. When this did not happen, they sought neither medical help nor adoption. A friend who worked in an obstetrician's office met Joy's birth mother and told Max and Olga; subsequently, a private adoption was arranged. "Joy seemed like a gift from heaven," the parents said. She was so unexpected and beautiful and clever. Since she also had a mind of her own

from the beginning, they followed her lead, doing everything they could to keep her happy.

When Joy matured, according to the mother, she "had a gorgeous figure that boys and men always noticed." The mother permitted her to go on dates from age 13, with young men as old as 22. But, Olga assured the therapist, this was permitted only if she knew the young men's families to be wealthy and prestigious within their ethnic group. By the time Joy entered high school, she was rebelling against her mother's directives about appearance, bathing, clothes, and dates. Occasionally she skipped a day of school or was out all night. Such events led to vigorous verbal battles between Joy and the mother. The father stayed out of the conflict, but remained supportive to both, separately.

Joy barely graduated from high school. During and after her senior year, she spent increasing amounts of time away from home "with her friends." Currently, her visits were only for the hour it took to eat a big meal and take a shower. When Joy was out of the house, the mother spent most of her time doing "detective work" about Joy's whereabouts and activities or consulting resources for advice. Meanwhile, Joy phoned her father every few days, telling him that she missed him and asking for money. This was provided with Olga's agreement, so that "Joy won't have to turn to prostitution."

The beginning of therapy was also a battle. The parents wanted a magic solution and resisted the idea that *they* had to *do* something. Finally they agreed to take responsibility, in large part because the therapist insisted that it was their responsibility as parents. With many false starts, a plan was worked out for handling Joy's phone calls to her father and visits to the house. Every contingency that Joy might try, or that could cause either parent to give in, was considered. The parents were coming to appointments biweekly; the plan was in place by the third meeting. Two weeks later, they reported that they had carried out the arrangements quite well. The father cited evidence that Joy was beginning to cooperate, even though she complained. The mother, however, said that there was no change and that father was being duped.

At the next (and last) session, the mother sadly reported that Joy "had caused" her to lose her temper. She had screamed at Joy, "Stop playing up to Dad to get around the rules — you are hopeless and you can just stay away for good!" Olga said that Joy was too far gone for *them* (the parents) to do anything, so she would not make another appointment. Instead, she planned to find a deprogrammer who would seize Joy and take her to some locked room or other situation where she could be forced to change. Max quietly said that he did not entirely agree with Olga, but he had to go along with her.

Interventions for Parent–Adolescent "Mismatch" Problems

When there has been a sense of parent–adoptee mismatch that has grown until the adoptee's adolescence, the presenting problem most often is a form of angry behavior by the adoptee. Long-festering feelings of not fitting in or being valued seem to explode. The behavior carries the message, which may or may not be in the adoptee's conscious awareness, "If you think I'm so bad or different, I'll just show you." Often the behavior is well designed to attack a particular vulnerability of the parents, embarrass them publicly, and/or show the community what bad parents they are. Externalized forms of this behavioral message may include public intoxication on any type of substance, drunk driving, getting caught with a stolen car or shoplifted merchandise, vandalism, or fire setting. Internalized forms of the message may include phobias, major depression, secret substance abuse, or eating disorders.

When this type of adoptive family first comes for treatment when the adoptee is an adolescent, almost always the symptoms are quite severe. Since the sense of mismatch is related to problems in attachment, the uneasiness in the relationships is further complicated by the life stage need for more distance and preparation to separate. Under these conditions, identity issues related to the adoption and the need to rearrange the dependency relationships become extremely complex. Generally, the conflict level of the family is high and pervasive, as accusations and blame fly among family members in hot or cold wars. Without projection of problems to forces outside the family, adoption is blamed as the source of trouble. There may be open threats that the adoptee will run away or be thrown out.

In assessing this type of family, a therapist's first clues may come from his or her own reactions. One such clue is a visceral reaction to the intensity of conflict or hatred and its focus within the family on the adoption; another is a sense that relationships in a family or the reactions between a parent and teenager are somehow "not right." Some clinicians are so well attuned to this that they accurately guess an adoption before they are told. As a means to take charge of a session firmly and interrupt conflict, a therapist can insist that family members talk only to the therapist. It may be useful to move those family members who are not to speak out of eye contact, to have them sit in the far corner of the room, or to place them so that their backs are turned. Sometimes the only way to stop conflict and to hear each person is to split sessions or a series of sessions into different combinations of individuals and dyads.

In any case, the question of the future of the relationships preferably follows from dealing with the present situation. When that is the sequence, planning for the future can be completed with healing and reconstitution of relationships on a more adult basis. More often, in these cases, the future is tangled with the issues of the present and past. All the issues are compressed into a push for an immediate decision about where the adoptee is to live. The therapist's goal is to guide them to the most reasonable decisions, in the best interests of all, that are possible.

> Junior, now 14, was born in Vietnam, the son of a native woman and a U.S. soldier. His father called him "my little Junior," a name to which his mother, and later he, clung.
>
> After his father went home, his mother eked out an existence for them for 2 more years. Then the mother brought Junior to an American service group for children, asking that they try to send him to "his father's country."
>
> When Junior was 3, he was flown to the United States for adoption by Jim and Marva. They were well-regarded high school teachers in a small city where there were few Asian people. When Marva and Jim first appeared with 3-year-old Junior, there were many questions about his origins. Frequently, people commented that they were just the kind of people who would rescue a child.
>
> Life at home was not so enjoyable, however. To the parents, Junior seemed stolid, unresponsive, and guarded. He resisted being held and stayed wherever put, quietly playing with toys he could reach. But he came to life when food was offered. Initially, he snatched the food and held it close to his body, taking quick, furtive bites. Some time later, he began hiding and hoarding food in his room. Junior also could get lively when there were other children around. He clutched toys to himself, punched at any child who approached, or suddenly swooped on another child, snatching away a toy.
>
> Within the year of Junior's placement, Jim and Marva were experiencing a painful paradox: Despite the public regard in which they were held as teachers, they felt rejected by a child in their own home and had new problems in the community. Junior

also was confused by experiencing his parents' frustration at home, while outside he heard them called "saints." When Junior began school, he seemed uninterested and did not learn well. His problems with other children continued. Now the increasingly frustrated teacher/parents were being called to school conferences, in the role opposite to which they were accustomed. Eventually there were periods when family life proceeded calmly and routinely, if not warmly; however, just when a period of quiet coexistence made the parents think that the problems were easing, some new incident always turned up.

When Junior began junior high school, he became close friends with another loner, Luke. The two of them dressed only in black and had a belligerent attitude toward peers and adults. By now Marva was in despair about the situation. Jim felt similarly but was still trying to relate to Junior. The turning point came about 5 months after Junior's 14th birthday. The incident began with the boys' raiding Luke's father's liquor cabinet. After drinking enough to be boisterous, they swaggered to the high school where four boys were shooting baskets. Junior and Luke called the boys obscene names; when this was ignored, Luke grabbed the ball and Junior shoved the boy who came after it. A fight broke out, stopped by police who were called by a passer-by. When the parents were called to the police station, Marva refused to go. Jim retrieved Junior and brought him home to bed. That evening, Marva said for the first time that she could not go on with Junior. She felt that the adoption had never worked for any of them, and that Junior did not even like them. Jim felt more mixed reactions and suggested therapy.

When the family came in, Junior wore a blue shirt and jeans. Although silent, he seemed more frightened than belligerent. He said little when the parents explained what had happened, even though both were quite open about their distress. But when Marva began to talk about her despair and the long history of difficulties, Junior erupted. He accused them of always picking on him and of feeling that other people's opinions were more important than his. With that opening, it was possible to get each of them to talk about the emotions and impressions they had about the meanings of their interactions. Over the next six meetings, the whole pattern of their relationships was reviewed, with misunderstandings, angers, and fears acknowledged.

As a result, they worked out a plan for a trial separation, which seemed necessary for Marva and Junior because of their accumulated anger with each other. During the separation, they all agreed to work to make an effort to rebuild their relationships and reattach in a different way. The parents located a group home for teenage boys run by their church in the nearest big city. While at the group home, Junior would finish high school and receive group and individual therapy. Also, he was to get help in contacting the Vietnamese community in the city. The parents agreed to continue in treatment as well. They would visit Junior on a regular schedule, and he would be invited home. The length of home visits was to increase as all felt satisfied with prior visits and ready for more.

Junior remained at the group home until he was 18. He finished high school, but never returned home to live on a permanent basis; instead, he was a regular, welcome visitor, particularly for holidays. The relationship between Junior and his parents never became demonstrative and close, but it did become cordial and comfortable.

Interventions for Families Adopting Adolescents

Some youngsters are placed for adoption just before or during adolescence. Placement at such a late date suggests that a youth has special needs or has only recently been freed for adoption by a court. The youngster may have been a ward of the state for some time, and often has had multiple foster placements. Sometimes, the young person has spent most of his or her life with one family — either a neglectful birth family or a long-term foster family.

When children are placed in adoption at about the time of puberty, the multiple levels and interactions of all the issues are confounding and often paradoxical. These children are of adolescent years but often function at much earlier developmental levels, as a result of deprivation, lack of stability, and/or abuse. So these are adolescent bodies containing the needs of much younger children. Moreover, these teens are entering families at a time when they would normally be involved with preparations to leave. Parents need to foster attachment at very the time at which increased distance is appropriate (at least between children and opposite-gender parents). In the face of these life stage issues for everyone, there is no common background or reservoir of good will to sustain relationships during difficult times.

Adolescents may be placed in homes where the parents are already experienced with adolescents, who may still be there or are launched. Some parents seem to resolve midlife issues by making a career out of their skills with teenagers, thereby in effect creating a group home. Others prefer one adolescent at a time in order to maximize nurture. Ideally, the needs of an adolescent should be carefully matched to the abilities of a family.

Parents who adopt an adolescent may seek therapeutic help during placement, as part of the placement plan. Otherwise, the request may come any time, but most likely early in the placement. Almost always, the assessment of a newly adopted adolescent leads to a recommendation for individual treatment for the adoptee. This individual treatment should be provided by someone other than the family therapist, but the individual and family therapists should coordinate their efforts. The teenager needs the extra time and a person just for himself or herself, because of all the paradoxical issues and difficult history. Individual therapy may be needed for some time, with eventual consideration of group therapy or a peer group related to adoption issues.

The central questions for the family therapist are how much to see the parents by themselves and on what schedule to include the new adoptee. Initially, it is advisable to see the parents mostly as a couple, because they need massive support and reinforcement for their individual and team efforts. An adolescent who is newly in adoptive placement soon engages in some sort of testing; parents may need help in sorting out the meaning of behavior and appropriate responses. From knowing a child's background, a therapist can educate the parents about the effects of deprivation on development and about lags that are discrepant with life stage. Mostly, however, the parents need the opportunity to report specific incidents with the teenager and to vent their emotions. Then they can look at what worked or not and consider alternatives.

These youngsters are likely to fluctuate between extremes of infantile behavior and bold attempts to act adult. Parents can be hard put to know where to draw lines between behavior to be accepted and behavior on which to put limits. Furthermore, there is great variety in what parents consider deviant behavior. Sometimes a therapist may have to help parents become more aware of the parameters of their tolerance and become more accepting. A therapist can also offer some general guidelines to new adoptive parents of an adolescent whose behavior fluctuates. Infantile behavior is to be confined to the interior of the home; behavior outside the home is to be age-appropriate. For example, the 14-year-old who likes to cuddle can do that at home, perhaps while watching TV. The teen is not to do that with parents on a city bus or to solicit the same from peers on the school bus.

The factor that makes nurturing an adolescent especially tricky is sexuality. Most youngsters who are finally adopted as adolescents have great neediness for nurture, while also experiencing sexual urges. Often they are confused about nurture, love, and sexual activity. If there is any history of sexual image distortion, early exposure, or abuse, the confusion can be severe. Thus an emotionally needy 13-year-old boy may try to touch his new mother's breasts or ask her to give him a bath. Or a 15-year-old girl may want to sit on her new father's lap, alternating between the behavior of a begging infant and a coquette. Most parents experience sufficient distress about such paradoxes to discuss them with their therapist. If not, the therapist must introduce the probable confounding of nurture and sexuality. If a therapist does not provide a vent, sexual steam can explode the family.

Mercidie was born to a teenage white mother and a black father who lived in the same poverty-stricken area of a big city. Mercidie's skin was light enough to make her stand out among her black relatives, while her hair made her noticeable among her white relatives. The first few years of Mercidie's life were spent with her mother in her grandmother's home while her father continued to visit.

By the time Mercidie was 4, however, her father was long gone and her mother had moved, frequently changing locations. For the next 7 years, Mercidie mostly lived with her grandmother, who continually tried to locate and persuade her mother to take the child. Sometimes the mother did keep Mercidie with her for a few weeks, but then left her with various of her own or the birth father's relatives. Eventually, Mercidie always returned to the home of her maternal grandmother. There she was fed, clothed, and not mistreated, but she was not given any attention either. The main message was "Stay out of the way."

Finally, the grandmother became ill and could not keep Mercidie at all, nor could her mother be located. She was then brought into the state's child welfare program. By the time Mercidie was 13, she was legally free for and was placed in adoption. She was adopted by Jack, aged 60, and Sarah, aged 52. They were a hearty couple who had successfully raised three children, the youngest of whom had just married and moved out of state. Both spouses felt good about raising their children and were motivated to continue. Mercidie's mixed racial heritage did not bother them, because they considered themselves "all American" and Jack was proud of a Native American ancestor.

At 13, Mercidie was an attractive girl who could pass for 15. She was happy to have a permanent home with two parents all to herself. She tried hard to please and not to get in anyone's way; on the other side, parents were delighted with such an agreeable child. Before 2 months had passed, however, Jack and Sarah consulted a therapist. In relating to Sarah, Mercidie often took the stance of an infant. She asked for help in getting dressed and for her food to be served to her, cut up, or even fed to her, while she sat as close to Sarah as possible. Also, she frequently said that she loved Sarah and that she would never grow up and leave her as Sarah's other children had.

With Jack, on the other hand, Mercidie's approach was quite different. She loved to parade in new clothes before him, especially shorts or tight jeans. Often she asked him to rub her neck and then wiggled her hips in front of him. Of even more concern was her flirtatious response to the attention she received from boys and men outside the home, and her apparent agreement to whatever was suggested. On one occasion, the parents intervened when an 18-year-old boy invited Mercidie into his car. He was shocked to hear that Mercidie was only 13.

The initial therapeutic plan was that the parents would be seen intensively for a while, while Mercidie began individual treatment. With help from the therapist to sort out the factors from Mercidie's background and her developmental confusion, these capable parents worked out appropriate responses that also protected Mercidie. They readily acknowledged that they had been disconcerted by behavior they had never coped with, but they also could laugh and say that it was never too late for parents to learn.

For the next 6 months there continued to be harrowing moments. After that, the parents came for an occasional meeting with or without Mercidie, who continued in individual treatment. By the end of the first year, they were enjoying a growing sense of being a family.

Interventions for Families Considering Adoption Dissolution

Paralleling the growing numbers of requests to family therapists for divorce counseling, there will be more requests for help from adoptive families regarding the question of adoption dissolution. In the last few years, there have been a number of research studies on adoption disruption with findings relevant to the clinician. Among these studies there is a fairly consistent report that special needs adoptions are disrupted at about the rate of 11%. Also, there is a consensus that higher rates of disruption are associated with children who are older at placement, have had more prior placements, and have larger numbers of problems. Festinger's (1990) study indicated that the adoptions of children placed between ages 6 and 10 were disrupted at the rate of 8–11%; the adoptions of children placed after age 11 were disrupted at the rate of 16–19%.

Barth and Berry (1988), as well as Partridge, Hornby, and McDonald (1986), found that the factor contributing the most to disruption is insufficient or misleading preparation of parents and adoptee. If either party has inadequate information about the other, a mismatch of expectations contributes to problems from the beginning. One recent finding has particular relevance to the family clinician: *Family factors are more important than the behavior or problems of the special needs adoptee.* Barth and Berry (1988) point out that even the best-functioning families need extra services and resources to withstand the stresses related to special needs adoption. When the most difficult children are placed with already vulnerable and poorly prepared families, the possibility of disruption soars.

Stein and Hoopes (1985) found that the quality of relationships in a family was the best predictor of disruption. Nelson (1985) also found that the *whole* family was important in the prevention of disruption. Most recently, an even more specific finding by Bourguignon (1989) indicates that the *quality of the parents'* marriage is the most important factor in whether a special needs adoption is disrupted. The most crucial aspect is the ability of spouses to work cooperatively as parents. This factor significantly distinguished placements that were disrupted from those that were not — not the behavior of the children.

The message is clear to the counselor faced with a family considering the dissolution of an adoption: The initial evaluation of the state of the relationships and the potential for repair *must* take the *whole* family into account. Furthermore, special attention must be given to the quality of the marital/parental coalition.

An adoptive family in which disruption may be impending usually seeks help in a crisis centered around the adoptee. Standard crisis theory supports interventions designed to get the family back to its precrisis arrangements (homeostasis). Such an approach may not be appropriate, however, when a family defines an adoptee as "the problem." It may reinforce the members' definition of the problem and lead them to return to their precrisis status by expelling the child.

Instead, when a family seeks help in such a crisis, a therapist needs to take the position that expulsion is not a simple solution. The focus is on eliciting ambivalence and considering which painful alternative is most tolerable: the daily struggle of dealing with the child, or grief and guilt over failing with a child who is no longer present. Parallel alternatives confront the adoptee as well. Thus, instead of accepting an "instant solution" of ejecting the adoptee, the crisis is generalized to the pain and losses involved for every person.

In the course of generalizing to the whole family, the positions of the parents and the strength of their marriage must be assessed. In particular, the parents' ability to cooperate must be weighed against the degree of conflict between them about anything, but especially about the adoptee. In situations where one parent is always the spokesperson while the other seems to concur, it is necessary to elicit a spoken opinion from the quiet one. In many cases, adoptive *mothers* of children with special needs instigate, promote, and handle the adoption and all the associated procedures. On the other hand, usually adoptive *fathers* finally declare that the youngsters must leave or the adoption must end. Therefore, it is necessary to trace the history, as well as the current position of *each* parent when an adoption disruption is under consideration.

Another factor for the clinician to consider while assessing the potential for adoption disruption is the stage at which therapeutic intervention is requested. Partridge et al. (1986) have identified six stages of disruption:

1. There is diminishing pleasure in the relationship.
2. The child is seen as *the* problem.
3. The family goes public (i.e., some one outside the family is told of the problem).
4. There is a turning point—disruption becomes a spoken possibility.
5. A deadline or ultimatum is laid down.
6. The decision is made to disrupt the adoption.

Awareness of these stages can help a therapist assess the state of the relationships. Educating a family about the stages may provide a structure that can help calm the situation. The earlier in the process the family has sought help, the better the possibility of working out the best plan for all members. The further along the process has moved, the less likely it is that disruption can be prevented, but even at stages 5 and 6 it is possible. Even if the family members decide that they cannot live together, even temporarily, the relationships may be salvaged (as in Junior's case, described above). A not-so-intimate adoptive family, whether living together or not, maintains its attachments in ways not so different from those of many birth families.

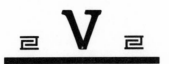

THE LIFETIME IMPACT
OF ADOPTION

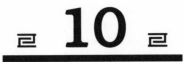

10

The Adoptee as Spouse and Parent

Themes and Issues in Marriage: A Review

The quality of any individual's formative attachments is proven in young adult relationships, especially relationships with the other sex and mate selection. According to the concept of equivalence, a person seeks a mate who is at a similar developmental level, in order to have a sense of familiarity and fit. Each mate looks for an exchange that enhances the self and promotes a sense of wholeness and well-being. If relationships in the family of origin have supported maturation, the person may look to marriage for a replication of the good aspects of those relationships. At the same time, there can be hope that the psychological exchange within marriage will provide restitution and growth in the inevitable areas of vulnerability. The particulars of the individual's experience bear directly on the psychological issues and associated behavior brought to dating and mate selection.

The typical psychological theme (from the schema in Chapter 2) for a marriage of young adults is competence. The young adult who has successfully emancipated himself or herself from, and gained adult status within, the family of origin can now turn to the next developmental stage. The task of the next stage is to develop adult competence in social roles, such as worker, intimate partner, friend, member of the community, and perhaps spouse and parent. Even the best-functioning young adult has anxieties associated with the major life decisions of choosing an occupation and a mate. After the big decisions are made, proficiency in the new roles must be developed in order to establish a sense of adequacy within them.

Young spouses whose psychological exchange is centered around this typical theme may relate to it behaviorally in several ways. They may support and enhance each other's competence, in an exchange that is satisfying to both as well as durable. Another possibility is that they compete in regard to some aspects of competence, vying to establish who is better at a particular role. In still another arrangement, they may develop a complementary role division in which each is valued for different areas of competence. Whatever the pattern of interaction, young spouses who enhance each other in the struggle for competence in adult roles subsequently move on to the theme of identity: They forge and then consolidate a secure sense of who they are as a couple and as individuals.

In contrast, for some other spouses, competence remains the theme of the marriage permanently. In such a case, the partners' sense of adequacy in social roles is fraught with anxiety from the past or from failures in the present. These individuals have probably come from less functional families and have undergone a skewed or partial emancipation process. Attachments to members of families of origin are overly strong, overly weak, or some of each; in any case, energy is still bound in the original families, so that it is not available for the individuals' further development. In a marriage where continuing anxieties about competence reinforce this theme, there is likely to be a negative cycle of failures, which feeds an increasing sense of inadequacy. Both spouses may participate in such a cycle, such as when both are repeatedly fired from jobs. More often, the increased sense of inadequacy leads to a complementary role division of the type that has sometimes been called an "overadequate–underadequate" relationship. In extreme form, one person sacrifices competence for the pseudocompetence of the other; this often results in a symptomatic spouse and a caretaker.

More severe attachment deficits or skewed alliances may have created developmental "stuckness" on the earlier themes of expressivity, behavior control, or nurture. At any of these levels, a spouse is likely to be more needy and to look to the mate for reparation of the original attachment difficulties. But since both spouses are at an equivalent level of development, they are equally needy and equally unable to give what is needed. Some of these relationships may be marked by conflict, but nevertheless may remain stable over long periods of time. In others, attachments may be constantly broken off and then resumed. In still other cases, individuals may have a series of partners.

Themes and Issues in Marriage for the Adoptee

The young adult who was adopted as an infant comes to the age of mate selection with additional formative pressures. These include not only the usual shaping experiences of the family dynamics, but also the interplay of adoption issues with the dynamics. The more functional adoptive family has coped with the anxieties and successfully launched the adoptee. With this family achievement as a foundation, the adoptee can move appropriately to focus energies on his or her development as a competent adult. This includes dating and the selection of a spouse with whom there is a good developmental fit and mutually beneficial psychological exchange.

The interplay of family dynamics and adoption can have a special effect for the long-awaited, highly prized adoptee who was raised as an only child. Such an adoptee may be doubly imbued with a sense of privilege and competence, which is based primarily on the ability to please the older generation. The outcome for actual adult competence may fall anywhere in the range of functionality. At the more functional end, the adoptee's employment and spouse continue to enhance the sense of privilege in exchanges that are mutually beneficial. At the less functional end, the adoptee fights with employer and spouse to gain a continual sense of being special. Or the adoptee may switch both employers and mates frequently, looking for the one in each case who will provide constant admiration.

In another form of interplay between family dynamics and adoption, the whole adoptive family may be organized around the theme of competence. The marriage may have been based on issues of competence, and subsequently anxieties may have been exaggerated by the inability to have children by birth. After a child is adopted, anxieties may shift to a focus on parenting, perhaps as measured by some standard of perfection. The adoptee may strongly sense such anxiety and respond by being a "good, achieving" individual so that the parents can be affirmed in their abilities. This "good" role in achieving the parental expectations may be carried into choices of career and spouse that please the parents. Another possibility is that the "good" adoptee rebels against the role during adolescence; then the effect on mate selection may be to find a "good" spouse who soothes or supports the rebelliousness.

Still another outcome related to a theme of competence is that parental anxieties may induce poor performance, thus setting up an escalating cycle of anxiety and focus on the adoptee. This type of cycle may also ensue when there is a sense of mismatch between one or both parents and the adoptee. A perceived mismatch, and self-blame about it, may cause either the parents and/or the adoptee to try harder in their roles with each other. Regardless of the source of a negative cycle related to competence, any type of symptoms can develop from such escalating anxiety. Usually these issues first show up in the adoptee's school performance. As the time for emancipation approaches, the family anxiety may become severe, inducing the adoptee further into a role of incompetence. Problems develop in regard to graduation from high school, dating, and planning for an occupation. As a result, if the adoptee marries at all, the relationship is likely to take an "overadequate–underadequate" form, with the adoptee taking either role.

The issues of adoption can also interact strongly with the next earlier psychological theme — that is, expressivity. Here there is a direct connection between the adoptive family's operating rules about expression of emotion in general and with the rules about adoption. The adoptive family may have suppressed most emotions, or anger or sadness in particular. In such situations there are often rules of secrecy concerning the adoption, which force the adoptee into an internal life of fantasy and/or depression. Such an internal resolution can become a major factor in mate selection. The adoptee may seek someone who provides understanding and comfort, or at the least tolerates depression. In a case where the internal load is too great, the adoptee may take little risk in new relationships with either gender. Another possibility is that the adoptee avoids peer relationships by putting all energy into the earliest one (i.e., fantasies about and search for the birth mother).

In an adoptive family whose issues are centered around the theme of behavior control, the adoptee may have grown up as an indulged child without sufficient limits. An adoptee raised in such circumstances may select a partner for a tempestuous relationship, before and after marriage. Such a relationship is fraught with demands for rights and blame over wrongs. Another alternative for mate selection related to a theme of behavior control is to find a mate who takes the role of firm parent; the spouse then provides the controls and struggles to keep the adoptee in line. Still another possibility is to find a mate with similar issues who has found the needed structure in some organization, such as a religious or self-help group. Whether the spouse first found the group or it is found together, the group provides the guidelines (sometimes very strict ones) for control of behavior.

Finally, the adoptee may have grown up in a family where there are issues of basic nurture. In such a case, the purpose of the adoption has been to serve the needs of the parents. The problems of role induction to the service of parental needs are often expressed early, through eating and attachment difficulties. The pattern may be set for continuing problems with eating and other forms of basic nurture, such as physical affection and, later, money. When the interplay of family dynamics and adoption is centered around early developmental issues, there is always some difficulty with emancipation. At best, the adoptee's attempts at emancipation are only partially successful. The result has a direct effect on whether the adoptee marries and what type of spouse is selected.

When an adoptee is raised in a dysfunctional family, the additional loading on attachments makes that adoptee worse off than if he or she had been born to the family. The outcome for an adoptee is also worsened if the family is severely dysfunctional and/or the adoptee has an inflexible role of symptom bearer. Other factors that contribute to poor outcomes are the adoptee's being older when adopted, having been in multiple homes, or having been abused.

When adoptees from such backgrounds do marry, they create dysfunctional marriages in which concerns about nurture and quality of attachment are central. Behavioral arrangements centered around these issues permit one or both to be openly dependent or counterdependent and distant. Often there is general conflict, as well as competition for allegiance between the spouse and the adoptive family. Some adoptees raised in dysfunctional families do not risk relationships at all, or do so only briefly. An adoptee may retreat to spend adulthood with the adoptive family of origin. Or the adoptee may only engage in serial brief encounters or back off to live alone in relative isolation.

In addition to the ways in which adoption can interact with specific types of family dynamics, there are some general issues that may affect adoptees' passage to adulthood. The extra emotional burdens of adoption (loss, dual heritage, identity issues) can cause adoptees to lag developmentally. Even when they are functioning well and on schedule in dealing with young adult role competence, adoptees may experience more anxiety than is typical.

Since adoptees are subject to bigger loads of grief and pain because of their early losses, they often have heightened longing for relationships in which they truly belong and that they have been equal participants in choosing. Such loads of emotion may weigh down energy, thus causing development to lag and keeping the adoptees in a position to enter relationships centered around the earlier theme of expressivity. One effect of such developmental lag is that young adult adoptees may function best at work and in other task-oriented roles. At the same time, they may be reluctant to test or have difficulty in testing social competence with the opposite gender. The teachings of the adoptive families about gender relations and loyalties to parents, as well as the adoptees' strong sensitivities to rejection and abandonment, come to bear on new attachments. Understandably, many adoptees are very cautious about permitting themselves to be emotionally vulnerable or to take chances of further rejection.

In a seeming alternative to caution about entering relationships with the other gender, some adoptees plunge into sexual activity very early. Here too, family teachings about relationships between men and women, sexuality, and anxieties about birth heritage may promote this form of response to approaching adulthood. However, when the sexual activity is promiscuous and without emotion, this is a desperate attempt to dispel anxieties about being an adopted adult. Such a solution is no more developmentally appropriate for gaining adult competence than the solution of withdrawal from relationships. The operating rules of the adoptive family determine what function such sexual acting out serves in dealing with anxiety about the adoptee's maturation. The rules also determine whether and how much difference there is in response to the sexual behavior of female and male adoptees.

Outcomes of Adoptees' Marriages and Families

Findings on Marriages

Very little research has directly examined the outcomes of adoptees' marriages and families. The few available findings come from the earliest research on adoption outcome, done by Jean Paton in 1953 (Paton, 1954). She solicited written responses to a questionnaire from 40 adoptees — 25 women and 15 men. These people, who at the time ranged in age from their early 20s to over 60, had been adopted between the years of 1893 and 1933. Over half were placed before the age of 2, and many did not learn of their adoption until adolescence or later. Of the 25 women, 8 (32%) were single or divorced. Of the 15 men, 9 (60%) were single or divorced. Although the numbers were limited and the research methods rather crude, significant clues about attitudes toward marriage were provided in the anecdotal material written by the adoptees. Several strong themes prevailed throughout, even though there were noticeable gender differences.

The comments of the single women about the effect of adoption on their relationships were of several kinds: Adoption had no effect on their single status; adoption had no part of the current choice to be single, but might be a factor if a woman decided to marry later; or lack of knowledge about background *was* the deterrent to marriage. One woman commented, "I am not normal according to society. . . . It could have been prenatal. I don't know" (Paton, 1954, p. 32). The comments of the single men also fell into several groups and were worded more emphatically than those of the women. The most emphatic group cited a negative relationship with the adoptive mother, who was described variously as a destructive person, a liar, and someone to be hated. Adoption, based on desertion by the birth mother, had made other men reluctant to trust, depend on, or even get close to women. Finally, there were comments about general aversion to women and marriage that may have had nothing to do with adoption.

The adoptees in the Paton study who did marry, although small in actual numbers, seemed to experience positive relationships in their adoptive families and in their marriages. Regardless of the age at adoption, there was open acknowledgment of adoption and the birth family, sometimes from the extended adoptive family. All spouses knew about the adoption. Several adoptees married other adoptees, apparently making a strong connection through their mutual understanding of this status. Most of the married adoptees either had or planned to have children, but they varied in whether they would tell children about their adoption.

Cumulative anecdotal evidence gathered by the authors from their own experiences, colleagues, and adoption literature also suggests trends and gender differences in how adoptees deal with adult attachments. Female adoptees are more likely to stay in relationships, even troubled ones. They may be enmeshed in marriages; they may be caught between parents and spouses; or they may engage in a series of short-term alliances. Male adoptees seem to take fewer risks and more readily opt to do without relationships. They may risk one relationship or none before backing off to stay alone, perhaps immersing themselves in work or some other interest.

Findings on Children

The question of children is an extremely important one for adoptees. Little is known about the rate at which adoptees have children or about the quality of their parental attachments. However, from adoptees' reports in informal discussions or in therapy with the authors, there are indications of the meaning and outcomes of children in adoptees' family relationships.

For any couple, the attachment experiences in families of origin are reworked, for better or for worse, in marriage. If marriage becomes a mutually beneficial exchange, children provide a natural outlet for further sharing and enhancing the general well-being. If the marital exchange is not satisfactory, children become another opportunity for resolving issues and getting needs met. While all this is also true for adoptees, the fact of adoption puts even more importance and more layers of meaning onto having children. First of all, the fact of adoption is highlighted once again by the very prospect of having children. Whether they have thought about it before or not, at this time most adoptees are quite concerned about their birth heritage — in particular, about the genetic and health history that will be passed on to a child.

Many adoptees have a great desire for a child by birth, as a result of a profound hunger to know a birth relative — someone they might actually look like. All the years of longing and fantasies come to fruition in the birth of a child. But these unknown aspects pull all the issues of two sets of parents to the fore again. Not only is there the renewed wish to know about birth parents, but also there is renewed identification with them in adoptees' becoming birth parents themselves. At the same time, there is heightened consciousness of not sharing a biological tie or a birth experience with the adoptive parents. Once again, now with the new generation, relationships must be reaffirmed through emotional attachments.

In her study, Jean Paton (Paton, 1954) did ask the respondent adoptees about their children. Only 15 (of 40) had children, and not all commented. Although the data certainly are inconclusive, Paton identified three distinct groups, almost equal in size, which suggest trends. The first group is described as "expressing continuity with adoptive family, and/or otherwise indicating security or continuity" (Paton, 1954, p. 35). Comments from this group indicated that they experienced open acceptance of themselves and adoption, and later of spouses and children, from their adoptive families.

The second group is described as "expressing use of children as a way of resolving adoptive problems" (1954, p.35). The comments by this group included many references to advantages and disadvantages. There were regrets about not knowing what heritage was being passed along, or wishes to do better for one's own children. Some commented about the fact that their children knew about their adoption and that they helped to make up for loss of the birth family. The themes are reminiscent of "the sense of disadvantage" experienced by adoptees, as described by Schechter and Bertocci (Schechter and Bertocci, 1990). Parents who are adoptees seem concerned that their sense of disadvantage could be passed on to their children, and they want it not to be.

The comments of Paton's final group (1954, p. 37) indicated insecurity about their relationships, sometimes with their own children; the respondents attributed this directly to adoption. Some of these respondents learned late and accidentally about their adoption, and many did not tell their children of it. Even when satisfaction was expressed about their children, that did not seem to mitigate the longing to know the birth mother.

There are no data on how often adoption becomes the means of parenthood for adoptees, whether because of infertility or by choice. It can be speculated that if the subject comes up between spouses one or both of whom are adoptees, there are no neutral or indifferent positions. An adoptee is probably either strongly for or against the adoption of a child.

Issues for Adoptees as Parents: Gender Differences

The general issues for adoptees who become parents have somewhat different emphases according to gender. For either gender, of course, the degree to which the issues become problematic is conditioned by the course of the person's development and general level of functioning. For an adopted woman, the physical aspects of pregnancy and giving birth intensify the bond between her and her birth mother. All during the pregnancy, the adoptee may think about whether each aspect was the same for her birth mother in carrying her. The act of giving birth allows the adoptee to know at the deepest level of human experience what her mother went through to give her life. Often, an adoptee mother speaks poignantly of holding her first child for hours after birth, studying the little face, not wanting to let go.

At the same time, the adoptee who is a blissful new mother may again be tormented by the question of how her birth mother could give her up. Through identification, she may become aware for the first time that her birth mother could have experienced incredible pain in placing her. Such an identification may lead to a new resolution that includes forgiving the birth mother. On the other hand, the adopted woman who is enthralled with her new child may be unable to imagine how her birth mother could have relinquished her. The contrast to her own emotions can reinforce a sense of abandonment, rejection, and anger.

However the new mother adoptee reacts emotionally to her birth mother, there are also ramifications for her relationship with her adoptive mother. No matter how good a relationship they have, the grief over not having a birth bond is always there. That grief can be reinforced by the inability to share and compare the experience of producing a new generation.

The way in which the adoptee mother resolves the duality and differences of connection with the two mothers has a profound effect on her relationship with her child. The adoptee mother can be expected to form an alliance with her first blood relative that is even more intense than typical for any first-time mother. But if there are substantial unresolved feelings of grief or anger with either of her mothers, all those emotions may be poured into the alliance with her infant. Sometimes there is awareness of such a transfer, evidenced by the adoptee's saying to herself that she will be a better, closer mother than either of them.

The result, in some cases, is a very strong mother–infant alliance that begins to exclude the husband/father. If there are more children, the alliance patterns may just proceed around the first triad, or there may be major realignments. It is speculated that the gender of the first child (and of subsequent children) makes considerable difference in the pattern of alliances. That is, if the first child is a girl, a very strong alliance between mother and daughter can be established and does not readily shift. However, if the first child is a boy, that first alliance may remain the strongest, but it may shift more easily if there is a daughter later.

The male adoptee who becomes a father may also be thrilled finally to have a blood relative and may feel the strain of having dual parentage. But since he does not experience the birth physically, his reactions must be on the emotional and intellectual levels. His initial response, especially if he has been present during the delivery, is usually to the physical process of his wife's becoming a mother. At the time of birth, just like the female adoptee, he probably thinks about his own birth and relinquishment in terms of his birth mother. There may be no sense of identification with the birth father, particularly if he does not know anything about that father's response to his birth.

There are several possible outcomes for the adoptee father, conditioned by the functional level of the marriage and his own developmental resolutions, particularly in regard to the adoption. In very torn in her allegiance to both males, she spoke to her priest about the situation. She was referred to the church agency for family counseling. Hans only agreed to go because the priest spoke to him in support of the referral. The parents were seen first, and then the whole family for a total of four times. Hans's attitude was that he had taken in this boy, and by God, the boy would respect him. Marianna was in a dither of upset feelings for Martin, but torn with concern not to alienate Hans. Greta just wanted to be left alone to do her own activities. Martin said that he got along fine with Mama, but Papa never liked him and never would.

In the few sessions, a different way of handling the dinner table situation was worked out. Marianna's concern for both males, and their wish to keep her good will, served as a lever for change. Doing it for her also gave the males a face-saving way to stop the standoff. With that, however, Hans declared he was satisfied and ready to stop therapy, to which Marianna agreed. The therapist pointed out that the reasons for the standoff had not been addressed and therefore the problems could return. Since Hans was not persuaded, they left treatment, despite the therapist's misgivings about how long the peace would last.

Twenty years later, the therapist had occasion to hear about the outcome. After the therapy, Hans and Martin did avoid direct conflict until Martin was 12, even though their relationship was never cordial. Then Martin took up with some late teenage boys and began a period of wild behavior. Hans threw Martin out of the house on Martin's 18th birthday. After that, Marianna kept in surreptitious contact with Martin, often bailing him out of trouble. At the time of the report, Greta had been happily married for some years and had two children. Martin, on the other hand, was just getting his third divorce. The longest of his marriages was the first, entered after his wife was pregnant; it lasted a year. The other two marriages were even shorter and produced no children.

Considerations in Treating the Families of Adoptees

The families of adoptees may come for treatment at any life stage or with any presenting problem which can bring any family. In adoptees' families, attachment and loss issues are always a part, if not a central part, of the problem. But, depending on the life stage or problem for which treatment is sought, family members may not make a conscious connection between the parental adoption and the

response to his pleasure at having a blood relative, the adoptee father may invest strongly in child care, saying how important it is for him to bond; in some instances, the adoptee father may compete with the mother or even take charge, becoming the primary caretaker of the infant. In other cases, the thrill for the male adoptee of having a first blood relative is mitigated by perceived loss of nurture from his wife. If the adoptee father has lacked secure attachments, he may compete with the infant, especially if it is a boy, for the mother. If the infant is a girl, the father instead may bid for a strong alliance: The baby may be viewed as the one female who cannot leave him and who can be a new source of nurture. Again, the alliance pattern that is set up within the initial triad may be reinforced or rearranged with the addition of more children.

The male adoptee may have an easier time resolving his identification with his two fathers than the female adoptee does with her two mothers. Without the physical aspect of pregnancy and birth to create the same deep bond of a mother, the adoptee father may be able to resolve his dual identity on an emotional basis by separating the two contributions. Thus he may identify simultaneously with his birth father's ability to reproduce and his adoptive father's ways of being a father and husband. However, his adoptive father may not have been emotionally available. Then the loss of his birth parents and identification with his adoptive father can lead to his becoming an aloof father who risks little in attachments. He may relate to his children intellectually rather than emotionally, laying down expectations for their performance. This transgenerational resolution is more likely to focus on sons, but daughters are not necessarily immune. Some adoptee fathers can become quite detached, conveying attitudes that their presence and financial support are stable and are all that can be expected from them.

Children of adoptees usually are well aware of their parents' adoption, or at least are very sensitive to issues of attachment and separation. In the way of children, they do what they can to keep their parents comfortable. That means that the children of adoptees tend to be affirmative and loyal in their relationships with parents.

In more functional families, children have full knowledge of their parents' adoption, and usually there is open communication about it. Older children may encourage or even participate in a parent's search for his or her birth parents. Still, the adoptee parent tends to be somewhat protective and to keep children close; children respond by staying closer, so as not to threaten parental security. None of these factors may ever become troublesome to a family, but they do increase the possibility of trouble when the children prepare to emancipate themselves. In a family where attachments and losses are highly significant, the need to rearrange relationships can be very painful or can even produce a crisis. The poorly functioning family of an adoptee has still more difficulty with the emancipation of children. But the type of difficulties vary, depending on whether the adopted parent is the mother or father.

A particular female heritage is illustrated by a three-generational family dynamic, established by the female head of the oldest generation. This first woman is very young when she loses her mother (i.e., her primary attachment) and then has no good enough substitute. The female adoptee who has not grieved for her birth mother and/or has not had an adequate substitute fits this dynamic. This woman marries as soon as possible, often without love, in order to escape her unhappy situation. She also wants children as soon as possible and they are inducted into close, even enmeshed alliances with the mother; thereupon, the marriage becomes very distant or ends. The mother's message to her children is that she cannot stand further losses, and so they are not to leave her. When the children are grown, they do not leave their mother; if they do depart, they are back before long. Even if they marry and have children, they remain close to the mother (perhaps even in the same house), and she holds the primary allegiance. The third generation of such a family becomes quite dysfunctional. Since there is no healthy way to emancipate, the members of this generation develops symptoms that permit them to stay, such as alcoholism or psychosis. Or there may be symptoms that symbolize the wish to get away, such as impulsive departures, arrests involving being taken into custody, or suicide attempts.

The adoptee father who has had severe deficits in his attachment experiences is more likely to become a remote figure, quite the opposite of the overinvolved mother. He may be distant or isolated within the home. In one extreme case we know of, the father lived alone in the basement of the home, coming upstairs only to get the plate of dinner set out for him and taking it back down. Or he may leave the family altogether, with or without notice or divorce. Whether or not he stays with the family, he may maintain his barriers to attachment through an addiction to work, an activity, or a substance.

The way in which the intricate interplay of adoption and family dynamics follow right into the adoptee's own family is illustrated by the following case.

Hans and Marianna adopted Greta when she Greta had been in only one foster home sinc received good care. When Greta was 5, the Martin, who was 2. Martin was removed by co young mother who lived with her mother and Martin's care (feeding and cleaning) was quite over, any adult who was around might decide to t or might slap or tease him at whim.

Hans was a severe man who liked a neat, or lavish attention from his doting wife. Both wante Hans was reluctant to adopt. He finally agreed Marianna's urgency, rather than risk the loss of he favors. When Greta entered their home, the s hardly affected the household. She and Marian days together. When Hans came home from greeted by two smiling faces, his dinner, and a nea before.

But when Martin came, he was very active, a word was "no." Many times he was deliberately unc mischievous. Martin competed so successfully fo attention that often when Hans came home, the hou and dinner was unprepared. After a few such oc intervened by strapping Martin in a chair, sitting ir to lecture, unmoved by Martin's sobs. If Martin tr Hans slapped him. After a few weeks of this treatr became more subdued, leading Hans to gloat ove However, when Hans was at work and Greta at l Martin clung to Marianna and wanted her total atte she gave. Frequently, she rocked him, gave him tr him to be a good boy so Papa would not be mad at

Gradually, the household settled back into a routine. However, almost every evening at the d Martin would say or do something well designed to ir By the time Martin was 8, the dinner table scene ha into a nightly struggle that began when Hans pil Martin's plate. Martin no longer said much, but he m rude noises over the food, or simply refused to eat. Ha waggling his finger, demanding apologies, and in: Martin clean his plate; thus they would spend 2 hours the table as soon as possible. Marianna alternate pleading with them both or leaving the room. After she offered Martin the alternatives of giving in or getting on his behind. Martin always took the three slaps. I rianna brought him some supper in his room, whi eagerly.

When Marianna became distraught about the situ

problem. Consequently, the adoption may not be mentioned until later in the treatment, when questions arise about the parents' background and growing up experiences.

Some adoptees request couples therapy for premarital problems or for help in deciding the question of whether to marry. In these cases, the struggles with affiliation are usually consciously connected to the adoption experience, which is mentioned early, perhaps even at intake. When adoption is consciously connected to the problems, the initial exploration of the situation should lead immediately into eliciting personal histories. The process of eliciting the histories should focus on the details of attachment and loss experiences, particularly for the adoptee, but for the partner as well. Then the earlier experiences must be connected to the problems and patterns in the current relationship. Once the individuals understand their differences in meanings and needs for affiliation, they are able to make a more informed choice about the future of the relationship.

An adoptee and spouse also may request treatment at the next stage, when the birth of a child has caused some dislocation in the marriage. In such cases, problems centering around the care of the baby are usually at the fore. Sometimes the spouses are not even aware that the adjustments required by the arrival of a wanted child are the cause of increased marital tension. Beyond that, adoptee parents also vary greatly in awareness of their emotions about adoption and about having a new relative by birth, sometimes the first one they have ever known. In these cases, the therapist must focus initially on helping the parents adjust to their new role in caring adequately for the infant. Education about inherent strain and about the need to realign the marital relationship can be offered, along with practical suggestions. If part of the dislocation results from an adoptee parent's strong response to having a relative by birth at last, this is interpreted and addressed at once. Otherwise, the therapist may first explore the meaning of attachment to an infant for each parent, taking up the special issues of adoption as soon as that fact emerges.

If an adoptee and family ask for help in regard to a symptom of a preadolescent child, the parent's adoption is often not mentioned during the whole phase of symptom focus. Only if there is resistance to change concerning the symptom, and the therapist inquires into the families of origin, may the adoptive status be told. Otherwise, the adoption may be mentioned when the presented symptom has shifted and the work turns to broader issues of family relationships. Regardless of the timing, when the fact of parental adoption is known, the therapist must examine closely its relevance to symptom formation and the family dynamics.

Just like any other type of family, the family of an adoptee most commonly requests therapy when the parents are at midlife and the child or children are adolescents. In these cases, the preparation for the younger generation's emancipation reopens and intensifies the adoptee parent's issues regarding loss of attachment. However, if an adolescent's behavior is dramatic or worrisome enough, the parental focus is strongly on the younger person, thus avoiding the parents' own distress. The teenager's behavior may not be viewed as at all connected to emancipation, much less to a parent's adoption. As the therapy moves from the presented problem into features of life stage and family dynamics, it is effective to ask parents about their own emancipation experience. At this point, the fact of the parental adoption usually emerges. When it does, the therapist may have the sense of finding the missing piece of the puzzle.

Tracing the process of the adoptee parent's emancipation (or lack thereof) from the adoptive family is the best diagnostic indicator of what is involved in the current family's launching of its young people. From there, the work can focus on the special connotations of attachment and loss, and the ways in which these affect the particular family's rearrangement of its relationships on an adult level.

The transgenerational transmission of the attachment issues of adoption can be seen in the following treatment case.

Gary and Joan requested therapy because of concern for Linda, aged 16. Linda had done well at home and school until a few months before, when her brother Christopher, 18, left for college. Suddenly Linda's grades plummeted; she also frequently violated curfew and seemed "boy-crazy" to the parents. Assessment indicated no particular elements of dysfunction, except that the family had been close and was quite disrupted by Chris's departure. During the fall when Chris left, Linda turned 16, became a junior in high school, and began talking about colleges.

Despite the obvious life stage issues, the therapist was hard put to find the key to the problems or to intervention. Joan seemed extremely tense about what Linda was doing with boys. Linda, in turn, vacillated between reassuring her mother and dropping hints that scared her. Gary felt lonely because he missed Chris and the former sense of the whole family. In addition he did not understand the tension between Joan and Linda or how to help them.

Finally, the therapist asked Joan how it was for her at age 16.

Joan began to cry and said that she had a horrible time. She was adopted. Almost all Joan knew about her birth mother was that she had been 16 when Joan was born. Her birth mother was forced to relinquish her in order to remain at home and finish high school. Joan had known of her adoption all along but only recalled being told the minimal facts twice. When Joan was 16, she and her mother never acknowledged that this was the age of her birth mother. Instead, Joan was aware of having very restrictive limits, being watched closely, and being questioned tensely about any interest in boys.

When Joan turned 17, her mother's vigilance eased a little; however, Joan did not feel free of being under guard or able to risk a relationship with a young man until she went to college. There she met Gary and married him right after college graduation. Tears rolled down Joan's cheeks all the while she talked, adding that she had never told this to anyone before.

Gary and Linda were riveted by Joan's story. Gary took her hand, saying that he wished she could have told him sooner, because suddenly he could understand a number of things. Linda said she knew about her mother's adoption, but just as a fact. Then she added softly that she felt watched by Joan and miserable about it, just as Joan had felt with Grandma. As the family went on to piece together the three-generational transmission of anxiety about the sexual behavior of 16-year-old girls, tension lifted rapidly. Linda admitted that while she had not yet "done it," she had come close and was considering it. She also had wondered whether she would be thrown out if she became pregnant.

The three of them went on to do some excellent work concerning their attachments, values about sexuality, and rearrangement of relationships. Linda was eased into more responsibility for herself, which would increase as she got closer to leaving home. Plans were made for filling in Chris about what they were learning, which culminated in his coming along for sessions during his holiday break from college.

When the family was ready to end treatment after a few months, relationships were cordial. Linda was again doing well at school and was cooperative in keeping mutually agreed-upon curfews. The final resolution of the family was that as Linda began to look at colleges, Joan would begin to search for her birth mother, and Gary would help them both.

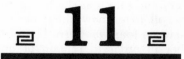

Search and Reunion

Because of its universal themes, adoption is a subject of popular interest, and the mass media have frequently chosen it for both factual and fictionalized presentations. Over the past 10 years, interest has been particularly keen in two adoption issues: "open adoption" and "open records." Both are related to the importance of confidentiality and secrecy that have traditionally been a part of agency adoption practice. "Open adoption" refers to the practices that encourage and support contact between the birth parents and the adoptive parents who will be rearing their child, with options for varying degrees of involvement at the point of placement and beyond. Open adoption has come about largely because of what those who participated in earlier confidential adoptions have said about their experiences (Campbell, Silverman, & Patti, 1991). For them, it is too late to experience an open adoption; what they seek now is information about themselves and about the others who were a part of their life before the adoption, and often contact with those people.

Many have felt strong pressure to engage in a search for those from whom they were separated by adoption. They want "open records" — that is, full access to the information included in agency and court records about themselves and the others who participated in the adoption in which they were involved. Most who are now adopted adults were adopted as children without their knowledge or consent. They feel discriminated against, and believe that they are entitled to early information that may be vital to their well-being. The factual information is all that some adoptees want, but many others view this information as a step toward locating and establishing contact with the others in their adoption triangle. Search and reunion are their goals.

"Open adoption" and "open records" are linked by a common concern about the secrecy in the adoption process and are historically related to each other. Since each presents its own clinical issues, however, each is explored separately. This chapter discusses the issues of search and reunion for adults whose adoption experience began in secrecy many years ago; Chapter 12 focuses on an approach that avoids that secrecy from the beginning of the adoption experience.

Open Records: Challenging the Validity of Secrecy in Adoption

Search stories featured by the media most often center on adult adopted persons who have searched for their birth parents, but there are searches by birth parents, siblings, and extended family members as well. The interest aroused by such searches and reunions reflects a natural response to the human drama that is inherent in the situations. It also reflects society's ambivalence about the secrecy that has been a part of the way in which adoption services have been historically defined and routinely delivered. The paradox is that people believe that "blood is thicker than water," and that a child always has ties and a sense of belonging to the family into which that child was born; however, they also believe that when a child is adopted, that child should "belong" to the adoptive parents as much as any child belongs to parents who have given birth.

Secrecy among the participants in an adoption has not always been a part of the plan. It came about as adoption changed from being viewed essentially as a legal transaction to being viewed as a social service. Adoption is regulated by state laws. The first adoption act in this country was passed in Massachusetts in 1851. There was no provision for confidentiality in that law or in any of the others that were passed in the next 60 years. The Minnesota statute in 1917 was the first to seal the court adoption records, and the purpose of such sealing was *not* to protect the participants of the adoption from knowledge of each other; instead, it was to protect all of them from scrutiny by the general public, to which court procedures are normally subjected. By the early 1940s most states had adoption laws, many of which provided for sealing of the court records to protect those involved in adoption from unanticipated consequences or deliberate exploitation by a general public that was not always sympathetic to those involved in the adoption process.

By now adoption agencies had developed the rationale and

skills that enabled them to lay claim to adoption as a service that could best be rendered by a social work agency. The essential belief underlying social work adoptions was that adoption should create a family that would resemble as closely as possible the family that the adoptive parents would have had by birth, had they had such a family. Agencies placed healthy infants, and the emphasis was on helping the adoptive parents view the infants as their children. The adoption process was viewed only as a means of creating this new family of parents and infant, with no awareness of the developmental impact of the experience on any of the participants. "Adoption" was a static event that happened. Sealing the records preserved the illusion that the new family was the same as any other family.

Agencies believed that adoption information should be confidential not only from outsiders but from the other participants. They supported legislation to seal records and began to close agency records, too. They took this position for both pragmatic and conceptual reasons. Pragmatically, adoption agencies were competing with independent adoption practitioners for healthy white infants, and the promise of secrecy was viewed as an added incentive at that time. Agencies offered participants the "guarantee" that the adoption would stand up in court, and that once the adoption was consummated, no one needed to worry about an unwarranted intrusion by any of the other participants. This was in keeping with what agencies believed to be in the best interests of those involved. Their conceptual rationale was (1) that adopted children would become more firmly attached to their adoptive parents if they were cut off from their original families; (2) that adoptive parents could more fully claim a child as their own when the birth parents were safely removed, both physically and psychologically; and (3) that birth mothers could best be helped to go on with their lives by making a clean break with the children they relinquished for adoption.

When a child was adopted, a new birth certificate was issued with the adoptive parents' names listed as the parents. The sealing of the adoption records meant for the birth mother who had relinquished her child that the infant to whom she had given birth no longer even existed. To the adoptive parents, the sealed adoption records meant that their adopted child's "other family" could be fully denied and that they were protected from the threat of intervention by any of its members. For adopted children, sealed records meant they were forever separated from information or contact with the families who gave them life. By midcentury, most states had laws sealing adoption records, and most adoption agencies were touting the promise of confidentiality as one of the advantages of adoptions arranged by them rather than by independent practitioners.

Jean Paton, an adopted person and a social worker, was the first to publicly challenge the validity of secrecy in adoption when she was denied access to the records of her own adoption. In 1953 she established the first search organization, Orphan Voyage, and in 1954 she wrote *The Adopted Break Silence,* the first public outcry for openness. (Some results from Paton's study of other adoptees have been presented in Chapter 10.) Almost 20 years later, Florence Fisher's (1973) book *The Search for Anna Fisher* dramatically brought the issue of secrecy in adoption to the public's attention.

The Pressures That Motivate Searchers

Three things drive adopted persons who search, whether their search is for information or contact: (1) the need to know why they were abandoned to adoption; (2) the unique genetic tie to their birth mothers and their need for continuity with their own history; and (3) the need to bring together the disparate pieces of their backgrounds in order to feel that they are whole and worthwhile beings. The birth mothers who search want to find out how their children have fared and to ease their loss. The pain, the anger, and the guilt generated by the surrender or termination have persisted.

Early research suggested that those adopted persons who search are people whose adoptions have not gone especially well (Triseliotis, 1973), and Schechter and Bertocci's (1990) summary of 12 studies between 1973 and 1980 indicates that one of the factors leading adoptees to search is a dissatisfaction with their adoptive parents' communication in regard to adoption issues. In a recent study (Miller-Havens, 1990) of 84 adopted women from a nonclinical population, however, an astonishing 98% of the women cited a desire to feel connected to their beginnings as a motivation to search.

It is our premise that much of the pressure for search comes from unresolved feelings about the earlier loss. Our experience is that almost without exception, this is the first issue addressed in adoption reunions. Within minutes (seconds?) into the initial reunion meeting, the adopted person asks, "Why did you give me up?" or the birth parent says, "Let me tell you why I could not keep you." Elisabeth Kübler-Ross (1969) has postulated that grief is a process with identifiable steps, and has offered a model for the mourning of death that has served clinicians well. Simply because death is the most permanent of universal losses, however, we cannot assume that it is the most difficult loss. In fact, losses in which there is the possibility of finding what one has lost may be more difficult, because the grieving process cannot be completed. When the loss is of something of sufficient value, the inability to go through the normal grieving process drives the search. The search for military personnel who have been reported "missing in action" is a case in point.

Although our intent is by no means to trivialize the importance of searches for those missing in action or lost in adoption, an everyday experience that most of us have had may suggest the power of that drive to search. We have a deadline to meet—perhaps to fill out our income tax forms—and have set aside time to complete the work. We have cleared our desks and our minds to work; we have put out the forms, the year's data that we need, scratch paper, and two or three carefully sharpened pencils. Things go well and then the telephone rings. We put the pencil down, push the scratch pad forward on the desk, answer the phone, and say we will call back later. We are ready to resume writing and reach for the pencil. It is no longer where we thought we put it. We look around the desk and do not see it. Nobody has entered or left the room; the pencil has to be there. We look again where we thought it was, and then in other places where it could have rolled or been placed. It is not in any of those places. We look at a watch and note that the time allotted for this project is quickly passing. We must get on with it. Do we calmly pick up another sharpened pencil and go on with the work? Or do we continue to look for the pencil that has somehow been misplaced? And if we do go on with the writing, can we focus our full attention on it, or do we find ourselves thinking of other places to look for the other pencil, or perhaps even giving up the writing for a full-scale search of the premises? For many of us, as long as we know of the existence of that first pencil, the perfectly good substitutes that are at our fingertips do not remove the pressure to search for that which we knew we once had—and have lost. Again, this analogy is not meant to equate parents and pencils, but merely to suggest the urgency that underlies the desire to reclaim something that is lost.

Many of those involved in adoption *must* search. Others are less interested, and some even find the idea of search and reunion unnecessary or offensive. Search and reunion issues, however, have become central for adoption agencies and therapists. Many of the service delivery questions are unresolved. To what extent does its prior involvement in an adoption place the responsibility for search and reunion services on an adoption agency? Who should serve those whose adoption was arranged independently of an agency or in some other state? Should adoption agencies devote time to this phase of adoption service while there are children now waiting for adoptive homes who need their time and attention? Do adoption workers have the knowledge and skill to assist in the actual search process? If adoption agencies do not provide the services, who should? Should there be mandatory intermediaries whose role it is to protect the rights of all involved and to ease the way for the emotionally charged reunion? Or should there be mandatory counseling for all who are embarking on a search, predicated on the knowledge that such a search is an attempt to resolve past unresolved issues and is certain to be a perilous psychological journey?

Five Steps in the Search Process

While these issues are being resolved, adoption workers, mental health practitioners, independent search consultants, and volunteers are all currently providing services. Several people have begun to conceptualize the clinical issues (see, e.g., Brodzinky & Schechter, 1990; Winkler, Brown, van Keppel, & Blanchard, 1988). Each searcher's story is different, but all searches are significant emotional experiences for those involved. Those who have chronicled the process of the search have identified some common characteristics (Gonyo & Watson, 1988) and some common steps in the search process itself (Gonyo & Watson, 1988; Lifton, 1979). Adopted persons are more frequently the searchers than are other members of the triangle or extended family members; more women search than men; the initial object of the search for most adopted adults is the birth mother; and most people who search are successful in locating the other party.

We identify five steps in the search process, each with its own issues. We have used the search of an adopted person for that person's birth mother in developing this model; other searches require some modification in the steps of the process. The five steps are (1) deciding to search, (2) learning the birth name, (3) locating the other person, (4) reunion contact, and (5) integrating the reunion experience. Most searchers decide to begin a search after a long internal struggle. The decision is frequently triggered by a significant event in a searcher's life or in the life of the one to whom the search is directed (e.g., a marriage, the birth of a child, the birthday on which the adopted person is legally recognized as an adult [emancipation birthday], or the death of a significant adoptive family member). Adopted persons usually take the first concrete step by calling the agency, the court, or a support group made up of others who are searching or have completed their searches. Most often they ask the agency or the court for medical information. This information is important, and the searchers may feel (probably correctly) that it is less likely to be refused. If they get the information or feel supported in this initial contact, they intensify the search process, which soon becomes obsessive and cyclical. During bursts of energy most searchers seem almost incapable of focusing on anything else, often including job and family responsibilities. After a period of frenzied activity, they push the search aside; either they must respond to demands from the rest of life or they are overwhelmed by the intensity of the experience. Sometimes they stop because of repeated failures, and sometimes because of the increased anxiety when success seems close. The pressure remains, however, and soon they resume the search activity.

The second phase in the process begins when a searcher learns his or her birth name (or when a birth parent learns the adoptive parents' name). At this point searchers must evaluate the decision to search not only in the light of their own needs and family systems, but also in terms of the anticipated impact on those to whom the search is directed and their family systems. Sometimes searchers are spurred on by learning their birth names; sometimes they slow down because the possibility of a dream becoming reality increases their anxiety.

When the searchers continue, and most of them do, they enter the third phase and try to locate the other persons. They sense that reunion is now really possible. Knowledge of one's birth name is an enormous asset, but finding a person can still be a slow process, especially if the name is common. Many searchers find this a period of great frustration. It is like the middle period of treatment — a time when hard work must be done and the results are not always quickly apparent. Then they locate the object of the search and the next phase, making contact, is at hand.

Unless a successful search has been brought about by matching through a registry, a person who has been found has no idea that anyone has even been looking. For the searcher, the first contact is the culmination of much work and a huge emotional investment. For the person who has been found, the meaning of the contact relates to the way in which that person has come to terms with the adoption experience of years ago; the potential for emotional upheaval is great. Searchers make contact in a variety of ways. Sometimes they employ intermediaries to make the initial contact. Intermediaries can confirm the match, ease the shock on the person who has been found, and provide support for both parties. The intermediaries are usually volunteers who have been through a reunion themselves or social workers from the adoption agency. Some searchers prefer to make the first contact themselves. If they do not call first, they usually try to choose a time when other family members are not around. Most prefer to make phone contact first. Usually a searcher uses the birth date or a first name, if it is known, to bridge the gap (see the case of Jennifer, described below).

The last step in the search and reunion process lasts the rest of the lives of those involved. Intimate strangers who are suddenly a part of each other's real world must negotiate their ongoing relationship. Reunion is one more step in a continuing process. It helps bring together some aspects of the participants' lives, but only to raise new concerns and open new options. Reunions do not simplify the adoption gestalt, but serve as a prelude to a postreunion phase. Even in "simple adoptions" the complexities abound.

> Keith had been adopted as an infant by a family with a birth son who was 4 at the time of Keith's adoption. By all indicators, Keith's adoption was a successful one: He was happy with his adopted parents, had a good relationship with his older brother, was popular with his peers, and went to college on an academic scholarship. He was also curious about his birth family and began an earnest search, with his adoptive parents' knowledge, when he was 23 years old. He said that he wanted to learn why he was placed in adoption and to see what his birth mother looked like.
>
> Keith found his birth mother, Beth, and traveled to her community for a visit. Although the reunion went well, Keith came away disappointed. Keith could see little resemblance between them, or between himself and a picture of Beth's adult daughter. Although Beth welcomed him, she was unprepared to introduce Keith to her husband, who knew about Keith, or to her daughter, who did not. Beth mentioned that Keith looked a lot like his birth father.
>
> Keith decided to find him. Although the birth parents had not been in recent contact with each other, Beth furnished Keith with a lead to locate Ron, his birth father. He lived in a town near Beth, and Keith found him within a few months and was invited for a visit. He was warmly welcomed into Ron's very large family and was delighted with this contact. Keith was invited back any time; in particular, he was urged to attend a family reunion the following month, when he would have an opportunity to meet 125

additional relatives. One of Ron's sons looked very much like Keith, and Ron's wife looked very much like Beth. In fact, the affair that generated Keith occurred when Ron and the woman who was now his wife were temporarily separated because of an argument. After meeting Keith, Ron's wife wondered what part she played in Keith's presence in this world.

Since he was in the area, Keith thought he would plan a second visit with Beth. Beth was cool to this idea, however, saying that since Keith had come to see Ron, he should perhaps confine his visiting to contact with him. The two birth parents told differing stories about the circumstances of Keith's conception and the adoption plan.

Keith's reunion plunged him into two new family systems with quite different perceptions of him and of his origins, and brought to the surface unresolved feelings between his two birth parents. He is now struggling to understand the four family systems in which he has membership and that he links together: his adopted family, Beth's family, Ron's family, and the family comprised of Ron, Beth, and himself.

Clinical Intervention in the Search Process

The searcher's request, and the particulars of that person's individual history and significant family systems, will shape any clinical interventions. A searcher may seek such help at any time in the search process. The request may be focused specifically on the resolution of adoption or search issues, in which case it is often directed toward an adoption agency; or the request for help may be related to other problems, with the adoption and search issues emerging in the course of the assessment or treatment planning. The role of the professional involved with clients addressing adoption search issues will be shaped not only by the service request, but also by the therapeutic orientation, experience, and personal beliefs of the clinician; by the policies and structure of the organization within which that clinician works; and by the adoption laws of the state. In this section, we suggest a general clinical framework for exploring the issues and offer some techniques for successful intervention.

Basic to effective assessment and intervention is the clinician's belief that an adoption triangle member's request for help with search and reunion issues represents a healthy response to a pathological situation, not a pathological response to a healthy situation. This runs contrary to the romantic myth that the legal act of adoption in and of itself is supposed to fix the problems of those involved. Our approach to adoption as developed throughout this book identifies it as a condition of the participants' lives that will make the normal developmental stages more complex, particularly in regard to certain issues that may reawaken the trauma of the original adoption experience. Just as the placement of the child in adoption did not "solve" for once and for all the crises in the lives of those involved initially and guarantee a happy ending, neither will more information or reunion do that. What it can do is provide an opportunity for triangle members to cope more effectively with the lives that their adoption has helped create for them.

Above, we have identified five steps or phases in the search process: making the decision to search, learning one's birth name, locating the missing person, making reunion contact, and integrating this experience into one's ongoing life. The clinician may be involved with any triangle member at any of the steps, and since the points are sequential, it is possible for the clinician to be involved throughout the process.

Deciding to Search

An adopted adult embarking on a search faces a venture that is frightening—because of the possibility of both failure and success. If the search fails to result in a reunion, the enormous physical and emotional effort it took is perceived as having been for "nothing," and the pain continues. If the search succeeds, the result may be rejection by the birth mother (and perhaps by the adoptive parents), and the pain may increase. Even a successful reunion leaves some earlier issues unresolved and adds immediate complications to the lives of those involved. There are no happy endings—only the increased options for becoming more whole.

Most often, those beginning to search show caution and ambivalence. The clinician's tasks in helping someone during this phase are to sanction the idea of search, to identify and help resolve the ambivalence, and to explore and develop the support base. Many adopted persons now struggling with search issues grew up feeling that they ought to be grateful for having been adopted, and that showing any interest in their birth families might be construed by the adopted parents as a sign of ingratitude or disloyalty. If an adopted person is married, this sense of disloyalty may be transferred to the spouse or children, especially if the searcher is aware

from the literature or from other searchers of the obsessive quality
of the search process.

The clinician should encourage the searcher's family to become
involved in the search. The impact of the search, whatever the
outcome, will be felt throughout the family, and the support of the
family system makes the search process itself far more bearable for
the searcher. Often, as the clinician explores with the potential
searcher the involvement of other family members, the issue of
adoption is opened up for the first time. Some adopted persons were
not told of their adoption as children and grew up either suspecting
the truth but not being able to talk about it, or learning about it as
adults in some traumatic way. Other adopted persons grew up
knowing about their adoption but getting clear messages within
their family systems that this was not a subject to be discussed in any
depth. And even for those adopted persons who grew up in families
in which the adoption was freely discussed, that "free" discussion
may have served to trivialize the importance of the adoption and
make the adopted children feel there must be something wrong with
them for having questions about birth parents, origins, or the reason
for the adoption.

Support groups are important to many who are searching.
People who were adopted, who were adoptive parents, or who were
birth parents initially formed support groups to meet their particular needs. They soon recognized that all triangle members faced
the common trauma of adoption, and that support was more
effective when groups included all members of the triangle. Now
most groups are open for any who are interested in support and
search, and most provide opportunities for both psychological
support and pragmatic help in the search process. Clinicians should
know the support groups that are available for referral, and their
active participation in support group meetings is mutually beneficial.

Clinicians must never lose sight of the importance of accurate
factual information. In a discussion of the reconciliation of cognitive dissonance, Schechter and Bertocci (1990, p. 81) cite examples
of dissonant elements in the adopted person's life—such things as a
birth certificate that offers inaccurate information; missing or faulty
information about ancestors or family medical history; and an
explanation of the circumstances of the adoption that equates love
with abandonment, since an adopted child may be told that the birth
mother surrendered him or her as an act of love.

Clinicians should foster discussion of these dissonant elements
and the pursuit of information about the birth family and the

circumstances of the adoption. Sometimes adopted persons get relief from the pressure they feel just by discussing adoption issues freely within their family systems and getting accurate answers to questions that have been buried in the world of make-believe and mythology in which they were reared. Accurate information is not always easy to come by. Many people were adopted independently, and the only information available may be sealed in a court record. Those who were adopted through agencies may have greater access to the facts. Many agencies provided "fact sheets" to adoptive parents at the time of the adoption; some adoptive parents may have destroyed or lost this information. In most cases agencies can share the circumstances that brought a child to adoption and any "nonidentifying" information about the birth parents. Unfortunately, agencies did not realize when the adults of today were adopted as children how important this information would be, and some failed to collect it or to preserve it.

Sometimes accurate information brings about cognitive integration, which suffices to relieve the pain of the potential searcher, and the decision to search is put aside (at least for the moment).

For example, Amelia was a 35-year-old woman who sought help because of a strained sexual relationship with her second husband and increasing anxiety about her capacity to parent her 3-year-old daughter. She married for the first time when she was 25, and the marriage was in trouble within a year because of her inability to respond sexually to her husband. She sought marital counseling at that time. Her wish was to preserve the marriage, but her husband was not interested in counseling and the marriage dissolved. She subsequently went into treatment for her "sexual disorder."

Amelia had been adopted at the age of 4 after spending her first year with her birth parents, followed by three foster home placements while her parents attempted to work out the problems that kept them from effectively rearing her. Finally, they voluntarily surrendered her. Her birth father kept a thread of contact with her until his death, when Amelia was 15. The birth parents had separated earlier, and Amelia did not know what had become of her birth mother.

In the treatment that followed the breakup of Amelia's first marriage, the therapist did not focus on the adoption, but chose to focus instead on Amelia's relationships with her adopted parents and her need to be a "good" child in a fairly moralistic environment. Amelia was seen in individual treatment, and her adopted parents were not told that she was in therapy. After a year, Amelia felt that the treatment had "loosened her up" sexually, and she left treatment. She had two serious affairs and then met Marvin, whom she subsequently married when she was 30.

Initially, Amelia and Marvin's sexual relationship was satisfying and they were both delighted when their daughter Amy was born. As Amy matured, Amelia began to feel increasing anxiety about her parenting capacity, and her sexual relationship with her husband began to parallel that with her first husband. She entered therapy (with a different therapist), wondering whether finding her birth mother might be a solution to her problems. The therapist immediately involved her husband in the sessions and focused on this idea. For the first time, Amelia began to share with Marvin what she knew about her adoption and to raise questions about why she came into adoption and what had happened to her birth mother. The perception that emerged was that she was surrendered by her birth parents because she was "bad," though Amelia could recollect nothing to reinforce that from her contacts with her birth father, who simply said that he and her birth mother were not compatible. A strong memory that Amelia had was of being moved rather quickly from her second foster home. This family was also the one that she remembered most fondly.

With the therapist's support, she contacted the adoption agency. Fortunately, they had a rather full history of Amelia while she was in care. Their record stated that the birth parents had voluntarily surrendered their rights. Their marriage had floundered because of the birth mother's alcoholism and her involvement with another man. The record also stated that Amelia was removed from the second foster home at the request of the foster mother because she suspected that her husband might have been sexually abusing the child. With this concrete information, Amelia was able to recall having "secrets" with this foster father and crying jags in the third foster home. With the support of the therapist and her husband, the anxiety about parenting her daughter and about her own sexual activity subsided. Amelia decided that she did not need to pursue the search for her birth mother, and, by plan, treatment was terminated.

The beginning points of effective clinical intervention with the adopted person who is contemplating search, then, are (1) a validation of the motivation to search; (2) the involvement of the potential searcher's family system in support of the search; (3) an exploration of the way in which the adoption was viewed and the issues dealt with within the adoptive family system; (4) the acquiring of information to work toward greater cognitive congruence; and (5) referral to a support group. All of this, of course, is done within the context of an understanding of adoption that recognizes the under-lying concerns about loss and rejection, diminished self-esteem, and an incomplete identity that prompts the search, and tempered by the dynamics of the particular searcher and the particular circumstances that bring that person to the clinician.

Learning One's Birth Name

Some adopted persons know their birth names as a result of information available from their adoptive parents or from their own memories. Most feel, however, that they take their first major step toward reunion when they learn their birth names. Now they no longer have external support for denying that they belong to two families, and ambivalence about their search mounts. Many question again whether their search is a good idea. Warnings about the unknown consequences of a successful search take on new meaning. Now that the odds of success are immeasurably improved, a searcher asks, "Am I sure that I want to go through with this?" The feelings about the original rejection and loss surge forth, and anxiety at the possibility of another rejection mounts.

When a searcher knows his or her birth name, the issue of identity comes to the forefront. This means a host of questions: "What does this name mean to me? Do I know anyone with this name? How many people with this name are listed in the phone directory? Might I be related to one of them or to someone that I know with this same name? What is the ethnic derivation? What do people with this name look like? What does my birth mother look like? Will I look like her? Will I recognize her? Will she recognize me?"

Since knowing their birth names clearly indicates to searchers that they are members of two families, many of them begin to set themselves apart from their adopted families. Differences that used to be overlooked in the service of denying the adoption are now accentuated in the service of defending the search. It is helpful if adoptive parents are involved in the search, so they can understand the rationale for this change in a child's relationship to them and not misinterpret it as a rejection. Adopted adults at this stage of the search process also begin to consider more carefully the impact of reunion on their family systems. They can be clearer about this impact on their adoptive families or on the families that they have created, but they must fantasize about the meaning their presence will have to their birth families. Fantasies flourish where facts are unknown. Sound intervention supports the gathering of facts and discourages speculation at this time.

Searchers seldom seek treatment because of pressures they feel at this stage of the search. Some are already involved clinically when the search process reaches this point, and therapeutic support can be useful. Although it may be necessary for a searcher to take a break to integrate the new name into his or her persona, discontinuing the search at this time is usually not easy for the searcher, nor is it helpful. Denial can no longer be as effective a defense as it may have been heretofore. Knowing the name empowers the searcher to proceed. Not to do so leaves the adopted adult feeling confused and inadequate.

Clinical interventions at this time, then, generally include recognizing the normalcy of the resurgence of ambivalence; engaging the adopted person's adopted family in the search process, both to provide additional support for the searcher and to help family members with the differentiation issue; continuing help with the loss and abandonment issues, especially in view of the fantasy (which could prove to be real) of another rejection; exploration of identity concerns, beginning with the meaning of the birth name; exploring with the searcher the impact of reunion on all of the family systems involved; and supporting the continuation of the search.

Locating the Object of the Search

As the search continues, a searcher must now actually locate the person he or she is seeking. Searchers alternate between high expectations and repeated frustrations. Leads are identified, explored, and discarded. They direct their energy toward pursuing sources of information not therapy. They spend time in libraries, courthouses, and newspaper offices, reviewing tax records, vital statistics, phone numbers, motor vehicle registrations, or anything that might help them with their search. Some rush to support group meetings, but others find these of mixed value now. Although they may learn some new search techniques that other group members have used, they may also hear of the success of people who began searching long after they did, or of others who have been searching unsuccessfully much longer than they.

This is a time when the cycle of search and inactivity is usually most apparent. Searchers seldom completely abandon their efforts, but often set the search aside. Following a period of frustration, they may become depressed and need a break from the active searching.

Then the pressure to search builds up again, and they begin another period of extensive activity. They may decide to put aside the search just after a big breakthrough. Sometimes a searcher will have located a birth relative who can say where the birth mother is, but the searcher does not pursue the question. Or an adopted person will have the telephone number of the birth mother that he or she has worked so hard to find, but holds off on making the call. The person is delaying now because of the fear of making contact.

Few searchers seek clinical assistance during this phase of the search process. Sometimes other family members will seek help on behalf of the searchers, either because of the obsessive searching or the depressive reaction to the lack of success. There is little clinicians can do at this point unless they have access to information that can be of concrete help in the search, which is sometimes the case with adoption workers. Should the search prove to be unsuccessful, or should it uncover information that a birth parent is deceased, clinical intervention can be directed toward helping resolve that loss.

Making Contact

Now the searchers are poised on the brink of an exciting yet emotionally perilous experience. Most searchers feel it is too late to turn back, yet many delay making the first contact. Fear of the unknown, concerns about rejection, unresolved feelings from the earlier adoption decision, a sense of losing control — all can cause a delay in decisive action. Yet the need to know, the power of the birth bond, the wish to look like somebody, and the sense of being incomplete propel the searchers forward. Questions about the longer-range impact of the reunion no longer seem important. The pressure for the immediate contact cannot be resisted.

Clinical services are not usually sought at this point unless they have been utilized earlier in the search and are viewed as supportive now. If an adoption agency has cooperated in the search, an agency representative may be asked to make the contact as an intermediary. Sometimes a search group member or community volunteer may fill this role.

> Andrea came into agency care as an infant. Her mother, Barbara, was a 22-year-old woman, an only child who was living with her parents when she became pregnant. The pregnancy was unexpected; the father of the child was a foreign exchange student who was soon to leave the country; and neither he nor Barbara was interested in marriage. Barbara's parents thought that she should

place the child in adoption, and made it clear that she could not continue to live with them if she kept the child. Barbara had a good job with prospects of advancement; she felt that she was not ready for living away from home or for motherhood. When Andrea was 1 month old, Barbara relinquished her, and she was soon placed in adoption with a family who changed her name to Jennifer.

Jennifer's adoptive parents subsequently adopted a boy, Danny, 2 years younger than Jennifer. As Jennifer grew up, she and Danny used to talk about adoption and speculate about their birth families. Was it possible that their parents were the same, or at least one of them? Did their birth parents have any other children? Jennifer was the more curious child and wondered whether, if Danny's birth parents had another child, she would be a sister to that child. And, of course, they wondered out loud what their birth parents looked like and why they had been given up. The children never raised these adoption-related questions with their adoptive parents. They were given the factual information about their birth families that the adoptive parents had been given.

Neither child presented "problems" until Jennifer, an honor student, surprised and disappointed her parents by refusing to go to college after graduating with honors from high school. (Her adoptive mother was a college graduate). Jennifer got a job, continued to live at home, and saved her money carefully. Within a year she had begun her search. Initially she told only Danny, but when the search stalled, she told her adoptive parents and enlisted their help. Although they were puzzled by Jennifer's interest, they knew and shared with her the name of her birth mother and the community in which she lived at the time of the adoption. It was a common name and a big community, so the search was slow. Jennifer persisted and finally located a telephone number for her birth grandparents, Barbara's parents.

Jennifer rehearsed what she planned to say and started to call twice. Both times she forgot what she had planned to say and hung up. When the third call was answered, she asked for Barbara. She was told that Barbara didn't live there and was asked who she was. She said, "An old friend," and inquired about Barbara's whereabouts. She was asked to leave her name and number if she wished Barbara to call her, and she did.

Jennifer felt sure that she was talking to her birth grandmother and sensed that the grandmother guessed her identity. She wondered whether her grandmother knew her adopted name. She did not think that Barbara would get the message and did not expect the call to be returned, yet each time the phone rang she was certain it was Barbara calling. After about a month, she called again. The same person answered the phone, recognized Jennifer's voice, and said that Barbara could no longer be reached at that number and had no other phone number. Jennifer was sure now that she had been identified and that Barbara had not been told of her earlier call. Two weeks later she called again and was asked by the same person not to call any more.

Jennifer deliberately waited until Christmas Eve, assuming that Barbara would probably be there then, and called again. The same person answered the phone and said that she must have the wrong number. She heard another woman in the background ask who was on the phone and whether the call was for her. Jennifer called right back, and a different woman answered the phone.

"Hello, is this Barbara White?"

"Yes. Who is this, please?"

"My name is Jennifer. We have met before, but I don't think you know me by that name. Does the date July 18, 1968 have any special meaning to you?"

Barbara immediately knew who was calling and, although initially taken aback, insisted on talking long into the night. She wanted to see Jennifer as soon as possible, and after a first emotional meeting they maintained regular contact. Adoption reunions, however, like adoptions, are not solutions to life's problems. They offer new opportunities but may open old wounds.

Jennifer wanted to know why Barbara had not sought her. Barbara responded that her pregnancy with Jennifer had been a constant source of friction between her and her parents and that she felt she could not search without their support. She had never married, and lived alternately at her parents' home and in an apartment by herself. Her parents were upset now with Jennifer's re-entrance into their daughter's life, and Jennifer was upset when they said they had no interest in meeting her.

Jennifer's birth father, however, wanted to see her as soon as he could. He had returned to this country several years ago, had subsequently married and divorced, and now lived in another state. He and Barbara had not seen each other since just before Jennifer's birth, but they had maintained telephone contact and Barbara had promptly called him to tell him the news about their daughter. At his suggestion, Barbara and Jennifer drove down to meet him for a weekend at a point midway between their city and his. That visit went well, but Jennifer later confessed that she had hoped her birth parents would find that they still loved each other, would then decide to marry, and that she would be the maid of honor.

Although Barbara had met Jennifer's adoptive family and everyone had liked each other, Jennifer's parents felt left out of their daughter's current life, which seemed focused on activities generated by the reunion. Much of Jennifer's and Barbara's energy was now directed toward the postreunion process. Gediman and Brown (1989) describe this process as developing "along two paths more or less simultaneously: the tangled path that leads backward to the past; and the newly laid track that is carrying birthmother and adult adoptee into their future" (p. 137).

Integrating the Reunion Experience

A searcher making the initial contact with the other person faces three possible responses: rejection, acceptance, or conditional acceptance. Although in time any of the responses may change to one of the others, each raises different clinical issues. Those who are rejected have their worst fears confirmed: Their adult attempt to redo a painful and inexplicable childhood experience in a way that will bring about a happier resolution has failed. The issues with which they may need clinical help are loss, abandonment, and self-esteem. They may also need help in weighing the risks and benefits of trying to make contact again.

Successful contact generates its own issues. When the found person welcomes the searcher, the first response is usually a flood of information and emotion that tends to overwhelm both parties. There is much feeling aroused by the reunion experience, and much factual information is shared. The most critical issues are usually addressed head on — the "explanation" for the adoption ("Why did you give me up?") and the search for common identifying characteristics ("Who do I look like?"). When the initial answers to these questions are unsatisfactory, either party may seek therapeutic assistance in assessing why this is so and what comes next. The answers usually lie in exploring the earlier adoption in the context of the current family system within which each party operates.

If the initial explanations are satisfactory and both parties want to move ahead, they are faced with negotiating a relationship that makes sense for them now. Clinical interventions at this point generally focus on problems of intimacy, family system homeostasis, and role definition. Each party independently has established a level of intimacy with which he or she is comfortable and has negotiated a network of relationships within that intimacy framework. Because of past history and the indissoluble bond between the two parties, this "new" relationship has the immediate potential for intimacy that may be perceived by either as inviting or threatening. Since each party is already functioning in a family system, probably with a defined role, the reunion has an immediate impact on the family systems of both. Family balances must be re-established, and both parties must determine the role each will now have in the other's life.

The interplay of the life history of both participants, the current needs of each, and their feelings about the adoption will shape these roles. What role does a "mother" play with an unknown adult child who has been reared by other parents, and what role does this adult child play with this old/new mother? How upsetting to their status quo is this new relationship, and what is it that each can gain from involvement with the other? What meaning does the adoption have to each, and what issues from the past have been reawakened and need attention now?

One frequent pitfall following reunions is the wish of one party or the other to make up now for the lost years of the relationship. This often takes the form of the birth mother's infantilizing her adult child while the adopted person, caught up in ambivalence about this "new" parent, may alternately welcome such dependency gratification and reject it. Such difficulties usually yield quickly to clinical intervention unless personal dynamics cause the birth parent to try to expiate her guilt through excessive generosity or the adopted person to express anger or control through manipulation.

Another stumbling block in developing this new relationship is what has come to be called "genetic sexual attraction" (Gonyo, 1987). When a birth mother confronts her adult child, she may see someone who embodies in looks and personality things that she sees and values in herself, or valued in the father of that adult child. Without the years of day-to-day parenting to confirm this adult as her child and to unconsciously reinforce the conventional incest barrier, she may feel a strong sexual attraction to this young person. Adopted persons may experience some of the same kind of feelings as they seek and find similarities between themselves and the new adults in their lives. Such feelings can be frightening if they are unexpected. Support group members or a sensitive clinician can help put this issue into perspective, and only rarely does it need prolonged attention.

Many searches result neither in outright rejection nor in immediate engagement in developing the new relationship. The acceptance is conditional. Not infrequently, this kind of situation comes about when the birth parent has not made a full disclosure of the existence of the adopted child. Although a birth mother usually tells the man she subsequently marries about a child who has been adopted, that information is not always shared with the husband's extended family or with their children. Adopted adults who have located their birth parents thus find themselves caught once more in a web of secrecy and denied contact with half-siblings. They face a dilemma: They do not wish to interfere with the birth parents' families, particularly if they feel that their involvement may be detrimental to the family members; yet they do not feel that they should be denied contact with their siblings. The question of allegiance to the birth parents surfaces. To what extent should they respect the birth parents' wishes? What do they owe the birth parents?

> May came seeking help in regard to this issue. She was an adult when she learned of her adoption, and 54 years old when both adopted parents were deceased and she felt free to begin her search. She found her birth mother when she was 59 and her birth mother, Sybyl, was 79. She learned then that she had three half-sisters, aged 53, 52, and 51, who were born to Sybyl in a later marriage. Sybyl was now a widow and a semi-invalid who lived in another state with her only sister, Rosemarie, and a single daughter who was not employed but served as a caretaker. The other two half-sisters were married and had adult children (as did May). Rosemarie was the only family member who knew of May's existence. Initial contact with Sybyl had been made through an intermediary, and Sybyl said she would see May only if May promised not to tell the other daughters of the visit.
>   A reunion visit was arranged. Sybyl said that she had expected May to search for her and was glad that she had found her while she was still living. However, she said that she thought it would kill her if her other daughters found out about May, and asked May to promise not to tell them. For the next 2 years May and Sybyl maintained limited contact by letter and phone. During this time May raised the possibility of contact with her siblings several times, but each time Sybyl said that any contact would have to take place after her death—or would be the cause of it. May's husband and grown children knew of the search and reunion, and were urging her to make contact with her half-sisters. It was when Sybyl's health began to deteriorate further that May became anxious and depressed and sought therapy.
>   The clinical focus with May was on exploring the power of her birth mother's wish to prevent sibling contact and the meaning of it in the context of the two family systems involved. May's

immediate family system was supporting her in an adult role in making a decision that she wanted to make. Sybyl, however, blocked her in making that decision by insisting that May's "other" family system could not sustain itself if her membership was recognized. To maintain the homeostasis of that other system, Sybyl extracted a promise of secrecy from May, complete with a threat should the promise be broken, much as one would do with a small child ("Step on a crack and break your mother's back").

Sybyl's family system would be radically altered soon by her death, and she felt that this would be time enough for the other daughters to learn of May. The price of May's compliance with Sybyl's demand was the disruption of May's immediate family system, the pain of learning of her birth mother's shame about acknowledging May's existence, conflict about the continuing secrecy, and the denial of contact with her siblings. In a series of therapy sessions that included her husband, May decided that this was too much to bear and that she would pursue contact with her half-sisters. She utilized Rosemarie and the pastor of Sybyl's church as allies in letting Sybyl know of her decision to move ahead and contact her sisters—with or without Sybyl's involvement.

There was a second reunion, this time involving May, Sybyl, Rosemarie, and Sybyl's three other daughters. May was accepted into that family system, and as one of her half-sisters said, "It is great to have you here to enjoy the family while Mother is alive, rather than to meet you at her funeral."

There are no happy endings, only new beginnings—each with the promise that those involved may become more fully themselves.

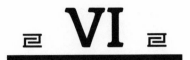

VI

TRENDS AND SPECIAL
CIRCUMSTANCES
IN FORMING FAMILIES

ㄹ 12 ㄹ

Open Adoption

Open Adoption and the Continuum of Openness

The term "open adoption" reflects the recent movement away from the secrecy that traditionally has enshrouded adoption. In 1976, Baran, Pannor, and Sorosky defined open adoption as "one in which the birth parents meet the adoptive parents, participate in the separation and placement process, relinquish all legal, moral and nurturing rights to the child, but retain the right to continuing contact and knowledge of the child's whereabouts and welfare" (p. 97). In a subsequent article in which they advocated for open adoption as standard agency practice, Pannor and Baran (1984) broadened their definition to include the exchange of identifying information as another characteristic and to suggest that "*Both* sets of parents retain the right to continuing contact and access to knowledge on behalf of the child" (p. 246; italics added).

Others who have been committed to an open process in adoption have suggested that a more flexible definition might be more useful. Watson (1988) wrote that "openness in adoption means supporting the members of the adoption triangle in doing away with as much confidentiality as they can [and] there should be degrees of openness so that the participants in an adoption can choose their own comfort level" (p. 24). Actual service has reflected such variations.

Open adoption has been practiced informally for many years in some adoptions that have been arranged independently of agencies. Agencies began to open up their adoption process in the 1970s. Among agencies subsequently identified with open adoption, the Children's Home Society of California started meetings between birth parents and adoptive parents in 1974; Catholic Social Services of Green Bay, Wisconsin, began to move from traditional to open adoptions in 1975; and in 1981, the San Antonio and Corpus Christi offices of Lutheran Social Services of Texas routinely offered the option of face-to-face meetings between birth parents and prospective adoptive parents.

Currently, agencies offer adoption service along a continuum of openness. At one end of this continuum are those agencies who believe that members of the adoption triangle are best served by the traditional emphasis on confidentiality. They make a genuine effort to protect the secrecy of the adoption transaction, in spite of mounting evidence that it is usually possible for any member of the triangle, with persistence, to find out information or make contact with another member. At the other end of the continuum are agencies committed exclusively to fully open adoptions. These agencies involve birth parents and adoptive parents in a mutual selection process, bring them together prior to the placement of the child, and expect the two families to maintain continuing contact beyond placement.

Most agencies' services range between these two points, because of their experience that offering choices about openness serves families better. McRoy, Grotevant, and White (1988) identify three points on an openness continuum: (1) closed adoption, in which all identifying information about the other parties involved is kept confidential; (2) semiopen adoption, in which there has been a mutual disclosure of information between the adoptive family and the birth parent, or a one-time meeting, or both; and (3) fully open adoption, in which the two families have continuing contact.

Some birth parents want to select the families for the children they are surrendering, and some do not. Some adoptive parents want to "choose" their children. Some birth parents and adoptive parents want to meet, but not all. Some birth mothers want to physically hand their children over to the adoptive parents (surely a good way to sanction the adopting parents' new role). Some parents want to stay in touch with each other; some do not; and others want to leave that option available as the children grow up.

There are many opinions about the value of open adoption, but there is as yet no empirical evidence to support or refute open adoption as a preferred adoption plan. Currently we are dealing with subjective experiences and theoretical formulations, not documented experience. There is no dearth of conceptual support for both traditional and open adoptions (see, e.g., Byrd, 1988; Chapman, Dorner, Silber, & Winterberg, 1986, 1987a, 1987b; Kraft et al., 1985a, 1985b, 1985c, 1986; Watson, 1988). Nor is there a lack of anecdotal reporting to support both positions (see, e.g., Byrd, 1988; Silber & Dorner, 1990; Sorosky, Baran, & Pannor, 1978).

In spite of agency resistance to modifying confidential practice, however, the trend has been toward openness. A number of new adoption agencies came into being in the 1980s, specifically directed toward meeting the needs of those who desired open adoptions and who were dissatisfied with the traditional agency approach. At its biennial meeting in 1986, the Child Welfare League of America, the standard-setting organization for child welfare agencies, endorsed the *Report of the National Adoption Task Force* (Watson & Strom, 1987), which supported openness in adoption (pp. 8–9); and in its revised *Standards for Adoption Service* (Child Welfare League of America, 1988), includes the following statement: "Adopted individuals, birth families, and adoptive families are best served by a process that is open and honest" (p. 4).

Open Adoption: Its Possibilities and Limitations

Throughout this book, we have stressed our belief that adoption creates a new kinship network that forever links together the adopted child's two families. Our approach to assessment and treatment is based on this premise. It should come as no surprise, then, that we argue here in favor of adoption planning that makes it possible for the two families involved to have access to each other as early as possible and to begin to create their new kinship network in as natural and comfortable a way as possible. It is too early in the history of open adoption to know yet whether greater openness will mean fewer disruptions or fewer situations in which subsequent clinical intervention is necessary. Our clinical experience with those who have been involved in confidential adoptions, however, consistently suggests that the most critical issues that surface in the treatment of members of the adoption triangle are (1) the unresolved loss by both adopted persons and birth parents; (2) the denial of the adopted child's dual family ties by all members of the triangle; and (3) the diminished self-esteem of adopted persons and birth parents. Although it may be true that the families or individuals involved in treatment represent a skewed sample of those who were unsuccessful in coping with some aspect of their lives—why else would they be in treatment?—the adoption population with whom we are in contact in a nonclinical context reflects these same issues— not as symptoms, but as concerns. All three areas appear to be ones that open adoption would make less stressful.

This is not to suggest that open adoption is possible or wise for everyone. For children who have been abandoned at birth, it is clearly not possible, at least initially. Some birth parents who have not abandoned their children may find the experience of caring for or surrendering their children so traumatic that they may be unable to enter into any kind of a relationship indicating that they continue to have parental significance to their children. Some adoptive parents, too, may find that their sense of psychological entitlement to their adopted children is blocked by the presence of the birth parents. Finally, there are children who cannot make a commitment to adoptive families if they are still in contact with their birth families. Other children may have experienced such trauma while living with their birth parents that they are fearful of their birth parents' even knowing where they are living; they cannot begin to consider contact with those parents until after they have experienced the security of a loving, nurturing, adoptive family and perhaps undergone some therapy.

> Marie, for instance was the daughter of a psychotic father and an alcoholic mother. During her first 4 years, she was physically and sexually abused by both parents. As a result of an abuse report, Marie was moved to a temporary foster home. Two nights later her birth father fired several shots into the foster home. No one was hurt, the birth father was arrested, and the foster parents asked for Marie's removal. After another placement for Marie and extensive efforts to rehabilitate her parents, the parents' rights were terminated. During that court hearing, the birth father went into an uncontrollable rage and vowed that he would kill anyone who adopted his daughter. Marie was placed in a confidential adoption in another area of the state. Marie has vivid memories of her experience with her birth parents, as she grows up she will need an opportunity to discuss them, perhaps in therapy, and she will probably need help in deciding whether or not to go searching for her birth parents.

There may be other situations in which openness would not be desired, but adoption agencies should provide it as an option. Sometimes it is difficult to assess whether the reluctance to pursue an open adoption should be respected because it is something that will make the adoption have a better chance of success, or whether the reluctance represents an attempted denial of the importance of the child's two families that, if respected, will make the placement problematic. Until there is more research on the results of open adoption and the factors that lead to its success, professionals involved in making placements should explore open adoption routinely, should help the participants understand the principle that adopted children always belong to two families, and should address the resistance that this concept may initially engender in the participants. Then they should allow the parties to make their own informed decision and should respect that decision.

Common Concerns in Open Adoptions

Because planned open adoptions are relatively new, the clinical data about the results or the problems that have been encountered are limited. At this point, the most common concerns of the families who have adopted openly are (1) defining parental roles, (2) defining family boundaries, and (3) broken contracts.

Defining Parental Roles

Adoption is a powerful emotional experience for adoptive and birth parents, and, of course, for the children. Semiopen adoptions, including those in which the two families are in contact and in which a birth parent may actually "give" a child to the adoptive parents, can serve to reduce some of the tension between the two families and make the placement a more satisfactory experience for both of them. Fully open adoptions, in which there is subsequent and continuing contact between the adoptive family and the birth parent (usually the birth mother), complicates the existing family systems of both, however, and may undermine the adoptive parents' initial claiming of the child or lead to confusion about the role that each is to play.

By the time that an adoption is legally consummated, the birth mother (and perhaps the birth father), the agency, and the court have all said to the adoptive parents, "You are now the parents of this child." Yet the child's "other mother" is still around. Although she has surrendered the child, the adoptive parents may feel that the birth mother still has a prior claim, or that she should be treated as a coparent. Whenever open adoption includes access to the adoptive family by birth parents, it must be clear that parenting tasks belong to the adoptive parents. The birth parents are important members of the child's extended family system, but they cannot be involved in the day-to-day parenting of that child. As part of the preparation for an open adoption, the agency reinforces the adoptive parents' claim to the child by discussing with the participants appropriate parental roles for each. The adoptive parents must assume responsibility for reinforcing their parental position at any time in the future if there is confusion.

Birth parents frequently assume a role similar to that of somewhat distant aunts or uncles. Their visits are infrequent, though usually scheduled, and often occur at holidays or on special occasions. Adoptive parents welcome the birth parent as one of the family, but also as a visitor. Visitors do not assume routine caretaking or disciplining responsibilities. Although this role resembles that of an aunt or uncle, the actual relationship of a birth parent to a child should be made clear. What to call the birth parent presents a problem to many families. Some use the term "your birth parent"; others use the term "your other mommy" or "your other daddy"; and some use the birth parent's first name—which is only appropriate if other adult visitors in that home are addressed by their first names by the children. Other children (with family help) invent a pet nickname, much as they do to distinguish grandparents. The term is less important than the comfort with which it is used and the understanding that it communicates to a child about the nature of the relationship between him or her and the birth parent.

Defining Family Boundaries

All parents with children function within two or three simultaneous family systems: one formed by the family they create through their parental roles, and the others formed by their relationship to their families of origins. In an adoption, the birth parents become a part of this family system, too. In forming the new kinship network, however, the members of the adoption triangle may be unsure where to draw the boundaries, or they may expect the new family system to meet some of their needs that have not been met in other family systems.

Members of this new family system may seek help if this boundary confusion causes difficulty to them. Depending upon when help is sought and the nature of the presenting problem, the adoption agency worker or therapist may become involved with the family. The clinician can help the family assess where the the boundaries of its family system lie, the roles each family member plays in the new family system they have formed, and the points of stress. Then decisions can be made about redrawing the boundaries, changing roles, or handling the stress in some other way. In families that are involved in open adoptions, all of the extended family system members need to understand the dynamic roles they are playing. That means that birth parents participate in family sessions with the adoptive family unit. Sometimes both birth parents may be involved, and possibly members of their extended family system as well.

A case example may illustrate boundary difficulties.

Yvonne was the second oldest of eight children who were reared by a mother who never married. While she was growing up, Yvonne and her older sister, Tammy, helped her mother care for the younger brothers and sisters. When Yvonne was 17 and Tammy was 19, Tammy left home; she went to live with her boyfriend, who was 5 years older, working steadily, and had his own apartment. Three months after Tammy left home, Yvonne became pregnant by her boyfriend, Andy, who was 16 and still in high school (as was Yvonne). Both Yvonne and her boyfriend wanted to finish high school, and they did not know whether or not they would ever marry. Yvonne's mother said that Yvonne could bring the baby home, but that she would have to take full responsibility for its care. Yvonne and Andy decided that adoption would give them an opportunity to finish school. Yvonne wanted an open adoption with the possibility of ongoing contact.

Michael and Theresa Chalmer, a childless couple in their late 30s, became involved with Yvonne and Andy in open adoption planning. Yvonne delivered a daughter with no complications. The Chalmers and she had discussed names as part of their earlier planning; the baby was named Elizabeth by agreement, and she was placed in the Chalmers' home. The Chalmers liked Yvonne and Andy and could understand why they had made their decision to place their baby. They had no difficulty in having them visit in their home. Andy made one visit about a month after Elizabeth's birth, and said that he was happy with the plan and might want to come to Elizabeth's first birthday party. Yvonne visited twice within the first month, and then started coming every Saturday afternoon, which was fine with the Chalmers. She said that she enjoyed seeing Elizabeth and that it was nice to get out of her noisy family. At first the Chalmers enjoyed Elizabeth's visits and spent a lot of time talking with her about her plans beyond high school. Yvonne began showing them some of her school papers, and sometimes would bring an assignment to work on while she was visiting.with them. She began talking about possibly going on to college, something that she said had not really occurred to her before. Then she began dropping in at other times in addition to her Saturday visits. She spent less time with Elizabeth on these visits than she did discussing school or her future plans or working on her homework. When she was at the Chalmers' at mealtimes she joined them, and sometimes in the evening after Elizabeth was in bed, Yvonne watched television with the Chalmers.

The Chalmers began to feel trapped. They recognized that Yvonne was viewing them in a supportive parental role. They wanted to help her finish school and go on to college, but they had agreed to adopt her baby, not her. They sought help. Initially, Mr. and Mrs. Chalmers met with a therapist to identify the problem and explore their feelings. They were reluctant to limit Yvonne's time in their home, both because they felt that they were helping her and because they did not want to jeopardize the ongoing contact, which they felt would be good for Elizabeth. With the therapist's support, Yvonne was invited to join them for several therapy sessions. The initial focus was on the impact of Elizabeth's placement on all of them and the roles each was now playing in the new family system. Yvonne said that she didn't feel like Elizabeth's mother, and at first wasn't quite sure what to do when she visited. Once she realized that the Chalmers were interested in her school work and her future plans, however, she relaxed and "began to feel like one of the family." She liked seeing her baby, but said that she had always had all of the babies she needed at home. What she didn't have was "peace and quiet."

The therapist used that comment to explore Yvonne's perceptions of her family system and whether or not it was meeting her needs. Yvonne's mother and her sister Tammy were invited (separately) to participate in the family counseling sessions, but neither accepted. Tammy did express interest in Yvonne's college plans and encouraged her to visit more often. The therapist referred Yvonne to individual counseling for help in working out her academic plans. The Chalmers decided that they wanted Yvonne to visit only once a week. In addition, they arranged to telephone her on another day to talk with her about school and her plans. Yvonne decided that as she thought more seriously about college, she needed time away from her family to study, and arranged to visit with Tammy on a regular basis. When treatment was terminated, it was with the understanding that it might be wise to get together to reassess the situation in about 6 months. Depending upon what the participants thought at that time, an annual "therapeutic review" could be considered.

Broken Contracts

Adoption establishes a new legal relationship between children and their adoptive parents. Most adoption laws make it clear that there can be no conditions attached to the adoption decree that mandate continuing contact between the two sets of parents. The courts have traditionally held that the adoption decree must not establish for an adoptive family any conditions that would set this family apart from a nonadopting family or that might be construed as restricting their right to parent their adoptive child in any manner that they choose, as long as they comply with the laws by which all parents must abide. There are, however, no legal restrictions *preventing* contact between the adoptive parents and the birth parents, except in some unusual circumstances when a special court order is issued independently of the actual adoption decree. The extent and nature of the relationships between the two families after consummation is left to the participants. Any agreements about ongoing contact must be extralegal, and compliance must depend on the good faith of those involved.

At the point of placement, any assessment of the value of such contact is based on conjecture about what the future will bring. The focus is on the immediacy of the experience. At the time of the adoption, the new adoptive family has had little or no opportunity to function as a family unit, unless the child has been in foster care in this family for some time prior to the adoption. The adoptive parents' feelings about the adoption are still very much influenced by the issues that have brought them to adoption and by their new role. Whatever their contact with the birth parents up to this moment, the adoptive parents are usually ambivalent toward the birth parents now. When they visit their child in the adoptive home, the birth parents, too, will feel a resurgence of ambivalence about their decision to surrender the parenting of their child.

Thus, the idea of a continuing relationship between the two families is viewed with mixed feelings by both. At the point of placement, it can be expected that all the parties involved will continue to grow and change.This means that the arrangement for an open adoption may at some time no longer meet the needs of any one of the parties involved. In the context of the pattern of meaningful relationships that we all form, this should not be surprising. Many of our most intimate relationships have meaning because of shared experiences that have significant emotional meaning to those involved. And many a sincere promise to keep in close touch is broken by physical separation, the lack of continuing common experiences, or shifts in life direction or focus. Sometimes plans to keep close contact are consciously re-evaluated and changed, but more frequently the changes occur by default.

The problem in open adoption is that to bind everyone into a

legal arrangement for continuing contact is to lay the groundwork
for possible adversarial procedures later, and not to do so is to leave
the openness plan in jeopardy. Baran and Pannor, two of the
pioneers in developing and implementing the concept of open
adoption, have become disenchanted with the idea. Recently they
have suggested that open adoption may not be the best route (Baran
& Pannor, 1990). Their experience, and that of others, is that the
original plan for continuing contact between the adoptive family
and the birth parents erodes with time. Baran and Pannor (1990)
have proposed instead a plan of permanent guardianship that they
feel provides the security of adoption for the child but leaves the
court involved to demand and monitor the involvement with the
birth family. However, there are three problems with such a plan:
(1) Continuing court involvement may lessen the sense of entitlement on the part of adoptive parents or the sense of security that the
child feels; (2) the likelihood of growth and changes in those
originally involved in the plan is held as the exception, rather than
the norm; and (3) court involvement by definition suggests the
possibility of future litigation and sets up a potential adversarial role
between the two families.

The difficulty about such changes in open adoption is that a
change that reduces or eliminates contact may leave members of the
triangle feeling that they have been betrayed. The child is particularly vulnerable to such changes and may feel that the contact has
been terminated because of something he or she has done. If the
adopted child is too young to have been initially involved with the
birth parent, later, when that child developmentally needs the
possibility of contact with the birth parent, that contact may not be
immediately available. Often triangle members seek clinical help at
such times.

When an agency arranges an open adoption, it assumes the
responsibility to be as certain as possible that the conditions of the
openness are clear and that all parties make a commitment to abide
by them. It is important to get the agreement in writing, not because
it is a legally enforceable contract, but because a written agreement
lends substance to the agreed-upon plan. Whether the agency is part
of the ongoing plan or not must be decided at the time that the
agreement is worked out. In some open adoptions, the agency is
invited to play some continuing role — initial letters may be exchanged through the agency, the agency may serve as a meeting
place, it may help arrange transportation for visits, or the like.

For instance, in the case of Joanne, Billy, and Adrian (discussed
in Chapter 5), both parents voluntarily surrendered the children

but wanted to maintain contact. The father, Ralph, visited the children in the adopted parents' home when he was not incarcerated. The mother, Anne, on the other hand, elected to visit them at the agency. She stated clear why she made this choice: "I want to see my children, but I do not want to be a part of their daily life in their adoptive families or communities." The agency served as a meeting place for Anne and the adoptive families twice a year. In the summer the adoptive parents and all of their children, only three of whom were Anne's, met Anne at the agency, and they all went for a picnic in a park near by; just before Christmas, the group assembled again at the agency for a holiday get-together.

Whether the agency continues its involvement can be a delicate point of negotiation. The agency should neither intrude into the lives of the families they have helped to create, nor remove itself from playing a role that those involved expect or want it to take. The surest way to handle this is by talking with all of the parties and identifying the options for agency involvement. If there is agreement that the agency has no further role, the worker should make it clear that should there be a change of mind in the future, anyone is free to contact the agency to see whether it can play a role.

When continuing contact is part of the agreement, the agency should help the participants structure the contact in a way that supports regularity. That means an early visit, concrete plans for future contact, and establishment of rituals that serve to reinforce the value of the visits. Although geography may not always make it feasible, a contact with a birth parent within the first 2 or 3 weeks of the consummation of the adoption is important. This helps to confirm the new roles that result from the adoption by providing everyone a chance to play them. A child is reassured by seeing that although the birth parent is still in contact, the child now "belongs" to the adoptive family. The adoptive parents are reassured by viewing the birth parent as a significant visitor who enters and leaves their immediate family system, and the birth parent is reassured by realizing an actual visit that had up until now had only been a promise.

Although flexibility is fine, nothing erodes an agreement for continuing contact any faster than a plan to get together "sometime in the future—date and time to be arranged." If the agreement is for ongoing contact, it is useful if at the end of each visit the next contact is tentatively planned and a date identified. Plans may have to be changed, but if a date has been set, someone has to take the responsibility to make the change. The idea that the contact will be rescheduled is implicit.

One of the values of rituals is that they help people focus

attention on things they consider important. Building rituals around contacts in open adoption will help maintain the contacts. The simplest rituals, of course, are those that incorporate existing or culturally accepted elements, such as the planned exchange of holiday greetings (or a regular holiday visit, as in the case of Anne, discussed above) or involvement in a child's birthday party. Altough a planned annual celebration of a child's adoption day is used as a ritual by some families, the value of this idea needs to be tempered by an assessment of how "special" adoption should be for a specific child in terms of where that child is, both in the developmental process and in the process of coping with adoption. The rituals do not need to be related to the child's adoption or to conform to the usual celebrations. Whatever is comfortable for the kinship network involved is what should be ritualized and institutionalized—such things as sending copies of the child's annual school pictures and photocopies of report cards to the birth parent; having a special picture taken each year that includes the adoptive family and the birth parent; or going on a spring trip to the zoo together. The actual event is less significant than the fact that it is given special importance and that it is established on a regular basis. Rituals need to be resssessed as new developmental levels are reached. Some children attach great value to the rituals of childhood as they negotiate adolescence. Others need to discard earlier rituals as they move along; however, it is good for them if they can accept new ones in the place of those that have been discarded.

Perhaps the most important device in keeping continuing contact is making sure that each family has the address of the other. In our transient world, some precautions should be taken to assure this. The best one, of course, is some sort of frequent, regular mail communication. Unless a party is deliberately trying to conceal his or her whereabouts, a first-class letter or greeting card will follow the recipient to a new address or will be returned to a sender. In either case, it alerts people to the need to take some action to maintain the contact. It is also helpful for each party to have the names and addresses of relatives who will be likely to know where the other person is.

> For instance, Alice was placed in an open adoption by her 18-year-old mother, Debbie. Debbie made regular visits until she moved to another community many miles away. Then she maintained contact with the adoptive family by telephone and letters. On Alice's birthday, she sent a small gift and in a note mentioned that she might soon be moving again. When the adoptive parents wrote to thank her for the gift, their note was returned as undeliverable: "Moved, no forwarding address."

Debbie's phone had also been disconnected. Although Alice was only 2 and there was no pressing need for contact, the adoptive family did not want to lose touch with Debbie. They sent a note with a recent picture of Alice to Debbie's mother, and enclosed another picture for her to send on to Debbie. Alice's birth grandmother knew about her adoption, of course. She responded to the picture promptly with a note to the adoptive parents, and sent along Debbie's new address. Debbie had moved in with her boyfriend and was using his last name. Contact with the adoptive family was quickly re-established; Debbie said she just hadn't gotten around to letting them know of her whereabouts. One can speculate, of course, that with Debbie's serious interest in a boyfriend, and the possibility of a subsequent marriage and children, maintaining contact with Alice no longer held such a high priority for her. Nonetheless, the pictures and the note reminding kinship members of their relationship to the adopted child helped to make sure that this adoption stayed open.

Sometimes the plan for continuing contact breaks down even when everyone's whereabouts are known. Usually this happens because one of the parties is no longer interested in maintaining contact. If the relationship has been comfortable and the communication open up to this point, the reason for the change in plans can be discussed, and perhaps a new arrangement can be negotiated. Professional assistance can often be useful at this point.

Sometimes the decision to modify the openness is arbitrary and unilateral. Usually such a decision is made in response to life or developmental changes in the adults or the child involved. Although clinicians can help assess the reasons for the change and evaluate how the kinship network can once again be made more functional, they are often not involved. Or perhaps they are insensitive to adoption dynamics and their effects on family systems.

Because the agreement for contact is not legally binding, and because too much pressure from the party seeking contact may end up hurting the child, sometimes little can be done other than staying in contact with notes and pictures. This is important, because it provides the option for the adopted child involved to make some choices about contact when he or she can accept adult responsibilities for making life decisions.

Unwanted "Open" Adoptions

There is another group of open adoptions that poses problems. These are those cases in which the adoption is "open," but not by the adoptive parents' or the community's desire. In such cases, the birth parents have problems that make it unwise for them to have ongoing contact with their children, but they may know the whereabouts of those children and seek contact. Sometimes contact is denied because of a fear that a birth parent's abusive behavior with a child will continue into the new family; in other situations the erratic behavior of the birth parent may necessitate limiting openness.

Adoptive parents confronted with such a situation need to be supported in an appropriate parenting role. Their first responsibility is to protect their own family and assure the safety of the child. Sometimes this can be done through thoughtful negotiation—either with or without the involvement of an agency. In other situations, it may be necessary to involve the police. In either case, it is important not to keep the experience secret from the adopted child. Adopted parents need to protect a child from the consequences of disturbed birth parent's actions, not from knowing about the reality of that parent's disturbance. Older adopted children should be made aware of the circumstances. Younger children need to know that a birth parent is having difficulty with the adoption plan, but that they themselves are safe and secure. There may be a need for clinical intervention at this point or at some time in the future when the adopted child questions the genetic implications of the birth parent's behavior or struggles with the issue of making contact with that parent.

The case of Marilyn and Frank illustrates this kind of situation. Eighteen-year-old Marilyn became pregnant by Frank, who was 25. Only after the conception did Marilyn realize that Frank had no interest in her, but had used her to conceive his child, on whom he now focused his attention. As the embryo developed, Frank's irrational obsession with the expected child became apparent; he insisted that the child was going to be a boy and the new incarnation of Christ. Marilyn now viewed Frank as psychotic and wanted to end the relationship with him as soon as possible. Marilyn delivered a boy, whom she called Tommy. She did not wish to rear her son, nor did she want Frank to rear him. She voluntarily relinquished her parental rights and moved to a new community. She said that she wanted to know when Tommy was "safe" — that is, placed in adoption — but wanted no further contact with him. Frank refused to relinquish his rights. It took months of court activity, two psychiatric evaluations of Frank, attempted outpatient treatment with him, and courtroom threats to the judge by Frank before his rights were involuntarily terminated.

Tommy had been in foster care during this time, and now at $2\frac{1}{2}$ was placed with a new family for adoption. By plan, this was a confidential adoption. Within 24 hours of the placement, however, the adoptive family had a call from Frank saying that he wanted to see his child and intended to get him back. He had followed them home after they had picked up their son. He accused them of being a part of a plot by the Antichrist to kidnap and destroy this new Christ Child. The adoptive parents, of course, knew the background history and refused to allow Frank access to the child; they also called their local police. After several days of telephone harassment and a couple of visits to the adopted home, where he was denied entrance, Frank was arrested and charged with trespassing and disturbing the peace. He was placed under a peace bond and threatened with more serious action if he persisted. After a few anonymous notes, he discontinued his contacts.

The adoptive parents sought agency help in handling this situation with Tommy. The emphasis of the brief treatment was on helping Tommy deal with the loss of the former foster family and to feel more secure in the adoptive family. This was done in family interviews, which were held in the home, to reinforce that this was where Tommy would stay and where he would be safe. Tommy's "life book" was used to review some cognitive data about both birth parents, whose pictures were in it. The information that was shared was limited, but accurate. At the termination of treatment, the plan was to continue to use the life book as a way of helping Tommy stay in touch with his past and gradually learn in more detail about the reasons for his placement and the absence of his birth parents in his life.

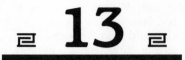

Treatment of
Variant Forms
of Adoptive Families

T hroughout the normal unfolding of the life cycle, every human being struggles with the universal themes of connection and loss. In addition, an individual's development may be affected by social arrangements that bear directly on these themes. With the steep increase of divorces and radical changes in adoption in recent decades, large numbers of adults and children undergo the confounding of normal developmental changes by socially created ones. Social engineering of this type includes marriage, adoption, divorce, remarriage, and the creation of stepfamilies. Each of these events has implication for variant forms of families and the development of the individuals within them.

As a result of divorce, many single parents and their children form households. The number of households with one parent has been further increased by unmarried birth parents who raise their children and by unmarried adults who adopt children. The membership of these families is sometimes unclear because of loyalties to, contacts with, or residence with members of extended families or other individuals. When a single parent marries for the first or second time, whole new sets of connections must be negotiated.

When one or more of these socially engineered changes converge with normal developmental stages, the potential for dissonance of experiences, overload, and distress is exponentially increased. Children are most vulnerable to such distress, because their developmental stages are compressed within fewer years. Furthermore, they have less understanding of the choices involved than adults do, and little control over them.

Interventions for Divorce in Adoptive Families

Socially arranged changes converge with heavy impact on all family members when adoptive parents divorce. Even though adoption is a means of adding family members, whereas divorce has to do with exits, the issues are parallel, loading on the issues of attachment and loss. Recently, Wallerstein and Blakeslee (1989) described divorce as not a single entity or event, but a lifelong process which has different effects and outcomes for adults and children. Outcomes for each person are affected by age, gender, developmental stage, and nature of prior family relationships. Very little has been written about, and there is no known research on, the outcome for adoptive families which undergo a divorce.

According to Wallerstein and Blakeslee (1989), there are two psychological tasks for adults in going through divorce: "The first is to rebuild their lives as adults so as to make good use of the second chances that divorce provides. The second task is to parent the children after the divorce, protecting them from crossfire between the ex-spouses and nurturing them as they grow up" (p. 277). The subtasks of divorce for adults, as described by Wallerstein and Blakeslee (1989, pp. 278-288), have additional layers of meaning for adoptive parents. The first subtasks are to end the marriage, as optimally as possible, and to mourn its loss. If mourning is aborted, the unaddressed emotions can go underground and can cause distortions in future interactions. A divorce may seem another bitter failure to adoptive parents, on top of their inability to produce children. In some instances, unresolved grief about infertility or difficulty in coparenting an adopted child may be the basis of the divorce. Without resolution, an individual may stay emotionally stuck or may transfer the emotions to the children or other relationships.

For adoptive parents, as well as any others who divorce, the prior family operating rules determine how separation is handled. The operating rules of a more functional adoptive family already include ways to deal with the loss and attachment issues inherent in adoption. Regardless of the type of marital difficulties or of whether the divorce decision was mutual or not, rules that permit openness about adoption aid discussions of divorce. Parents in a family with open regulation are able to acknowledge the pain for everyone and to cooperate on plans for separation and for care of children.

The operating rules of more dysfunctional adoptive families usually limit the expression of issues and emotions centering around attachments and loss. In the most extreme cases, needy parents who have adopted form a rigidly regulated arrangement. If one parent is left out by a coalition between the other and a child, or if the parents vie for the child's affection, the situation can escalate to divorce. In either case, the separation probably occurs in a destructive fashion, paralleling the prior process. For example, a parent who has been left out may depart without warning, perhaps just leaving a note. When there has been competition over the adoptee, the precipitant to separation is often a fight that has exceeded the usual limits, sometimes becoming physically violent. Thereupon, one parent may be thrown out or may flee, with or without the child.

Working through the emotions associated with the separation leads to a sense of detachment or decoupling, which furthers the reclamation of identity as an independent person. The culminating task of the divorce process is for adults to rearrange relationships, so that future interactions benefit all family members, particularly the children. The multiplicity of loss issues may overload even those adoptive parents who generally function well, so that they become anxious and cope more poorly in relationships. For a person who entered marriage, and subsequently adopted, in order to have a dependent relationship, establishing independence under the duress of divorce is particularly difficult. The divorced person who is unable to establish a separate identity may not risk another adult relationship or may plunge into another that replicates the former marriage. In either case, the parent may either cling to or detach himself or herself from the adoptee.

Wallerstein and Blakeslee (1989, pp. 282–294) also delineate the psychological tasks of children during the divorce process. The need for attachment and fear of abandonment underpin all of a child's responses to the divorce situation. When parental conflict and divorce converge with developmental vulnerability, fears can soar. Very young children are not yet equipped to understand either adoption or divorce, and so may be protected from a doubled load of concern; still, they may respond to the divorce with fears or fantasies of abandonment or parental destruction. They may assume that their "bad" behavior or angry wishes have caused the divorce. Young children also are unable to take in lengthy explanations or long-term plans. They must be reassured frequently, in simple terms, and prepared in detail just before any change takes place.

The grade school child is more able to understand both adoption and divorce, but that awareness may heighten fears of abandonment as well as grief, anger, and often guilt. A child of this age who is in a close alliance with one or both parents can easily be burdened by parental needs beyond his or her ability to cope. An adoptee in a role of distractor or caretaker may feel guilty for not carrying the role well enough to prevent the divorce. Furthermore, the adopted child who is aware of having lost one set of parents is likely to try harder in rescuing adoptive parents. The adoptee can feel even more upset when those efforts are not successful, creating more potential for symptom development.

The adopted adolescent whose parents divorce may suffer from the convergence of three major transitional processes. The adolescent adoptee already has the problem of how to select values and incorporate them into an identity when there are two sets of parents. When divorce impends at the same time, it may seem that no parents are reliable or safe objects of identification. Having the family dissolve leaves such an adolescent without a secure launching pad.

Older children and adolescents need to understand the reasons for the divorce and the implications for their own future security. Adoptees especially need assurance that divorce is an adult responsibility, even when the children or the adoption is somehow involved. Adoptees may be angry that parents have chosen to adopt and then divorce without seeming regard for the children's security. They may not express such feelings directly, out of deference for the parents' pain and needs, so they need permission to put these emotions into words.

Children of grade school or high school age may also withdraw from family relationships, as well as from divorce and adoption issues. They need to get back to their own normal activities as soon and as well as they can. Withdrawal from the family may be a sign that a youngster is reassured that the adults can handle the divorce and still provide security. Or it may be avoidance or denial of turmoil, which may include the fantasy that parents will get back together. Some children do not really accept the permanence of divorce until they themselves are ready for independent living. Whether or not this is a real resolution is shown then, in how willing these young adults are to risk intimate, sustained relationships. An adoptee who finds the confluence of life stage, adoption, and divorce overwhelming is likely to make this known very early in the process. The resulting symptoms are usually severe and difficult to ignore.

Adoptive parents may seek help from a therapist at any point in the divorce process — while making the decision, during the throes of negotiations and changes, or afterward. The presenting problem may focus on the marital interactions, an adopted child, or the

whole family. The form of the presenting problem is an important
clue to the stage of the divorce and the level of family functioning.
Even well-functioning adoptive parents may quaver under the
additional burdens of divorce. They may fear the effect on the
adoptee and/or family attachments. These parents may voluntarily
seek a therapist for another opinion about their process and for
assistance in making optimal arrangements. Divorce and adoption
issues can be discussed and reworked together, so that attachments
are affirmed within the new arrangements.

More dysfunctional adoptive parents who divorce usually
present in regard to, or are referred about, the severely symptomatic
behavior of the adoptee. Often there is a rigid focus on the
youngster's behavior, which is signaling the distress of multiple
transitions as well as dysfunctional family dynamics. A therapist
must try to move the focus to the adoptee's behavior in relationship
to alliance patterns and probable changes in these patterns after the
divorce.

When a therapist is exploring the presenting problem of an
adoptive family in a divorce process, items for assessment include
the following:

1. The connection between the presenting problem and divorce, adoption, and life stage.
2. Status of the divorce decision (under discussion, change-
   able, definite, in process, or complete).
3. What part adoption plays in the divorce decision, or what is
   attributed to the adoption or adoptee.
4. The age of the child(ren) at the time of adoption and
   divorce.
5. The status of family relationships before and after the
   transition points of divorce, adoption, or life stage.
6. Most important, the extent to which fears of lost attachments and abandonment are central and strong in the
   family dynamics.

When the assessment has taken form, the therapist must decide
how to use the information in combination with grief work, in a
treatment plan suited to the particular family. Sometimes the issues
of loss can be addressed in orderly sequence from the presenting
problem, to divorce stage, to life stage and adoption. But most
often, multiple layers of loss-related fears and pain surge back and
forth from all the issues and from all the family members.
Maximum flexibility is required of a therapist regarding content

and membership at sessions. A therapist helps most by maintaining a steady, nonreactive stance that includes two features. One is that grief, fears, and anger are at the bottom of the trouble, and that *these emotions are legitimate for every member*. The other is that the therapy offers a safe place to express these emotions; the therapist keeps each person speaking for himself or herself and prevents attacks on anyone.

Then, to the extent that the family operating rules allow, the therapist guides the family through the stages of divorce. Even though the facts may have been covered in the assessment, at this point the whole process is redone with more detail and especially with more depth of emotional expression from each person. The process may begin with what led up to the divorce decision, why and how it was made, and how each member learned about it. Care must be taken that terms are kept appropriate to the age of the children and that no one is left out of the process. Even very young children should have some opportunity to participate and react. A therapist can interpret a child's behavior as a reaction to grief, loss, and change. Parents may need the therapist's help with appropriate words for talking to young children about divorce and reassuring them about the future.

As the family members vent and work through their emotions concerning the divorce decision, the therapist picks up consistently on any references to adoption. Repeated affirmation of the double (at least) load of grief and loss issues validates the reality of these issues . A therapist must make sure that parents address an adoptee's fear of abandonment by a second set of parents and that they assume full responsibility for the divorce decision.

If parents are already in separate households, each person is encouraged to express how the actual changes have been experienced. Any plans being tried for shared child care and visiting are carefully reviewed as to outcome for each person. During this phase, fears and grief are often covered by anger; unspoken assumptions, broken promises, misunderstandings, or hostile retaliations may heat up the sessions. At these times it is essential that the therapist hold the ground of acceptance of each person's *emotions*, but not of judgments or attacks on another. It may be necessary to split sessions so that different combinations of parents only, children only, or parents and children are seen.

During this phase, very difficult realities sometimes emerge and must be addressed. For example, an adoptee may learn that the adoption was meant to reinforce a shaky marriage but did not. A child may learn through a parental slip or in direct anger that parenting in general, or parenting him or her in particular, has not lived up to expectations. Whatever bitter or hostile positions come forth, almost always they are already known or suspected. By promoting an open discussion, a therapist can hope to enable the least destructive handling of a painful reality.

The final phase of treatment with the divorced adoptive family focuses on plans for the future arrangements of relationships. The plans should detail the responsibilities of each parent, how they will communicate in behalf of the child(ren), and what exactly the child(ren) can expect from each parent. At this point, some sessions are held without children present, but are focused strictly on parental cooperation in child care and are not allowed to revert to refighting marital issues. Children should be included sufficiently to have the opportunity to voice their wishes and concerns, and later to hear the outcome of planning.

Members of more functional families complete the process, despite the storms of renewed grief; they are likely to come through the process with parent–child roles and relationships affirmed, and as sadder but stronger individuals. The members of less functional adoptive families go through the divorce process haphazardly or in some truncated manner. The most extreme possibility is that a whole adoptive family comes apart—that *all* relationships, both marital and adoptive, are dissolved. In a case where the outcome of an adoptive family's divorce process is potentially very negative, clues from intake continue throughout early sessions. The best possibility of modifying such an outcome is to point out the potential or even predict it as soon as the therapist sees it. When it is not possible to forestall a negative outcome, the family members have probably reached a similar conclusion about their future relationships and the end of therapy.

> Sven and Marta met in an office where both had promising business careers. They dated for 5 years, punctuated by conflict whenever Marta mentioned marriage and children. Sven liked their life style as it was. They married after Marta turned 30 and delivered an ultimatum that either they would marry or she would find someone else. Even after the marriage, however, Sven kept deferring the question of children. After another 5 years, Marta announced that she had not been using birth control and wanted to adopt. Again, if Sven did not agree, she would leave him.
>
> Eventually they adopted siblings, Eric, 4, and Ingrid, 2, who were removed from a birth home in which an older sibling had been badly beaten. Initially both children were timid, fearful, and clingy, but Eric was protective of his sister. Marta quit work to

devote herself to the children, claiming that she was finally fulfilled. Soon Sven worked longer and longer hours. When he came home, he often smelled of alcohol and complained that Marta was no longer a companion or interested in sex. At home he usually sat alone and drank more, ignoring the three of them, or muttering to Eric about "that freezin' female."

When Ingrid started first grade, Marta went back to work. After school, the children went to the home of Marta's wealthy parents, where there was a full-time housekeeper. If Marta did not arrive until the children were asleep, all spent the night there. Meanwhile, Marta's father discovered through business contacts that Sven was having an affair with his secretary; at that point Marta requested divorce counseling "for the sake of the children." Sven reluctantly agreed, but only if the children, now aged 7 and 9, were present.

In the first meeting, Marta kept the children close and hinted that her real agenda was to have Sven give up his parental rights. Sven played to the children, particularly Eric; he emphasized that no matter what their mother said, he intended to remain their father.

When urged for the sake of the children, the parents agreed to a second session alone. Therein, Marta made it clear that she wanted the children to herself. Sven made it equally clear that since she gave them all the attention that she used to give him, he would fight. Comments about the children's welfare or symptoms (bed-wetting by Ingrid and aggressiveness by Eric) led to vociferous mutual blaming between the parents. But when confronted, both parents said that the children were the true priority.

This couple was seen on an irregular schedule in various combinations with the children. Each parent seemed to make a genuine effort to understand and help the children when the other was not present. But when the adults were together, each one's anger about the perceived deprivation to himself or herself led to mutual blame, which overcame concern for the children.

After 2 months, all four had agreed on a plan. Marta and the children were to move into her parents' huge home; Sven was to visit with the children for an afternoon every other weekend, taking them back to the apartment where they all had lived. After two visits, however, Sven did not come for the children, nor did he show up for his next therapy appointment. When the therapist phoned him, Sven said that his girlfriend had moved in with him, so he no longer had time for visits with the children or therapy. He said that he might as well give up anyway, because the children were totally engulfed by Marta and her family. In a separate conversation with the therapist, Marta agreed with a more benign version of Sven's statement: She and the children were just fine at her parents' home, and they had no further need for therapy or for Sven.

Interventions for Single-Parent Adoptive Families

The single adoptive parent either is divorced or has chosen to adopt alone. The divorced parent typically adopted the child as an infant with his or her ex-spouse and experienced the usual developmental sequences in the family setting, at least until the divorce intervened. The single parent who has chosen to adopt alone is usually somewhat older and has adopted an infant or older child with special needs. If a single adoptive parent in either situation applies for therapy, the following factors are important to consider in making an assessment:

1. Is the problem presented in terms of the child, difficulty in a transition (recent placement or divorce), or the relationship between parent and child?
2. What is the sequence of the decision to be single and the adoption in relation to the life stages of both child and parent?
3. How is the role of the absent parent filled, in belief as well as in reality?
4. How are the child's birth parents perceived, and what is their role, actual or in fantasy?
5. What support system is available to the parent, the child, and their relationship?

When a recently divorced parent who adopted a child soon after birth applies for help, the presenting problem most likely derives from the changes caused by the divorce. But the changes have also stirred up the family loss issues in regard to the adoption. Whatever the quality of the parent–child relationship before the divorce, it tends to intensify afterward; the two become even more strongly allied, conflictual, or distant. This shift may serve the needs of and may be acted upon by both parent and child.

However, because adopted children are particularly vulnerable to being assigned roles and needing to fulfill these roles, an adoptee may try harder to meet the needs of both divorced parents. A youngster may try to mediate or bring parents together, may side with one against the other, or may be very angry with both for loss of a second family. The adoptee's reaction can be complicated by developmental issues, particularly those of adolescence. If a teen has needed distance from a close relationship with the parent of the opposite sex and is now living alone with that parent, the need for distance may escalate. Such a need may be served by increased fantasies about birth parents and sometimes leads to running away.

How a custodial parent is reacting to his or her own experience of the divorce conditions the parent's attitude to the child's pain. A therapist can interpret that both are coping with loss and that although the emotions are valid, the behavior may contribute to misunderstandings. If the noncustodial parent is available, his or her direct involvement is requested. If there is more than one child in one parental home, or children are split between the homes, all the children should be included as well.

Regardless of the availability of the noncustodial parent, other supports to the household are important and may also need to be invited to a session. These may include members of the extended families, friends, or lovers who have a special relationship to one or more of the family. When parents of an adopted child divorce, each person has an original family whose members might be helpful. Invitations to others to join sessions should include a specific reason based on helping the household, but the issues of divorce, adoption, and loss need to come into the discussion.

When the request for therapy comes from an adoptive parent who has chosen to adopt alone, issues of attachment are often primary. This parent (most often female, but not always) has usually chosen to adopt after becoming established in employment. She can provide for a child but is nearing the end of her child-bearing years, and has chosen adoption as the best way to have a family. Most such adoptions take place through agencies serving infants and older children with special needs—that is, children who have medical or emotional problems, who are of mixed racial heritage, or who have been in multiple homes. A longitudinal study by Shireman and Johnson (1973, 1986) indicated that children adopted by single parents generally fared as well as others. The development of gender identity did not suffer. The exceptions in outcome were the children who had the most difficult prior experiences.

The request for help with attachment issues in such a case comes soon after placement and/or at adolescence. The original placement may occur at a time that is out of phase with the development of both child and parent. In an extreme example, an inexperienced parent at midlife adopts an emotional "baby" who in age and physical maturity is an adolescent. Although most placements are not so extreme in developmental discrepancies, placement and attachment issues are complex. Even if the initial placement goes smoothly, the issues of attachment tend to be resurrected during adolescence.

When the placement is recent, a therapist emphasizes that attachment takes time and is a process that must be negotiated. Emotions are elicited and supported; in addition, education is provided about the issues, and alternative behaviors are suggested for both parent and child. (For an example, see the vignette at the end of Chapter 2). In working with attachment, a clinician must take care not to assume knowledge about what quality of relationship and degree of closeness are most desirable in a particular case. Sometimes the backgrounds of both the child and the parent cause them to prefer relationships that are not overly demanding of intimacy. A child may be well served by having the exclusive attention of one adult.

Even when an adoptive parent has never married, the ways in which the parent and child define the meaning of the empty role are significant. However, sometimes the levels of meaning and reality must be considered separately. For example, a parent and child may believe themselves to have an exclusive attachment, when in fact particular other people are very important. The role of the other parent may in fact be filled by the parent's relative, friend, or lover. Often the caseworker who has arranged the placement takes on or is invited into the role of second parent, whether any of them realize it or not. Sometimes a child promotes an attachment between parent and someone important to the child.

Sometimes the definition of the parent–child dyad has other implications. For example, claims that their arrangement is just what they want may indicate a potential for closeness that will become too much for them. Or the single parent and the child may shut out the need for a second parent by joining in rejecting potential spouses for the parent or the child's former foster or birth parents. The beliefs and realities about the role of second parent are discussed in session; if this is thought to be appropriate, *de facto* occupants of the role can be invited to participate. The creation of shared, mutually acceptable beliefs about the meaning of their arrangement fosters attachment. In order to arrive at shared understanding, past experiences in family relationships must inevitably be discussed and compared.

Regardless of how a single adoptive parent and child work out their beliefs and realities about their arrangement, they need ample supports. If they already have a network, keeping up contacts is encouraged. If there is not a sufficient social network, or if there is no awareness of resources, a therapist can help locate what is needed. Resources may include various services, such as special educational or recreational programs, adoption support groups, individual therapy for the child, medical resources, or respite care.

The following case illustrates the complex interplay of single-parent–child dynamics with life stage issues.

Georgia, at age 36, was an established pediatric dentist who concluded that she wanted a child of her own even though she did not plan to marry. She adopted Jenny, then 5, whose parents were Chinese and Native American. At 5, Jenny was a tiny child who looked "Chinese with a tan."

Jenny's birth parents had not married, but lived together on and off for over a year after Jenny was born. When the parents were not together, the birth mother and Jenny stayed with various relatives or friends. After Jenny passed her third birthday, her parents split up for good. The mother had no money and wanted to go on the road with a new boyfriend, so, she applied for foster care for Jenny, "just until I can get on my feet." Instead, she disappeared. When she was finally located and her parental rights were challenged, she said she could not possibly care for a child and signed the relinquishment. Jenny meanwhile had been in two foster homes, the first briefly and the second until the adoption. In both homes she had a reputation for being a quiet, timid child who was extremely cooperative. But she rarely showed any emotion and preferred playing by herself.

Georgia and Jenny seemed to like each other right away. They soon settled comfortably into their well-appointed home and established a very regular routine. The routine included their separate time at work and school, as well as time at home together and meals. On weekends, they spent a lot of time in proximity to each other, but usually involved in an activity rather than chatting. Neither was very demonstrative or emotional, but things seemed to go along well. Georgia marveled over what an agreeable "little doll" Jenny was. Jenny, meanwhile, learned how to smile and to play with a best girlfriend she met at school.

When Jenny was 14, Georgia brought her to a therapist. Jenny had become sassy in every exchange with her mother. She was rebelling against attending school and against the schedule for meals and coming home. Her long-time girlfriend had been rejected in favor of smoking cigarettes on street corners with older boys. Georgia said that when Jenny passed puberty at $12\frac{1}{2}$, she seemed to change radically. Nothing Georgia tried seemed to work, and she felt frantic but did not know what to do. Moreover, she was afraid of what could happen.

Separate meetings with Jenny led the therapist to conclude that adolescent changes had taken the lid off all the emotions she had been storing. Jenny was furious at all three of her parents for not "really loving" her; at the same time, she had some awareness of feeling that she needed to distance herself from her mother's care in order to grow up. This assessment was delivered to the two of them, with the result that Jenny went into individual treatment with a second therapist. The first therapist alternated between meetings with Georgia alone and joint sessions. For a while the situation became much more difficult, because of the extent of Jenny's rage and her mother's distress with it. Then, at the end of a year, Jenny became pregnant.

This event led to the turning point between them. Sharing the pain of this circumstance and working out the decision about what to do gave each another way to relate. Jenny gratefully allowed her mother to take care of her, while Georgia was grateful to have a role in which she knew what to do. They decided together on an abortion, which was arranged by a plan that suited both of them. Thereafter, they worked out new ground rules for how they would live together. They planned a limited amount of time together, which would mostly be centered around meal preparation. But there was a prescription for 15 minutes after dinner in which they would check in with each other by talking. Now, when they did talk, both Jenny and Georgia were better at expressing their opinions and emotions.

Interventions for Marriage or Remarriage in Adoptive Families

When a single adoptive parent marries or a divorced parent remarries, there is a convergence of still more levels of attachment and developmental issues. In both instances, the parent–child relationship precedes the marriage; also, both situations include at least two sets of parents, and maybe more.

About 65% of remarriages in the United States involve children from a prior marriage and result in the establishment of a stepfamily, according to Pasley and Ihinger-Tallman (1988, pp. 204–205). From 7% to 12% of remarriages include children from both adults' former marriages. Only about 3% of remarriages have the most complex stepfamily structure, involving his, her, and their children. Since mother–stepfather households are the most common, they are described most often here in order to simplify the discussion. The other forms are recognized as well, and the issues can be transposed as appropriate.

Considering the numbers of stepfamilies and adoptive families, huge proportions of children have dual sets of parents. The biggest difference between these groups is in personal knowledge of the two sets of parents. A child adopted just after birth has no memory of his or her birth parents. In contrast, a child in a stepfamily almost always has memories of and often continuing contact with the nonresidential parent. The experience of a child in an open adoption or an older adoptee who remembers the birth family can be quite similar to that of the child living in a stepfamily. But when adoptive parents remarry, the adoptee can have three sets of parents. When the issues are multiplied by six, the situation can be enormously confounding for all parties. A review of the areas that concern remarried families, described by Visher and Visher (1988b, pp. 225–236), quickly shows how these concerns overlap with those of adoption (for therapeutic strategies with stepfamilies, see Visher & Visher, 1988a).

Themes related to attachment and loss are central and already heavily loaded when an adoptive parent remarries. The way in which these issues were handled in the first marriage and through the divorce affects the needs and fears brought to the new marriage. The new spouse must find a role with a child who already has two other parents of the same gender, with whom there are real or fantasied relationships. The child may feel abandoned by three other parents and may approach the stepparent with grave misgivings. Or perhaps the pain of earlier losses is mediated or denied through unrealistic hopes and beliefs for the new stepfamily. Either an adult or a child may attempt to disregard the prior experience and force the new family into the mold of ideals or fantasies. Such wishes may be reflected in the expectation that nuclear family names be used at once; for example, the stepfather may be expected to become "Dad" immediately.

Commonly, misunderstandings center around the stepfather's role in a household shared with a custodial mother. He may have come on strongly as the "new father," in an effort to make a role for himself or in response to the mother's request for him to take over. Children resent too quick an assumption of a parental relationship, and may cling to the mother and/or the noncustodial father. For her part, the mother can feel torn about keeping good relationships with her new husband and with the children, especially when the others are in conflict. The stepfather also may experience exclusion when the mother deals with the children or with their father, the ex-husband. Children, especially adoptees, can feel left out because of the intensity or priority given the new marriage.

During the negotiation of stepfamily relationships, the additional vulnerability to loss embedded in adoptive relationships can produce a shift in degree in prior alliances. The alliances either weaken further or intensify, perhaps to the point of virtual symbiosis. The direction of such shifts often has less to do with who lives together than with the prior alliances and attempted defense against loss. The operating rules of the prior family in regard to the adoption set a precedent for what will happen in the stepfamily. For example, if there was an open, positive attitude toward birth parents, that can ease the adoptee's acceptance of stepparents. If the prior rule was that the adoptee's loyalty must be exclusively to the adoptive parent(s), that may pose difficulty in relating to a stepparent. Conversely, whatever is worked out in the stepfamily relationships may set a helpful precedent for an adoptee's subsequent interest in search, reunion, or ongoing contact with the birth family.

Regardless of the nature of the power arrangements in first marriages, the potential for stepfamilies, at least initially, is that previous alliances hold more power than the newer ones. If an adoption held special meanings in the earlier family, the adopted child may be overly powerful in some way and may use that power to assuage guilt and fear. The behavioral manifestations of jockeying for power in the stepfamily are closely related to loyalty issues (i.e., the underlying emotional attachments). When adoptive parents in separate households continue to compete for the affection of a child, the child can be confused or conflicted about loyalty to both. Nevertheless, an adoptee probably tries harder to meet parental expectations, even when his or her assigned role is to serve as arbiter, messenger, or character assassin.

When an adoptee lives with his or her adoptive mother in a stepfamily, loyalty to the adoptive father, even when he has disengaged, can have a major impact on relationships. A child's verbal or nonverbal grief can increase the mother's indulgence or ambivalence toward the child. Similarly, a child's loyalty to the father may interfere with attachment to the stepfather, even when the child likes him. Finally, if an adoptee's loyalty to and grief about a second missing father is not recognized, the layers of loss and conflicting emotions can be internalized. The result can be long-term difficulties in relating to adult males or superficial relationships.

As the adoptive stepfamily struggles through the rearrangement of attachments, households, power, and loyalties, redrawn boundaries should emerge; these are necessary to secure the new family structure. An important but difficult part of this is that while new spouses try to develop a secure boundary around their dyad, each must manage a different level of relationship with the child(ren). At the same time, the schedule of visitation and financial responsibilities of the noncustodial parent are an ever-present reminder of the previous family structure. There is a need for new boundary definitions for those relationships as well.

Former spouses, even when there is optimal investment in continued coparenting, must determine what privileges the former spouse has in relation to the new home and stepfamily. The two new stepfamilies of former spouses can draw the boundaries between them in various ways. At one pole, there is spontaneous, friendly visiting back and forth; at the other pole, contact is only by telephone or at the doorway. Remarried adoptive parents, as a result of the intensification of early arrangements, are likely to be closer to these poles.

Misunderstandings can be rife during "changeover periods," the times when children move between households. Most children react to the change itself with some sort of unsettled behavior. Often an adult assumes that a child's upset results from something the other parent said or did. The solutions of boundary issues must be especially clear and reliable for the adopted child. The upset of changeover time should be accepted and acknowledged, and a way to ease the particular child's transitions should be found. Some examples are quiet time alone, extra time and attention from the welcoming parent, and/or agreement not to discuss the other parent or visit unless the child wishes.

The final issue for stepfamilies—one that, like the others, is more difficult when adoption is involved—is the potential for discrepancies in life stages. Each spouse may come to the new marriage with different amounts and types of life experience. Commonly, this occurs when an older man with half-grown children marries a younger woman who has no children but wants them. Such an event puts the family into at least two life stages simultaneously: Children are both being added and preparing to leave.

Under such circumstances, the father often feels torn or guilty about the need to spread his resources between two sets and stages of children.

The adoptive parent whose ex-spouse was infertile may indeed have another chance to have a child by birth. But when adoptive parents have children by birth in second marriages, feelings of concern, guilt, or ambivalence toward the adoptees may heighten. Conversely, an adopted child may be terrified that if a parent has a child by birth, the adoptee will lose still another parent; therefore, he or she may be hostile to the stepparent (who is viewed as abetting potential abandonment) or to a new child.

On the whole, research evidence on the outcome for children living in stepfamilies indicates that no difference in general functioning is predictable by family structure alone. Pasley and Ihinger-Tallman (1988, pp. 216–217), suggest that both male and female children fare better in stepfamilies than in single-mother households. There is some indication that levels of withdrawal and depression decrease with the remarriage of custodial mothers for both male and female children. But while antisocial behavior decreases for boys following parental remarriage, such is not the case for girls. Girls who seem to adjust well immediately after the divorce may erupt during adolescence (see also Isaacs & Leon, 1988).

The results for adoptees in stepfamilies are likely to be similar but somewhat more negative. The observation about a delayed reaction for girls after divorce closely parallels observations about "good" female adoptees in adolescence. Especially relevant is that both adoptive families and stepfamilies often have heightened anxiety about a weakened incest barrier. When a family has both features, anxiety and pressure on the incest barrier may greatly increase. An adopted son who lives with his mother may be greatly relieved at the presence of a man when she remarries, especially if he is in or near adolescence. On the other hand, an adopted daughter who lives with her mother probably became closer to her during the stress of divorce, solving for a time the problem of which mother to identify with. A stepfather, then, is a threat to her relationship with her mother and to her solution of her dual heritage. In addition, if the daughter is in or near adolescence she has the problem of how to relate to a new father figure, who has a sexual relationship with the mother, with whom the girl identifies. If the daughter is able to manage all this anxiety during adolescence, it may surface later as difficulty in establishing enduring, intimate relationships with men.

When a stepfamily that includes an adoptee applies for treatment, most often the remarriage figures prominently in the initial request; concern for a child or for particular relationships is cited. Right from the initial contact, it is useful to select one pressing aspect of the complex set of problems as a place to begin. All along the treatment of stepfamilies requires quick judgments and considerable flexibility about who to see and in what sequence. Assessment of a stepfamily is more complex because the family structure is often in a state of flux. The broader range of individual developmental stages adds to the general confusion, particularly when these individual stages are discrepant with the affiliation stage of family life. Under the stress of all these factors, a child's adoption may not be mentioned very early.

From the initial selection of one issue, a therapist can set up an interview plan that seems most likely to enhance assessment and begin intervention. Each dyad of the household, adults together, children together, or the whole household may be seen in whatever sequence can be agreed upon. The noncustodial parent is included as soon as doing so is seen as relevant to the problem and as feasible. Usually it is best to see the noncustodial parent alone for the first appointment, so as to hear that side of the story without contamination from present or past spouses. From that interview, it should be possible to decide whether next to see the noncustodial parent with his or her new partner, with the children, with the ex-spouse, or in some combination of adults and children.

The focus on the first problem serves as a bridge into the complexities of the stepfamily — in particular, to the most recent structural event, which is probably the remarriage. Each person should have ample opportunity to express opinions and concerns about how the new arrangements are working. The therapist may need to do a great deal of supporting and educating about normal reactions of each person according to age and position, so as to cut into misunderstandings, assumptions, and blame. In particular, it may be necessary to counteract the wish for an instantaneous, ideal family by insisting that family relationships must be built slowly. It is necessary to stay with these structural issues until there are changes in the problems and more comfort is experienced by all.

In the course of addressing the issues of reorganization, emotions relating to loss, loyalty, and new attachments emerge. At this point the divorce and prior family experiences can be reviewed, including those of the stepparent. The therapist must take care that each person has an opportunity to talk about prior experiences, with all the pain, fear, and hope brought along to the stepfamily. During this phase of treatment, misunderstandings that stem from lack of shared meanings about behavior can be cleared up. In instances where there has been conflict about the stepfather's role, the mother must be encouraged to assume the main authority with the children. The stepfather's position evolves most positively when he begins by supporting the mother in her authority while staying out of discipline. At the same time, he makes overtures to develop friendly relationships with the children.

In working backward through a stepfamily's history, it can be useful to do a time-line genogram. (Chapter 8 discusses the use of this technique with adoptive families with young children.) This chart, usually done on large sheets of paper so that it can be easily seen and saved, depicts all parts of the stepfamily. Such a chart is particularly useful for assessing these complex structures, as well as helping the family members (and the therapist) organize and clarify their experiences. Furthermore, for a family whose members have never talked about these matters or have difficulty in doing so, a chart aids and eases discussion. The drawing of the chart begins with the current stepfamily and moves backward in time through all the events of affiliation and change. In turn, each change is reviewed, including dates of and impressions on first meetings, prior life situations, dates of and reactions to divorce, prior family experiences, and original affiliations. As persons and events are added to the chart, all family members are asked about their experiences in regard to each one. Adjectives that reflect attitudes are selected from these descriptions and listed. If the adoption has not been mentioned long before, it emerges here; either way, it is added to the chart and the whole adoption story is elicited.

People with the ability to build a well-functioning stepfamily go through the whole therapy process and emerge with new arrangements that are workable and secure for all members. But most families go through the process with many steps forward, backward, and sideways, reflecting the reverberations of issues related to attachments and loss. Stepfamily members who are having great difficulty negotiating a new family structure, often do not stay long in therapy, and the new spouses may also decide on another divorce.

> Maria phoned for help with 10-year-old Peter, who refused to attend school. Each morning he claimed an upset stomach and cried for his mother to stay with him. When he did get to school,

he was preoccupied and not learning. Maria mentioned that she had recently married Juan.

Seen alone first, Maria gave the background. She came from a Hispanic professional family and had met Steve, an Anglo, at graduate school. They married after 6 months, finished school, launched careers, and generally enjoyed life together. After Maria passed 30, they agreed to start a family. Within 2 years, a diagnosis of infertility led quickly to a decision to adopt. Through a contact of Maria's family, they were able to adopt Peter, who was half Hispanic and half Anglo, at 6 weeks of age. Both parents continued their careers and had daily child care in the home.

Looking back, Maria realized that both parents were enthralled with Peter (whom she fondly called Pedro sometimes), but no longer had time as a couple. When Peter was 3, she won a much higher-level job, while Steve seemed stuck in his position. Because her new work required longer hours, Steve spent more time with Peter alone, and they became "buddies." Maria felt excluded even when she was at home, because Peter's refrain was "I want my daddy." Eventually, Maria confronted Steve about the serious gap between them, and they went into marital therapy. After 3 months it seemed clear that their marriage was beyond the point of repair, so they decided to divorce. They were enabled to go through the divorce with little rancor and to commit themselves to joint parenting. Peter never attended a session.

Steve moved to a nearby apartment, while Maria and Peter stayed in their home. Maria took Peter to day care early in the morning. In the afternoon, Steve picked up Peter and stayed with him until Maria came home. Often he stayed for dinner and put Peter to bed. For over 2 years this plan continued, ironically providing the ex-spouses with more pleasant time together than they had had before the divorce.

Then Maria met Juan and wanted to bring him home some evenings. So she suggested that Steve take Peter to his apartment and then bring him home later. Steve was coldly angry about this, but complied; however, when he brought Peter home he stalked throughout the house, seemingly checking whether anything had been changed. When he came across Juan, Steve glared at him silently. Peter also watched Juan but refused to talk with him. On occasions when Juan stayed overnight, Peter banged on the bedroom door in the night, hollering, "Mom, I'm sick!"

Over the next 2 years, Steve and Peter gradually seemed less angry. Peter still went to Steve's apartment after school, but by then he could walk home alone. When he was alone with Maria, he wanted her undivided attention, but they began to have good chats. Meanwhile, Peter was no longer overtly hostile to Juan, but still competed with him for Maria's attention. Just before Peter's 10th birthday, Maria agreed to marry Juan because she thought Peter could handle it now. After the wedding, Peter wanted more attention from Maria, but he also asked more frequently about "living with Dad." As tension built, Maria finally said that maybe Peter should live with Steve.

From the first day of school, about a month after the wedding, Peter complained that he had an upset stomach and wanted to stay home with Maria. Maria tried staying home a few times and took him to the doctor. When no physical problem was found, she began forcing him to go to school, but then she received several calls to come and get him because he had thrown up. Every day there was a struggle; not knowing what else to do, she phoned for help. The initial appointment was with Peter, Maria, and Juan. Subsequently, the sequence of attendance was as follows: Peter and Maria; Maria and Juan; Peter alone; Steve alone; Peter and Steve; Peter, Maria, and Juan; and then Steve, Peter, Maria, and Juan. During these sessions, each person's reactions to and emotions about the remarriage, the divorce, and the predivorce period were aired.

The main theme that emerged for Peter was that as much as he wanted a close connection with Steve, he feared that Maria would let him go. If she was content with Juan, she might become a second mother who did not want Peter. Maria hastened to assure him that she had thought he *wanted* to go to Dad's, but she did not want him to leave.

She also told him that she wanted him to get along both with Steve and with Juan. Steve, having vented his anger about the divorce, reaffirmed that he wanted what was best for Peter and would adjust his behavior accordingly. Juan told Peter that he wanted to be friends but that Peter had to meet him halfway.

When all this was clarified, Peter's stomachaches cleared up and he was back in school regularly, doing his work. The four of them cooperated in working out new arrangements for Peter's evenings and weekends. There were several further monthly meetings for all four wherein the only topic was following up on the arrangements for Peter. In the second of these monthly meetings, the therapist brought up that Peter's adoption was a complicating factor in the situation. When Maria and Steve told about the circumstances of Peter's adoption and how glad they were to have him, both Peter and Juan learned a great deal. Finally, the therapist introduced the idea of normal curiosity about birth parents. Their conclusion was that they had enough to do to keep the new arrangements going without adding the complication of search for birth parents.

The boy announced his resolution for the present by saying that he wanted Maria and Juan to call him Pedro, but only in the house. He wanted Steve to call him Peter, but also only in the house. At school and otherwise, he would be known as Pete. They all also agreed that if Pedro/Peter/Pete ever wanted to know more about his origins, he was free to bring up questions and pursue his interest.

Interventions for Stepparents
Considering Adoption

Although exact statistics are not available, stepfamily adoptions are generally cited as the most prevalent type, reported at rates between 40% and 75% of all adoptions in the United States (Cole & Donley, 1990, p. 273; Wald, 1981, p. 168). Yet very little is written about this type of adoption. In their books on remarried families, Wald (1981) and Visher and Visher (1982) devote a few pages to stepfamily adoption. They counsel that this is an extremely complex matter about which little is known, but which is best reviewed in family therapy.

The stepfamily situation in which the question of adoption is most likely to arise is that of a remarried mother whose children live with her. The father of the children has died, disappeared, or stopped contact and financial support. Adoption is not as likely to be a question when a child is actively involved with both parents. When adoption is mentioned in the latter situation, it may just be a new weapon in ongoing wars.

Since it is the most common type, stepfather adoption is used here as the basis for discussion; again, however, the issues can be transposed to other kinds of stepfamilies. A variety of reasons for wanting the stepfather to adopt may be expressed. One may be to symbolize or to solidify his position and relationship to the child(ren). Also, it is the only way he can have any legal authority over children he is raising, should something happen to the mother. Other times, adoption may be intended to enhance a child's sense of permanence, security, and belonging by giving him or her the same surname as the rest of the family.

Whatever the reasons of the mother and stepfather, the legal process of ending the parental rights of any other living parent usually produces reactions. Even a disconnected birth father may contest the adoption. Wald (1981, p. 169) gives such an example. A father who had been depressed and unemployed after the divorce used his wish to resume contact with his son as an incentive to pull himself together. Just as he felt prepared to do so, the petition for adoption arrived. His protest and his son's preference to keep the father's name and involvement led to shelving the possibility of adoption.

Even when the father has died or disappeared, the question of adoption by the stepfather is a highly charged issue for children. At best, it is fraught with ambivalence. On one side is the universal wish to hold onto roots, even when the realities must be mitigated by fantasy. On the other hand, a child whose original father is gone may welcome a secure, legal tie, as well as the name of the man who is providing a home and fatherly relationship.

Since most parent–child relationships include mixed experiences and emotions, these feelings add to the confusion. The child who has felt the loss of the first father grievously may stifle ambivalence, out of fear of further loss and rejection by the mother and stepfather. Such a child may seem to agree readily to adoption by the stepfather, out of self-protection. But the suppressed feelings for the birth father may well be released when the child reaches adolescence. For the child who was adopted after birth, adoption by a stepfather means that the previous father is being displaced for the second time, and thus all these concerns are even more intense.

When a therapist is confronted with adoption in a stepfamily, it is important to begin by focusing on the two sides of the issue. If two sides are not being discussed, the therapist must introduce and normalize them. Especially if parents are pressing for adoption as a symbol of family unity and legal protection, the therapist must suggest the other side. At the least, a child's mixed feelings must be legitimized and underscored as not constituting a commentary on the stepfather.

The child should have freedom of choice about the adoption and surname, but this is no easy matter with all the loyalty, attachment, and loss issues involved. If the child is old enough to be able to think through the issues with assistance (age 8 or over), ample time should be taken without rushing the decision or its acceptance. A child may need individual appointments for help in addressing these complexities. If there is more than one child, both individual and collective sessions for the children about adoption are advisable.

There are instances where parents feel compelled to arrange a stepparent adoption without a child's consent. A child may be too young to understand and/or may have experienced only the stepfather as a father. If the mother contracts a life-threatening illness, she may request adoption by the stepfather so that he can provide continuity of care and family life for the child. In such circumstances, a therapist can be helpful in reviewing all the pros and cons of the decision in the present, as well as later implications for the survivors. A seriously ill parent can be encouraged to talk directly to the child, as well as to write a letter of love and explanation for future reference.

An optimal stepparent adoption occurs when a child freely wishes, along with the rest of the family, to have legal affirmation of securely attached family relationships. Regardless of the presenting problem in the treatment of stepfamilies, adoption may play a part in the closing ritual. For some families, the decision or fact of adoption may be the vehicle for the celebration of stepfamily attachments.

Like any other adoptions, those that occur in stepfamilies are likely be re-examined by the adoptees when they become adolescents. This may come as more of a surprise to a stepfamily than to a family in which both parents have adopted a child. Although an adopted stepchild may only have three parents, instead of the four of the full adoptee, nonetheless there are questions of origins, identification, names, and possibly search. Adolescent reworking can led to a better resolution for a child badly wounded by the parents' divorce. The affirmation of attachment to mother and stepfather can provide the solid base needed for launching.

Such positive affirmation can occur even when the stepfamily is created after children have already become adolescents. Wallerstein and Blakeslee (1989, pp. 252–254) give the example of a girl who was 12 when her parents divorced. She was angry and estranged from both, spending most of her time with a tough leather-wearing crowd. The group rarely attended school and indulged in a variety of petty delinquencies. Ten years later, this young woman was transformed into a well-groomed, confident college senior. She credited the difference to the good man who became her stepfather. He had taken her aside many times, pointed out her self-destructiveness, and offered her the opportunity to go to college, paid for by him. Just before she turned 18, *she* asked her stepfather to adopt her, because she wanted to recognize their relationship by having his name. He was very pleased, and both were very proud of the young woman's achievements.

The most potentially damaging stepfamily adoptions are those instigated by one or both of the adults and accomplished either without consent or with pressured consent of the child. Sometimes the adults in a stepfamily, struggling in therapy to work out family relationships, casually suggest adoption as a solution to problems and a way of creating instant attachment. After a 5-minute discussion, they consider the decision made because no one has voiced objection. The therapist should object and insist that the decision is complex and warrants thorough discussion.

> In a stepfamily whose relationships were fraught with conflict, misunderstandings, and loyalty issues, the birth mother had urged the adoption of 11-year-old Diane by her husband. The mother hoped that this would ease tensions in her new marriage and between Diane and her stepfather. When the stepfather finally agreed, Diane was told in passing. Being a rather timid child, she did not dare question the decision for fear of being thrown out. Secretly she harbored memories of some happy times with her birth father, whom she had last seen at the time of the divorce, when she was 5.
>
> As an adolescent, Diane did all right as a student and socially, but stayed away from home as much as possible. When Diane turned 18, during her senior year of high school, she announced that she had located her father in another city. She intended to go to college near that city and to take her father's surname back. She said that her decision was based on her missing him and his needing her. Her mother had a husband and could continue to share his surname.

Interventions for Adoptions within Extended Families

In the early part of this century, adoptions within the extended family probably were by far the most common type, even though most were not legalized. When a young woman "got in trouble," often she was sent away during the pregnancy. Later, some story was concocted so that the infant and girl could return home and be raised as siblings. Another alternative was that a married sibling or other relative of the girl took in and raised the infant. Because of the moral climate of the times, an "out-of-wedlock" pregnancy occasioned secrecy and family rules limiting who could know, sometimes even excluding the adoptee.

In contrast, in those days, when a child's parents died or were incapacitated, extended family members took in the children and raised them openly. If there were no available relatives, the children went to orphanages often sponsored by churches. In the black subculture, which had little access to white child welfare institutions, children whose mothers were single or unable to care for them were generally absorbed openly into the extended family. Most of these arrangements were informal, and although a child might stay in only one household (perhaps with his or her grandmother), until grown, sometimes a child was frequently moved among relatives. In other cases, even arrangements that were handled informally by the birth mother were made legal and permanent.

> A middle-aged black professional woman reported that she had been adopted as an infant. Her birth mother, who already had a number of children for whom she could not provide, sought out the adoptive parents.' The birth mother had met these people only once during a visit to another city, but she knew that they had a good home and were childless. The mother placed the baby, and a legal adoption was arranged. The adoptee reported that every year or so, her birth mother came for a pleasant visit and a meal. She knew who the birth mother was but claimed there was never any question among the three adults or herself about who her parents were. This birth mother created an open adoption!

At present, there are still many adoptions within extended families of all ethnic groups (Hoopes, 1990, p. 147). Most of these are arranged informally but with open knowledge of all parties. If the parents are gone, or if relatives become guardians through a court order, usually the adoption is eventually made legal. The fact that the child and adoptive family already know each other and have a blood tie is both the major advantage and the major disadvantage of such adoptions (Strizak, 1990). The fact of common heritage and relatives may mean that family values, connections, and even operating rules are known in advance, thereby easing a child's entry into the family. On the other hand, the child's parent may be the "black sheep" of the original family. In such cases, the child may have had no socialization similar to that of the adopting relatives, or may receive projections of "black sheep" characteristics.

Likewise, previous experience in the extended family relationships may make openness about the adoption more easy or more difficult. If adoptive parents have a positive attitude toward the birth parent who is their relative, and consequently toward the child, the child may have permission to speak openly and fondly about that birth parent. But if even one adoptive parent has a negative attitude toward even one birth parent, that can transfer to the child and have a negative effect on his or her care. Another possibility is that relationships between the birth parent and original family members deteriorate when neglect or abuse of a child is discovered.

For example, consider the following hypothetical complexities (the gender of any character may be transposed, of course). If a man adopts the son of his deceased, drug-addicted sister and a man he despises, he may have trouble differentiating any negative behavior of the boy from that of the birth father. Similarly, if the man takes in his beloved sister's daughter and transfers affection to the girl, the man's wife may feel resentful of his indulgence, especially if the wife must cope with difficult behavior. Finally, a man may take in the child of a younger sister whom he resented when they were growing up, because she got more attention while he got more responsibilities. This man may now resent his sister even more and worsen her image in the original family, while being either indulgent or resentful of the child.

For a child, too, having relatives in the role of adoptive parents can be supportive or confusing. If the child is very young when adopted by relatives, the usual explanations about adoption must be offered along each developmental step. These explanations are more complex because they must include not only the past situation of the birth parents that led to adoption, but also what is known about the birth parents currently, as well as the child's dual relationships to members of the extended family.

Whatever the child's age at the time of adoption by relatives, the definite advantages include the potential for openness, as well as for the child's knowing his or her birth identity and knowing relatives he or she may resemble. In addition, there is the possibility of continuing contact with at least the birth parent who is related to the adoptive parents. When extended family relationships are positive, this can eventuate in a benign and comfortable open adoption situation. But there is also more potential for conflict and mixed loyalties affecting the entire extended family, especially when the birth parent is not cooperative with the adoptive parents regarding the care of the child.

All the issues of dual heritage, even when they overlap as in this instance, become active issues during adolescence. Then the sorting of the issues of dual heritage is complicated by the fact that the birth parents are known in reality, not fantasy. The youth's issues in regard to loyalty and identification can be complicated by the attitudes and real relationships between adoptive and birth parents. Openness about adoption may be assured, but the adolescent's identity development can still be skewed.

A therapist seeing members of an adoptive family who are

relatives of the adoptee still begins with the presented problem. But in the phase of working into family dynamics, a detailed focus on the dual relationships is essential. The details should include the nature and quality of the relationship between the adoptive and birth parents; the way in which the placement and adoption came about; the age of the child at the time of placement and adoption decisions; and the extent of the child's participation in these decisions.

Again, a time-line genogram is helpful in these complex situations. In this instance, charting begins with the original family and moves forward in time. The initial chart should show the connection between the birth parent who is the relative of one of the adoptive parents. Then, in sequence, events and emotions as they actually happened are added. If the adoptive parents were married before the adoptee was born, their marriage and the spouse's family are added to the chart. Sometimes both birth parents already appear on the chart. If only one does, then the other birth parent and family are added. Lines and adjectives are added showing the quality of the relationship between the birth parents and all other relatives. Finally, the circumstances of the adoptee's birth, placement, and adoption are charted.

Such a time-line genogram may depict a fairly well-functioning family network in which some event of development, loss, or accident led to the adoptee's birth and need for a home. As the members of such a family tell their story, through a genogram or in some other way, whatever emotion they identify as pivotal to the adoption is the key to treatment. Possibilities are loyalty, sympathy, grief, or rescue of the birth parent. For example, let us assume that a young boy lives with the married female cousin of his birth mother, who was the same age as the cousin and was a close friend of hers. At 17, the birth mother ran off with a member of a rock band, and 2 years later she died as a result of complications of childbirth. When the musician brought the infant to the birth mother's family, the cousin immediately volunteered to take him, citing her closeness to his mother. If such an adoptive family comes to treatment later, citing the boy's behavior as the problem, the circumstances clue the therapist to the need for all of them to do grief work.

The more dysfunctional family of adoption by relatives distinguishes itself while discussing the presenting problem or the time-line genogram. Problems of rigidity or disorganization in the original family can be directly traced to, and are still active in, the dynamics centering around the problem presented for treatment.

Here the treatment focus must remain on behavioral change—not just in the immediate adoptive family, but also in the dual relationships of the extended family. The degree of change possible in the patterns of interaction provides the gauge for when and how much the emotions and meanings can be directly addressed. The members of such a family tend to be clear in notifying the therapist about the limits of their tolerance for change.

> Ian applied for therapy for his adopted son, Paul, aged 7, and quickly noted that Paul was really a nephew. The problem was that Paul continually fought with children and complained to adults at home and school. Ian and his wife, Margot, had an older son and a younger daughter by birth. Ian reported that the rest of the family was fine; he only wanted therapy for Paul.
>
> When Ian was persuaded to come only with Margot to the first session, they told Paul's story. Ian was the oldest in a family of four, followed by two sisters and the youngest, Derek. Ian was always a responsible caretaker and buffer to his parents and the other children. His father was an alcoholic and for years stopped at a pub after work, coming home only to sleep. His mother was long-suffering and passive.
>
> Derek, a lively youngster, had a tempestuous adolescence marked by truancy, alcohol and drug abuse, and brushes with the law. When Derek turned 18, the mother told him (strongly supported by Ian) that she had to put up with his father but not with him. She gave Derek an ultimatum: "Shape up or leave." Derek threw blue language at her and left. Ian tried to mediate, but both the mother and Derek insisted that things had gone too far and they were finished. Derek was not heard from for over 6 years. Meanwhile, Ian married Margot and they began their family. In addition, Ian's father died and his mother went to work, where she met a "friend who was a real gentleman."
>
> One day a disheveled Derek turned up at his mother's house with a 5-year-old son named Ringo Starr (after the Beatle); the two had hitchhiked from California. Derek had gone right to California and gotten a job in a pizza place, where he met Cindi, whom he soon married. The young couple lived in a trailer and had a good time, hanging out at bars where there was dancing. A year later their son was born, to whom they gave "a classy name" but the fun soon came to an end. Cindi complained of being cooped up with "a kid who was always yelling and who had spoiled her figure." Money was always scarce because Derek frequently quit or was fired from jobs. The couple's stormy relationship continued on and off for some years until Derek came home one day to find a note from Cindi, saying, "I'm outa here—Ringo's at the neighbors'." Derek claimed he had tried to take care of Ringo

for a while but just could not do it, so he brought him home to the mother.

Derek's mother said, "No way. When you left, that was the end, and I'm not taking your child either." She did consent to feed them and let them stay one night. In the morning, Derek was gone but Ringo was still there. The mother called Ian immediately and said they should hand over Ringo to the state child welfare department. Ian could not agree, because "the boy is family." Apparently he also suffered unacknowledged guilt over the way Derek had originally left. Since his sisters were in no position to help, Ian persuaded Margot to take in Ringo. Margot was quite reluctant because she was about to have a second child. When she finally agreed, she told Ringo that he could not keep that name but could take some other Beatle's name, so he chose Paul.

A full assessment of Ian's family and a psychological workup of Paul was done. Ian's mother and sisters refused to take part. The test results on Paul showed that he was indeed a deprived, angry child who saw adults as hostile and withholding, and other children as competitors for scarce supplies. Margot truly had her hands full in trying to provide care for three small children, one of whom she had not planned and who was hurtful to the two she had. Ian was very torn between his responsibility to his own family and his long-standing role of caretaker to his original family.

A plan of parent conferences and individual treatment for Paul was begun. Before the adoption became final, Paul began going through still another phase of aggressive, testing behavior. He pushed Ian and Margot's daughter violently, causing her to fall and break an arm. At that point Margot had had enough and Ian concurred, seemingly out of concern that Margot might leave him otherwise.

Paul was removed by the state child welfare workers and placed in a temporary foster home, pending further testing and possible placement in residential treatment. Ian and Margot came for two more sessions, in which they discussed the outcome. Both were very relieved to have Paul out of the home, but only Margot could openly acknowledge these feelings. Ian could only focus on the need to make it better for his family and for Paul by getting Paul into a treatment milieu that Ian could not provide. When the therapist raised the possibility of future connection or visits with Paul, Margot said she might consider it in a year or two, but only if there was definite evidence that Paul had changed. Ian looked miserable but refused to comment.

Interventions for Families with Various forms of Open Dual Parentage

We conclude this chapter by given consideration to the several newer forms of families where there are two sets of parents. In these families, there is knowledge about and contact among all the parents and child(ren). The three types of such open dual parentage are stepfamilies; families created through open adoption procedures; and families that adopt older children (whose other known parents may be birth parents and/or foster parents). Of the three types, stepfamilies are best known to therapists at present.

Although the adoption of older children by nonrelatives is not new, much larger numbers of parents are adopting older children in recent decades. Placement workers are devoting much effort to, and learning rapidly about, promoting the development of a sense of family in these cases (see Gill, 1978; Katz, 1990; Triseliotis & Hill, 1990). Nevertheless, with larger numbers of people engaging in this fragile process, no doubt more will seek family treatment.

Families created through open adoption in its varying degrees have not existed long enough to provide much information on outcome for adoptees. There is not yet a cohort of adults raised in open adoption who can report on their experiences into the life stage of founding their own families. Early reports (Baran & Pannor, 1990b; Siegel, 1990) from parents who have adopted infants through an open process are on the whole, favorable, even though difficulties are acknowledged. Nor is there yet a body of accumulated practice knowledge to guide procedures or degrees of open adoption. With little to guide such intricate processes, it can be predicted that there will be difficulties for many families. Family therapists can expect to see more adoptive families and/or birth families that are participating in open adoption. In addition, questions related to open adoption can come from any part of the dual extended families. Eventually, family therapists may have more opportunity to try their skills in working with the whole network of dual extended families.

The main issue for all of these families is the variance between the two sets of parents in the kind and degree of their attachment, contact, legal authority, and personal authority with the child. In remarried families, the parents with the legal and personal authority are in separate households and must negotiate from different bases. Parents by open adoption of an infant have complete legal and personal authority. But when there is continuing contact with the birth family, there may be discrepancies between attachments and legal authority which are confusing for the child and all the parents. At least initially, the adoptive parents of an older child have all the legal authority, while the child's stronger attachments may still be to the prior family. In all these family types, the issues of dual parentage surface when the child comes into contact with the noncustodial family. Adult attitudes are reflected in how visits are arranged and in what happens. Perceived threats to adults' relationships with the child must be negotiated or will be acted out through conflict.

In any family with two sets of parents, there is the possibility that the parental authority structures will be blurred. This is most likely to occur when the two sets of parents have no clear boundary agreements between them and freely move in and out of each other's homes and lives. This sometimes happens when each ex-spouse in a divorced couple remarries a former friend of both. Other examples of blurred boundaries occur when adoptive parents seem to take in the birth parents along with the children. There are instances of open adoption where a teenage birth mother comes to be considered a member of the adoptive family. (For an example of the difficulties that can arise in such a situation, see the case of Yvonne and the Chalmers, described in Chapter 12.) In other instances of open adoption or adoption of an older child, the two sets of parents become friends or family members to each other.

To date, there is no reason to say that any of these arrangements are not viable. But if they are to be viable, there must be clear agreements about the differences in parental roles and authority, and the boundaries between the two sets of parents . Although there are as yet no models for developing such agreements, without them, there is ample potential for confusion and misunderstanding among the adults. Whenever there are problems among multiple parents, there are more errors, anxiety, and insecurity for a child.

When family members come for treatment in regard to issues of dual parentage, the presented problem either is connected directly to the double structure or is expressed in terms of a child's behavior. Adults may or may not be conscious that the child is reacting to confusion and stress about the dual parentage. The assessment of the problem and its function must follow from a very careful structural analysis. Attention must center on the child's experience as regards attachments, changes, and who holds legal authority. The history of family changes must be noted, including prior and current attitudes and alliances between every dyad, and especially any discrepancies between emotional and legal ties.

The therapist's task is to support the parents who hold the legal authority. Usually this is the set of parents who seek help, and so they are seen first. Their dyad is strongly reinforced by encouraging both their teamwork and the exercise of their authority for the best interests of the child. However, not only the child's current needs must be respected, but also the attachments to other parents; thus, in various combinations with the child, the views and emotions of each person must be elicited and considered. Nonetheless, the parents in legal authority have the final responsibility and are in the best position to make the judgments. They have the child in care and see reactions on a daily basis. Such judgments are difficult at best, especially since children often signal needs or distress through nonverbal means. Judgments are even more difficult when a child is reacting to some or all of the parents, thereby stirring up parental emotions even while the parents try to make a sound judgment. A therapist can help the parents understand a child's signals, and then can offer suggestions of alternative responses designed for the situation.

When confronted by a family where there are blurry boundaries and confusion of roles between two sets of parents, the therapist must maintain a calm, rational approach. Such an approach is supportive through conveying confidence about knowing how to help in the midst of confusion, and it also models clear personal boundaries. During the initial work with the custodial parents, the therapist must emphasize appropriate parental authority and teach about a child's need for clear structure in order to feel safe. At the same time, the parents are helped to strengthen their attachments to the child without expecting change in any prior and coexisting ones. When parents and child meet together, each should be encouraged to consider how any of the dual relationships clash and what enables comfortable coexistence. As household members develop understanding, the other parents and family members may be invited to sessions.

Noncustodial parents and other relatives must be included in sessions in a carefully planned sequence. The timing and combination of participants should be geared to support clearer structural arrangements. All members of a family with dual parentage should be brought together in session only when there is a specific goal that the therapist is relatively sure can be reached. Sometimes such a gathering serves as a closing ritual that acknowledges and affirms improved boundaries around subsets of the family. The therapist needs to resist the notion that simply bringing everyone together early on, without assessment or goals, will benefit the situation; on the contrary, a premature gathering is more likely to worsen the already existing structural problems.

Here are examples of two types of these cases.

A couple selected by the birth mother had also been her main support prior to and during the birth. Although surnames and addresses were not to be exchanged, the information came out in the course of such intimate contact. Later, the adoptive parents wrote and sent pictures of the baby (whom they named Mindy), through the agency, on schedule as promised.

Shortly, they began to get letters and handmade gifts directly from the birth mother, who also asked for more pictures and reports of the girl (whom she still called Kate). The adoptive parents were dismayed by these contacts, which they experienced as inappropriate. But they were also torn by gratitude for being selected and by their previous supportive relationship to the birth mother. With the help of the social worker, who also maintained contact with the birth mother, they wrote a kind but firm letter. In it, they affirmed their gratitude and best wishes to the birth mother; they also restated that they would continue the agreed-upon schedule of pictures, but only through the agency, and urged her to do the same.

Jeff had been removed from his single birth mother when he was 9 years old, because he was malnourished and badly neglected. Thereupon he spent a year in a genial foster family with a number of older children who liked him. Then he was adopted as the only son and youngest child of a family that already had two girls by birth. Jeff formed his strongest attachment to the younger sister.

The placement arrangements for Jeff and the family included follow-up services. Support to the parents enhanced their ability to stay firmly in charge of decisions and planning for Jeff. Therapy also enabled then to allow Jeff access to the people to whom he was previously attached.

At the beginning of placement, Jeff wanted to phone and visit his foster family frequently. His new parents were understanding and permitted unlimited phoning, but kept visits strictly limited to the previously agreed-upon schedule. As Jeff settled into the new family and school, he phoned the foster family much less often; at the 6-month visit he told them, "Thanks for everything, but I won't need to come back any more."

About the same time, Jeff began to talk about his birth mother, and subsequently a visit was arranged at the agency. Afterward, Jeff seemed shaken. He said that although it was nice to see her, all she talked about was how good he has it now and how bad things were for her. She even asked whether he had any money with him. Nevertheless, he asked and was permitted to phone her every week or so. After each call, he went to his room and sat in silence for an hour or more.

When Jeff turned 12, he asked to see his mother again at the agency. After that visit, he announced that he told her he would not call or visit again for a long time. He had decided to get on with growing up and could not take care of her. Later on, he would think about it again. Jeff seemed a little angry, but mostly resigned, that his birth mother's response was to shrug and say, "OK."

This action with his birth mother seemed to be a pivotal step for Jeff. It signaled his growing security in the adoptive family and his readiness to put his energy into his own development. As Jeff entered adolescence, he tested his parents at intervals, mostly by distancing them and stubbornly refusing to talk. In fact he had nothing to hide, since he was attending school regularly, getting average grades, and maintaining a heavy schedule in athletics.

Continued therapy enabled the parents to withstand the testing and to reaffirm their commitment, regardless of Jeff's need to be separate. The parents sought conferences as needed, for several years. As Jeff approached the end of high school, they identified behavior related to his reluctance to leave home. They realized that this behavior was related to the early neglect, so they were the ones to suggest and then arrange individual therapy for Jeff.

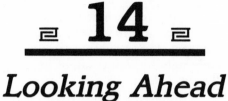

Looking Ahead

Two trends that will clearly affect adoption thinking and practice in the foreseeable future are (1)the marked decrease in the number of healthy white infants who are being relinquished for adoption, and (2) the sophisticated reproduction technology that has vastly expanded the ways in which babies can be made. The implications of the former are already apparent; those of the latter are beginning to be recognized.

Implications of the Shortage of Healthy White Infants

The perception of parenthood as a norm in our society, and the ease with which most people achieve it, supports the common belief that parenthood is an inherent right. When people have been denied that right as a result of their infertility, many have turned to adoption to fulfill their parental expectations. Understandably, they have sought to adopt an infant who is healthy, who has "good potential," and who physically resembles them. They have assumed that somewhere a birth parent is looking for a home for a child that exactly matches their fantasies. The problem for such prospective parents has been locating that child and negotiating the legal and agency processes that would make the child's adoption possible.

There has never been an adequate supply of children available for adoption to match the fantasies and meet the demands of all of the white couples who wanted to adopt. It has always been true that families with enough money or influence could use one or both to locate children, and they and others with access to children (either through personal friendships or through professional intermediaries) often adopted independently of agencies. Until recently, the rest of the prospective families approached agencies, and if they measured up to intake criteria, they were offered a chance to be "studied." Once "approved" as adoptive families, they were placed on waiting lists. Although the wait could be long and stressful, most families eventually got a child.

This is no longer the case. The number of healthy white infants relinquished for adoption has been declining for several reasons. Birth control techniques have improved and are more generally utilized. Abortion has also become a legal way to terminate pregnancies. And, finally parenting a child born to one outside of marriage is now much more acceptable. Today the largest numbers of children available for adoption through agencies are those of minority races; those who suffer from physical, mental, or developmental difficulties; and those who have come into the child welfare system not as infants, but as older children who have been abused or whose developmental needs have not been met by their birth families.

This change in the availability of infants for adoption for a large group of potential adoptive parents has had a number of repercussions. It has encouraged an increase in the number of adoptions arranged outside the adoption agency system (both legally and illegally). It has spawned a number of new agencies that specialize in helping prospective adoptive parents and birth parents "find" each other. And it has caused established adoption agencies to review and modify their programs.

Changes in Agency Structure and Procedures

Traditionally, most of the white birth parents who were interested in relinquishing their infants for adoption did so either independently of an agency or through a voluntary, not-for-profit adoption agency. The cost of the service was supported by fees charged to the adoptive parents, or by contributions made either directly to the agency or to central fund-raising organizations such as the United Way. Since adoptive parents bore all or part of the costs of adoption, the funding of an adoption program was dependent on providing those parents with children whom they wanted to adopt.

Most families were not interested in adopting children who had genetic or congenital liabilities or who had suffered deprivation during their early years. Such children were referred to the public agencies for possible adoption or for foster care. A report prepared by Westat (1986) and submitted to the U.S. Department of Health and Human Services documents what adoption agencies have long recognized: minority children available for adoption wait longer for adoptive families. Generally, minorities have not been well served by the private adoption agencies. Minority families were deterred from pursuing adoption, because agency standards and practices were not culturally sensitive and because these families held lower-paying jobs and were less able to pay the fees. Within their subculture, children might be informally adopted and reared within kinship networks, but there were biases against formal adoption or against established institutions. Minority birth mothers, too, had less opportunity for good prenatal physical care or for counseling about the options available to them. Voluntary adoption agencies were reluctant to accept minority children for adoption because there was less likelihood of a prompt placement with a fee that covered costs. Many children ended up in the care of the public agencies, where some were adopted, but many others grew up in foster care.

Beginning in the 1970s the focus on permanency planning helped identify the large number of children adrift in the child welfare system for whom adoption might be an appropriate plan, and the emphasis on placing "special needs" children in adoption followed. Special public funding was often made available to voluntary agencies to help get these children adopted. This emphasis on the placement of minority and special needs children in adoption occurred at about the same time as the number of white infants began to decline appreciably.

Faced with a decline of healthy white infants available for adoption, many adoption agencies changed their programs. Those that offered adoption as one of a range of child welfare services reduced or modified their existing adoption programs. Some agencies offered only adoption services, and their existence relied heavily on fee-paying adoptive parents. If they wished to continue to offer adoption services, they had to make adjustments. Some decided to expand into the area of special needs or minority adoption, and sought money to finance such programs by soliciting special grants or by accepting contracts with the public agencies that had these children in foster care. Others developed international adoption programs. When white infants for adoption became scarce, they discovered that some potential adoptive families were interested in adopting foreign-born children. Some of these families were able to pay the expenses of such adoptions, including transportation costs and fees to the agency to sustain its program.

Still other agencies recognized that even though the number

had declined, there were still white infants available for adoption, as well as prospective families who wanted them badly enough to pay whatever it cost to get them. These agencies began to specialize in finding infants for families that could afford the service. Other agencies developed what they called "identified adoption" programs. Such programs encouraged families wanting to adopt, or women wishing to relinquish their babies, to locate (or "identify") each other independently of an agency. Then the families and the birth parents came together to the agency for the services they needed.

Problems with the Split between Public and Private Adoption Services

Each of these variations on adoption has introduced new complications in terms of ways in which adoption is viewed and services delivered, and raises important clinical considerations. The very fact that the number of healthy white infants available for adoption is decreasing makes each of these infants more valuable within the community — more valuable to the couples who are seeking to adopt; and more valuable to those in the community who have the skills, the knowledge, the resources, and the commitment to place them in adoption. In the baldest terms, these infants have become a valuable commodity on the adoption market. Inevitably, some such children are "sold" to the highest bidder or offered to those with the power to demand them, and the "seller's market" affects service in all areas.

The service fee that is charged to prospective adoptive parents has increased. Some nonprofit agencies that charge fees have attempted to determine the average actual cost of an adoption and to set their fees accordingly; such attempts are difficult, however, and the results often are not comparable. Agencies do not agree about what expenses are to be included in the fee. If, as agencies usually say, the fee is intended to cover the expense of the service to adoptive parents, is it legitimate to include the expense of caring for an infant after birth? The hospital expenses of the birth? The prenatal expenses of the birth mother? How far back should the expenses go? And if the fee is for service to the adoptive parents, should those prospective parents who either withdraw along the way or do not receive a child pay the same fee as those who do? If the fee is different, is it based on an hourly rate for service?

Adoptions that take place independently of agencies pose another set of complications. State laws define and limit independent placements in a variety of ways. Even when the law prohibits such placements, however, there are usually ways in which the identification of a family for a child can be done legally through some intermediary, or in which the required agency assessment can be done after the child is already in the new adoptive home.

Public funding for the placement of minority and special needs children has not kept pace with the need. More and more voluntary agencies have had either to close out their adoption programs or to turn to one of the variations discussed above. The result is an increasing conceptual and programmatic split between the public adoption programs and the voluntary sector. Minority and special needs children are in the public agency caseloads, while the private agencies, for the most part, are serving healthy white infants coming in for adoption.

New agencies offering services to white families wanting to adopt healthy white infants have been springing up, and offer a number of justifications for their existence. The most common ones are that traditional agencies are too slow in making placements; that agency secrecy limits decision making by the families involved; and that agencies do not fully reimburse costs to the birth parents. Those statements are grounded in historical fact. Existing agencies defend their practices by suggesting that they are slower because they take necessary precautions to do a better job; that they are now moving toward openness and the involvement of birth and adoptive parents in mutual decision making and possible continuing contact; and that the costs of full service to birth parents cannot legitimately be charged to adopting families.

There are four essential questions to be addressed in considering adoptions that are altogether independent of agencies (or those that begin independently and end up with agency sanction). The first is whether or not those involved in independent and identified adoptions get service equal to those being served by agencies; the second is the extent to which these adoptions establish wealth or influence as the primary criterion for adoptive parenthood by restricting those without one or the other from even being considered; the third is whether the exchange of money in an adoption, no matter what the explanation, is not always really the selling of a human being; and the fourth is the wisdom of relegating all of the special needs adoption services to the public agencies.

Adoption agencies do not have a monopoly on skills or commitment. Many established and fully competent adoption agencies are now doing identified adoptions, and independent practitioners generally have to meet standards in most jurisdictions. However, if we accept that adoption encompasses a range of services, from helping newly pregnant adolescents to sharing information with someone with whom one's organization was involved 50 or 60 years ago, the chances that an agency can do this better increase.

The rising costs of adoption and the increasing value of a healthy white infant bode ill for infertile couples who want to adopt and who would be good parents, but who do not have the money or the position to get service. Money and power do not make a person a bad risk as an adoptive parent, but neither are they the most important criteria for rearing an adopted child.

The relationship between money and adoption is an interesting one. Selling people is illegal. However, as long as we expect adoptive parents to pay for the adoption services that they receive, but do not charge the birth parents of the children for the services they receive, logic suggests that the payment is actually for the children safely delivered. If we believe that adoption exists primarily to make certain that children have secure, nurturing, permanent, and legal parents while they are growing up, then those children are the real recipients of our service and ought to pay for it. Since they are usually dependent minors who cannot pay for services offered them, and often do not even know about these services until long after the fact, society must cover the costs of the services they need. It does this as it covers other expenses for the indigent, through the use of tax monies or voluntary contributions for those who believe in the value of the services. When it becomes illegal for money to change hands in any adoption transaction, the exploitation of children and families will cease or be dramatically reduced.

The split between the public and private adoption services is one from which both will ultimately suffer. Nothing has brought more life to adoption or has had greater impact on opening up the adoption process than feedback from special needs adoptive families. From them, we have learned more clearly how to assess the strengths of families for the unique tasks of being adoptive parents; we have also learned the importance of services to families beyond legal termination. If we are to reconceptualize adoption to have it make more sense, and if we are to provide services that all members of the adoption triangle need, we are going to have to utilize all of the experience and knowledge of those working with the range of adoptive families.

Potential Problems of Independent, Identified, and International Adoptions

The potential problems of the increasing numbers of independent, identified, and international adoptions are apparent both from of the families that are now seeking therapy and from our present knowledge about what is important for an adoption to be successful. Adequate and accurate information is one important ingredient. Pragmatically, for all three of these kinds of adoptions, there is the possibility that critical background information may not be available to the adoptive parents and subsequently to the child. In some independent adoptions and in identified adoptions, the potential for *more* information is available because birth parents and adoptive parents "know" each other and have the opportunity to ask questions and to share information. The questions are: What information is shared? How important is the sharing of information in meeting the immediate needs of the adults involved? And how accessible will this information be when it is needed in the future? Will adoptive parents and birth parents discuss information that may be critical to the developmental needs of the child, or will their exchange be predicated on their own immediate needs?

Identified adoptions within traditional agencies stand the best chance of developing and sharing important information. Even here, since the parties to the adoption have already found each other and agreed to move ahead, they may see agency involvement as a necessary procedural delay rather than as an opportunity to improve the chances of the success of the adoption. In many independent adoptions, the focus on merchandising means that critical information is withheld or distorted, in order that the birth parents or the adoptive parents can present themselves in the best light and thus be chosen. Background information that is useful (and may at some time be essential), is not carefully documented, or there is no certain method of storing this information and having it available at some future point.

There are children the world over whose families have been lost to them as a result of war, natural disaster, or social and psychological dysfunction. Some such children are living in institutions, with little hope of growing up in families unless they are adopted. Many prospective parents who are interested in adopting internationally are motivated not only by their own desire to parent but by their wish to rescue such children. There are legal and psychological complications in bringing these children to this country, however. Among other things, parents adopting internationally may find that they cannot get critical information on the child they are adopting. Either the child's history is unknown, or the problems of language and the lack of standard international practices make it unavailable.

All international adoptions are by definition transcultural, and many children who are adopted internationally look racially different from their adoptive parents. Becoming an adoptive family, then, is made more complicated by the absence of background information, by geographic limitations in developing the new extended kinship network, and by the child's physical and psychological cultural isolation. Not surprisingly, some international adoptive families begin to experience difficulties with their children during the early school years, when the children become aware of their racial differences. They are often helped in gaining this awareness by unkind schoolmates. Even culturally sensitive adoptive parents experience difficulty in helping their children cope with this issue. Culture is not something that is taught; it is lived.

In most instances, transcultural adoptive families make efforts to help their children understand and accept their heritage. That does not allow a racially or culturally different child full access to the adoptive family system, however. Neither can a family take on the culture of such a child. In order not to deny that culture to the child and yet integrate the child into the family system, the family must develop a new cultural context — one that includes only their own family. Successful transcultural and transracial adoptive families blur the differences between family members and view themselves as somewhat "special" families; they take pride that they have managed to do in a microcosm what should one day be accomplished in the macrocosm.

The problems come when the outside world in which these families live fails to share the families' values or recognize their cultural context as within the norm. Children are asked about their racial background. Answering that they belong to the "human race" may not be acceptable, especially on application forms. The questions must be faced: How well does such a unique family culture work, and how long will it last? The answer may be that it will last, only through childhood. Like children who are born in one country to parents who have citizenship in another country, these children may claim "dual citizenship" while they are minors. When they reach their majority, however, they must declare what country they wish to be citizens of, and renounce their citizenship of the other country. Evidence suggests that at some point children who grow up in transracial homes are going to have to decide what ethnic or racial heritage they will claim. In many instances, if they have racial attributes that are recognizable, the decision will be made for them.

The problem of establishing identity will be harder for many of the children adopted from faraway countries, because the adoption isolates them from the culture of their genetic origins. The best way to help these children is to search out others of their culture to provide a support group for them. Also important is accurate factual information about their country of origins, about their family history, and about the circumstances of how they came to be adopted in a country so far away.

Implications of the New Reproduction Technology

Nearer to home, sophisticated reproduction technology has vastly expanded the ways in which babies can be made. The technology has also generated a whole set of new issues to be faced by those who choose to make babies in these new ways, and for the children who will be produced. It is important to discuss these issues in a book on family therapy and adoption. Many of the families that will be utilizing the new technologies are families that otherwise might adopt or that have perhaps adopted already. Some of the reproductive techniques will produce a baby who is biologically related to only one parent, and the other parent will then have to adopt that child legally. And although it is too early to know what problems these "high-tech" children and their families will face, we do know about the complications of adoption, and this can provide some important clues.

The new technologies raise a number of legal and ethical questions that are not addressed here. Rather, we focus on areas of psychological concern and suggest responses based on our experience with similar concerns in adoption. We must begin, however, by suggesting an underlying philosophical dilemma that this subject poses for those working in the fields of family therapy and adoption. We are all too familiar with the complexities of families and with the number of things that can go wrong. From our experience, we know of the additional complications that families built through adoption face. And we sadly know how many mistakes we have made in adoption in the past, largely as a result of rushing ahead into what appeared to be a marvelous solution to a problem without thinking through the potential new problems our "solution" would generate. We know that there really are no "solutions" to human problems — only the possibility of exchanging a set of conditions that pain people for another set with which they can live more comfortably.

We thus approach the world of the new reproduction technology with concern based on our past experience, and with a wish to anticipate the results and manage the process from the beginning in order to reduce the negative consequences. At the same time we believe that people who are not suffering from some ailment that impedes their judgment, if given accurate and adequate information, can make decisions about their own lives and well-being better than other people can make those decisions for them. If new technologies exist to produce children for people who might otherwise not be able to have them, those interested ought to have equal access to the available resources and to make their own free choices about whether they wish to avail themselves of those techniques to have their families. Unfortunately, our experience with adoption suggests that often the people who are the most driven, and who have the resources to pursue their drive, are the most successful in achieving their ends; it also suggests that these people are not necessarily the ones who are best equipped to fill the unique parenting roles that adoption requires.

Our major reservation about the new technologies, then, is that an adult's need to be a parent may jeopardize the long-range best interests of the child whose role it is to meet that need. There are now more than 15 different ways to make a baby, using different combinations of eggs, sperm, and initial environments. Those in which all three of these involve only the two parents who end up with the baby (such as the insemination of a woman with her husband's sperm in some manner other than traditional sexual intercourse) do not concern us here. We focus only upon those children whose biological existence depends upon the contribution of one or more people other than the person claiming to be their biological parents—in other words, children similar to the children who have routinely been adopted.

Perhaps the greatest evil is the potential for exploitation that the new technologies make possible. When it is possible for a poor but fertile woman to make $10,000 by carrying to term a baby (no matter how conceived) and delivering that baby to someone who has staked a claim to it, there are going to be women willing to do it. Whatever the circumstances of the genetic origin of such a child, or whatever rationale is advanced on behalf of allowing free choice to the woman and those who are paying her, she has sold either her reproductive facilities or her baby. We need to acknowledge that fact and either accept or reject it. And if there is a shortage of women willing to perform this service for $10,000, someone will (or has already?) offered more. If our experience in adoption is any indicator, unethical people will engage in "bidding wars" for the "best" babies available.

The implications of this sort of exploitation of those who become birth mothers for money seem tragically obvious. As we already know, children bring into the families in which they grow up their genetic heritage, their uterine experiences, a bond to the "mothers" who gave them birth, and questions about their origins and identity. This raises the question of what will be shared with these children about their origins. Again, our adoption experience suggests that anything short of the truth will interfere with family openness and ultimately complicate the children's lives. An immediate problem is the real complexity of some of the procedures that are involved in generating these children, and the difficulty of explaining what has happened to children whose cognitive skills are not yet fully developed. If we fall back on our adoption experience, we know that factual information can be shared with children in response to their developmental capacity to understand and process it. We also know that more important than this factual information is the comfort of a nurturing parent with the questions, as well as that adult's capacity to accept a child's feelings about the "painful" way the child has joined this family and the sense of loss of the parts of the child that he or she could not bring along.

The circumstances of these babies' origins and the feelings of the nurturing parents about them would seem critical to the success of these new families. The kinds of issues that are explored in adoption are relevant — the circumstances of the infertility, what has been done up to now; whose idea this potential solution was; the degree of commitment of both parties to the plan; the differences the parents foresee in the family as a result of the peculiar way it is being formed; and what they will do if this current attempt is not successful. Especially critical are the feelings of the prospective nurturing parents about the method of generation and about the other parties involved. In an effort to deny the pain of their own infertility, the technological aspect of the generation of a baby may be accentuated, so that the child's creation becomes a scientific operation rather than a human transaction.

Unlike conventional adoptions, in many of these technologically created families one of the nurturing parents will have a special claim to the child as a result of a genetic tie. The nature of the relationship between the two parents and the shifts in the family system when the baby arrives are significant. Does the genetic ownership of the child give one parent more power or decrease the self-esteem of the other? What happens at points of disagreement, or at the time of a contested divorce?

Extended family involvement is also complicated by bringing a child into a family this way. Whatever the unique aspects of a particular family system, parents are always interested in the fertility problems of their offspring. This interest reflects in part their wish for family continuity and immortality beyond the next generation, and in part the pleasure of having grandchildren. Infertile couples may or may not have shared the details of their difficulties in procreating with their families. In either case, the utilization of one of the newer techniques raises new questions. The issues of "blame," genetic mixing, family integrity, and sexual values will all surface. Ultimately, the question is the extended family's degree of acceptance of the process and of the child, and the difference that this makes to the nurturing parents.

We do not yet know the difficulties that children who are generated by new technologies will have. It was only recently (Baran & Pannor, 1989) that any systematic attempt was made to examine the results of donor insemination, although this technological means of achieving a child has been available at least since 1890 (Baran & Pannor, 1989, p. xi). The experiences chronicled in the present book suggest that these nonconventionally generated children will face issues that parallel many of those faced by adopted persons. Genetic confusion, difficulty in identity formation (especially, perhaps, sexual identity formation), and poor self-esteem seem three areas of greatest potential difficulty.

The questions of the child who is the result of modern technology will be these: Who am I? How did I get here? Who will take care of me? Who loves me? What will I be like when I grow up? Am I of value? These are the questions of all children. But for the children reared by parents other than those whose genes they share, the search for answers is more difficult. It is our hope that this book will make that search a little easier for some.

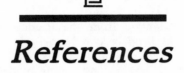

References

Ackerman, N. (1980). The family with adolescents. In E. Carter & M. McGoldrick (Eds.), *The family life cycle: A framework for family therapy* (pp. 147–169). New York: Gardner Press.

Adoption Assistance and Child Welfare Act of 1980, rel. L. No. 96–272, 42 U.S.C., 670 et seq. (1988).

Baran, A., & Pannor, R. (1989). *Lethal secrets.* New York: Warner Books.

Baran, A., & Pannor, R. (1990). It's time for sweeping change. *The Decree* (American Adoption Congress), *7*(2), 5.

Baran, A., Pannor, R., & Sorosky, A. (1976). Open adoptions. *Social Work, 21*(2), 97–105.

Barth, R., & Berry, M. (1988). *Adoption and disruption: Rates, risks, and responses.* New York: Aldine/DeGruyter.

Beavers, W. R. (1976). A theoretical basis for family evaluation. In J. Lewis, W. R. Beavers, J. Gossett, & V. Phillips (Eds.), *No single thread: Psychological health in family systems* (pp. 5–20). New York: Brunner/Mazel.

Beavers, W. R. (1982). Healthy, midrange, and severely dysfunctional families. In F. Walsh (Ed.), *Normal family Processes* (pp. 45–66). New York: Guilford Press.

Beavers, W. R., & Voeller, M. (1983). Family models: Comparing and contrasting the Olson circumplex model with the Beavers systems model. *Family Process, 22,* 85–97.

Boszormenyi-Nagy, I., & Spark, G. (1984). *Invisible loyalties.* New York: Brunner/Mazel.

Blacklidge, M. (1989). *Bonding.* Workshop presented at the Region V Conference of the American Adoption Congress, Indianapolis.

Bourguignon, J. P. (1989). *Toward successful adoption: A study of predictors in special needs placements.* Springfield: Illinois Department of Children and Family Services.

Bourguignon, J. P., & Watson, K. W. (1987). *After adoption: A manual for professionals working with adoptive families.* Springfield: Illinois Department of Children and Family Services.

Bourguignon, J. P., & Watson, K. W. (1990). *Making placements that work.* Evanston, IL: NBI Press.

Bowen, M. (1978). *Family therapy in clinical practice.* New York: Jason Aronson.

Brinich, P. (1990). Adoption from the inside out: A psychoanalytic perspective. In D. Brodzinsky & M. Schechter (Eds.), *The psychology of adoption* (pp. 42–61). New York: Oxford University Press.

Brodzinsky, D. (1990a). A stress and coping model of adoption adjustment. In D. Brodzinsky & M. Schechter (Eds.), *The psychology of adoption* (pp. 3–24). New York: Oxford University Press.

Brodzinsky, A. (1990b). Surrendering an infant for adoption: The birthmother experience. In D. Brodzinsky & M. Schechter (Eds.), *The psychology of adoption* (pp. 295–315). New York: Oxford University Press.

Brodzinsky, D., & Schechter, M. (Eds.). (1990). *The psychology of adoption.* New York: Oxford University Press.

Burns, L. (1987). Infertility as boundary ambiguity: One theoretical perspective. *Family Process, 26*(3), 359–372.

Byrd, A. D. (1988). Open adoption: Defining the terms and psychological issues. *Public Welfare, 46*(4), 20–23.

Campbell, L., Silverman, P., & Patti, P. (1991). Reunions between adoptees and birthparents. *Social Work, 36*(4), 329–335.

Carter, E., & McGoldrick, M. (Eds.). (1980). *The family life cycle: A framework for family therapy.* New York: Gardner Press.

Carter, J., & Carter, M. (1989). *Sweet grapes: How to stop being infertile and start living again.* Indianapolis: Perspectives Press.

Chapman, C., Dorner, P., Silber, K., & Winterberg, T. (1986). Meeting the needs of the adoption triangle through open adoption: The birthmother. *Child and Adolescent Social Work, 3*(4), 203–213.

Chapman, C., Dorner, P., Silber, K., & Winterberg, T. (1987a). Meeting the needs of the adoption triangle through open adoption: The adoptive parent. *Child and Adolescent Social Work, 4*(1), 3–12.

Chapman, C., Dorner, P., Silber, K., & Winterberg, T. (1987b). Meeting the needs of the adoption triangle through open adoption: The adoptee. *Child and Adolescent Social Work, 4*(2), 78–91.

Child Welfare League of America. (1988). *Standards for adoption service* (rev. ed.). Washington, DC: Author.

Clemmons, M. P., Gora, K., Moline, B., Mulryan, R., & Saunders, R. (1989). Unpublished notes from committee meetings and lecture series, entitled *Family life after adoption,* Chicago.

Cole, E., & Donley, K. (1990.) History, values and placement policy issues. In D. Brodzinsky & M. Schechter (Eds.). *The psychology of adoption* (pp. 273–294). New York: Oxford University Press.

Cole, E., & Duva, J. (1990). *Family preservation: An orientation for administrators and practitioners.* Washington, DC: Child Welfare League of America.

Conway, P., & Valentine, D. (1988). Reproductive losses and grieving. In

A. (1985a). Some theoretical considerations on confidential adoptions: Part I. The birth mother. *Child and Adolescent Social Work, 2*(1), 13–21.

Kraft, A., Palombo, J., Mitchell, J., Woods, P., Mitchell, D., & Schmidt, A. (1985b). Some theoretical considerations on confidential adoptions: Part II. the adoptive parent. *Child and Adolescent Social Work, 2*(2), 69–82.

Kraft, A., Palombo, J., Mitchell, J., Woods, P., Mitchell, D., Schmidt, A., & Tucker, N. (1985c). Some theoretical considerations on confidential adoptions: Part III. the adopted child. *Child and Adolescent Social Work, 2*(3), 139–153.

Kraft, A., Palombo, J., Mitchell, J., Woods, P., Mitchell, D., Schmidt, A., & Tucker, N. (1986). Some theoretical considerations on confidential adoptions: Part IV. Countertransference. *Child and Adolescent Social Work, 3*(1), 3–14.

Kral, R., & Schaffer, J. (1988). Treating the adoptive family. In C. Chilman, E. Nunnally, & F. Cox (Eds.), *Variant family forms* (pp. 185–204). Newbury Park, CA: Sage.

Kübler-Ross, E. (1969). *On death and dying.* New York: Macmillan.

Lax, W., & Lussardi, D. (1988). The use of rituals in families with an adolescent. In E. Imber-Black, J. Roberts, & R. Whiting (Eds.), *Rituals in families and family therapy* (pp. 158–176). New York: Norton.

Lederer, W., & Jackson, D. (1968). *The mirages of marriage.* New York: Norton.

LePere, D. (1988). Vulnerability to crisis during the life cycle of the adoptive family. In D. Valentine (Ed.), *Infertility and adoption: A guide for social work practice* (pp. 73–85). New York: Haworth Press.

Lifton, B. J. (1975). *Twice born: Memoirs of an adopted daughter.* New York: McGraw-Hill.

Lifton, B. J. (1979). *Lost and found: The adoption experience.* New York: Dial Press.

Lindsay, J., & Monserrat, C. (1989). *Adoption awareness: A guide for teachers, counselors, nurses and caring others.* Buena Park, CA: Morning Glory Press.

Mason, M. (1987). *The miracle seekers: An anthology of infertility.* Fort Wayne, IN: Perspectives Press.

Maxtone-Graham, K. (1983). *An adopted woman.* New York: Remi Books.

Mazor, M., & Simmons, H. (Eds.). (1984). *Infertility: Medical, emotional, and social considerations.* New York: Human Sciences Press.

McCullough, P. (1980). Launching children and moving on. In E. Carter & M. McGoldrick (Eds.), *The family life cycle: A framework for family therapy* (pp. 171–195). New York: Gardner Press.

McRoy, R., Grotevant, H., & White, K. (1988). *Openness in adoption: New practices, new issues.* New York: Praeger.

McVoy, J. (1987). Family fat: Assessing and treating obesity within a family context. In J. Harkaway (Vol. ed.), *The family therapy collection: Eating disorders* (pp. 70–83). Rockville, MD: Aspen.

Melina, L. (1986). *Raising adopted children: A manual for adoptive parents.* New York: Solstice Press.

Miller-Havens, S. (1990). *Connections and disconnections: The birth origin fantasies of adopted women who search.* Unpublished doctoral dissertation, Harvard University.

Moley, V. (1987). Brief therapy and eating disorders. In J. Harkaway (Vol. ed.), *The family therapy collection: Eating disorders* (pp. 40–54). Rockville, MD: Aspen.

Nelson, K. (1985). *On the frontier of adoption: A study of special-needs adoptive families.* New York: Child Welfare League of America.

Olson, D., McCubbin, H., Barnes, H., Larsen, A., Muxen, M., & Wilson, M. (1983). *Families: What makes them work.* Beverly Hills, CA: Sage.

Pannor, R., & Baran, A. (1984). Open adoption as standard practice. *Child Welfare, 63*(3), 245–250.

Pannor, R., Massarik, F., & Evans, B. W. (1971). *The unmarried father.* New York: Springer.

Partridge, S., Hornby, H., & McDonald, T. (1986). *Learning from adoption disruption: Insights for practice.* Portland, ME: Human Services Development Institute.

Pasley, K., & Ihinger-Tallman, M. (1988). Remarriage and stepfamilies. In C. Chilman, E. Nunnally, & F. Cox (Eds.), *Variant family forms* (pp. 204–221). Newbury Park, CA: Sage.

Paton, J. (1954). *The adopted break silence.* Cedaredge, CO: Life History Study Center.

Powers, D. (Ed.). (1984). *Adoption for troubled children: Prevention and repair of adoptive failures through residential treatment.* New York: Haworth Press.

Reid, W., & Epstein, L. (1972). *Task-centered casework.* New York: Columbia University Press.

Reitz, M. (1982). *Model building for marital assessment: A study of new marriages on systemic dimensions.* Unpublished doctoral dissertation, University of Chicago.

Roberto, L. (1987). Bulimia: Transgenerational family therapy. In J. Harkaway (Vol. ed.), *The family therapy collection: Eating disorders* (pp. 1–11). Rockville, MD: Aspen.

Roles, P. (1989). *Saying goodby to a baby: Vol. 1. The birthparent's guide to loss and grief in adoption.* Washington, DC: Child Welfare League of America.

Roles, P. (1991). *Saying goodby to a baby: Vol. 2. A counselor's guide to birthparent grief and loss.* Washington, DC: Child Welfare League of America.

Rosenthal, J. (1990). Race, social class, and special needs adoption. *Social Work, 35*(6), 532–539.

Sager, C. (1976). *Marriage contracts and couple therapy.* New York: Brunner/Mazel.

Salzer, L. (1991). *Surviving infertility: A compassionate guide through the emotional crisis of infertility.* New York: HarperCollins.

Sandmaier, M. (1988). *When love is not enough: How mental health professionals can help special-needs adoptive families.* Washington, DC: Child Welfare League of America.

Schaffer, J., & Kral, R. (1988). Adoptive families. In C. Chilman, E. Nunnally, & F. Cox (Eds.), *Variant family forms* (pp. 165–184). Newbury Park, CA: Sage.

Schaffer, J., & Lindstrom, C. (1989). *How to raise an adopted child.* New York: Copestone Press.

Schaffer, J., & Lindstrom, C. (1990). Brief solution-focused therapy with adoptive families. In D. Brodzinsky & M. Schechter (Eds.), *The psychology of adoption* (pp. 240–252). New York: Oxford University Press.

Schechter, M., & Bertocci, D. (1990). The meaning of search. In D. Brodzinsky & M. Schechter (Eds.), *The psychology of adoption* (pp. 62–90). New York: Oxford University Press.

Schmidt, S. (1968). Special treatment applications: United front, acting-out-adolescent, and only-adopted-child families. In C. Kramer, B. Liebowitz, R. Phillips, S. Schmidt, & J. Gibson, *Beginning phase of family treatment* (pp. 39–51). Oak Park, IL: The Kramer Foundation.

Schmidt, S., & Liebowitz, B. (1969). *Adolescents and their families: A treatment model combining family and group treatment.* Paper presented at the annual meeting of the American Orthopsychiatric Association, New York.

Shireman, J., & Johnson, P. (1973). *Adoption: Three alternatives.* Chicago: Chicago Child Care Society.

Shireman, J., & Johnson, P. (1986). A longitudinal study of black adoptions: Single parent, transracial, and traditional. *Social Work, 31*(3), 172–176.

Siegel, D. (1990). *Open adoption of infants: Adoptive parents' perceptions of advantages and disadvantages.* Unpublished manuscript.

Silber, K., & Dorner, P. M. (1990). *Children of open adoption.* San Antonio, TX: Corona.

Simon, B. K. (1960). *Relationship between theory and practice in social casework.* Silver Spring, MD: National Association of Social Workers.

Slipp, S. (1984). *Object relations: A dynamic bridge between individual and family treatment.* New York: Jason Aronson.

Sorosky, A., Baran, A., & Pannor, R. (1978) *The adoption triangle: The effects of the sealed record on adoptees, birth parents, and adoptive parents.* Garden City, NY: Doubleday/Anchor.

Stack, C. B. (1974). *All our kin.* New York: Harper/Colophon.

Stanley v. Illinois, 405 U.S. 645 (1972).

Stein, L., & Hoopes, J. (1985). *Identity formation in the adopted adolescent: The Delaware family study.* New York: Child Welfare League of America.

Strizak, M. (1990). *Relative foster homes.* Unpublished manuscript.

Talen, M., & Lehr, M. (1984). A structural and developmental analysis of symptomatic adopted children and their families. *Journal of Marital and Family Therapy, 10*(4), 381–391.

Tansey, B. (Ed.). (1988). *Exploring adoptive family life: The collected adoption papers of H. David Kirk.* Port Angeles, WA: Ben-Simon.

Terry, L. (1987). Ordering a therapeutic context: A developmental interactional approach to the treatment of eating disorders in college counseling center. In J. Harkaway (Vol. ed.), *The family therapy collection. Eating disorders* (pp. 55–69). Rockville, MD: Aspen.

Triseliotis, J. (1973). *In search of origins: The experience of adopted people.* Boston: Beacon Press.

Triseliotis, J., & Hill, M. (1990). Contrasting adoption, foster care, and residential rearing. In D. Brodzinsky & M. Schechter (Eds.), *The psychology of adoption* (pp. 107–120). New York: Oxford University Press.

Valentine, D. (Ed.). (1988). *Infertility and adoption: A guide for social work practice.* New York: Haworth Press.

Visher, E., & Visher, J. (1982). *How to win as a stepfamily.* New York: Dembner Books.

Visher, E., & Visher, J. (1988a). *Old loyalties, new ties: Therapeutic strategies with stepfamilies.* New York: Brunner/Mazel.

Visher, E., & Visher, J. (1988b). Treating families with problems associated with remarriage and step relationships. In C. Chilman, E. Nunnally, & F. Cox (Eds.), *Variant family forms* (pp. 222–245). Newbury Park, CA: Sage.

Vogel, E., & Bell, N. (1967). The emotionally disturbed child as the family scapegoat. In G. Handel (Ed.), *The psychosocial interior of the family* (pp. 424–442). Chicago: Aldine.

Wald, E. (1981). *The remarried family.* New York: Family Service Association of America.

Wallerstein, J., & Blakeslee, S. (1989). *Second chances: Men, women and children a decade after divorce.* New York: Ticknor & Fields.

Watson, K. W. (1986). Birth families: Living with the adoption decision. *Public Welfare, 44*(2), 5–10.

Watson, K. W. (1988). Open adoption: Defining the terms and psychological issues. The case for open adoption. *Public Welfare, 44*(2), 26–28.

Watson, K. W. (1989–1990, December–January). Infant bonding and attachment: A helpful distinction. *Stepping Stones* (Illinois Council on Adoptable Children), pp. 2–9.

Watson, K. W. & Strom, J. (1987). Report of the Child Welfare League of America National Adoption Task Force. Washington, DC: Child Welfare League of America.

Watzlawick, P., Beavin, J., & Jackson, D. (1967). *Pragmatics of human communication.* New York: Norton.

Watzlawick, P., Weakland, J., & Fisch, R. (1974). *Change: Principles of problem formation and problem resolution.* New York: Norton.

Westat, Inc., (1986). *Adoption services for waiting minority and nonminority Children.* Rockville, MD: Author.

Whiting, R. (1988). Therapeutic rituals with families with adopted members. In E. Imber-Black, J. Roberts, & R. Whiting (Eds.), *Rituals in families and family therapy* (pp. 211–229). New York: Norton.

Winkler, R., Brown, D., van Keppel, M., & Blanchard, A. (1988). *Clinical practice in adoption.* Elmsford, NY: Pergamon Press.

Winkler, R., & van Keppel, M. (1984). *Relinquishing mothers in adoption* (Monograph No. 3). Melbourne, Australia: Institute of Family Studies.

Wynne, L., Ryckoff, I., Day, J., & Hirsch, S. (1967). Pseudomutuality in the family relations of schizophrenics. In G. Handel (Ed.), *The psychosocial interior of the family* (pp. 443–466). Chicago: Aldine.

Young, L. (1954). *Out of wedlock.* New York: McGraw-Hill.

Ziegler, R., & Musliner, P. (1977). Persistent themes: A naturalistic study of personality development in the family. *Family Process, 16*(3), 293–305.

Index